Asbestos in Australia

Asbestos in Australia

From Boom to Dust

Edited by
Lenore Layman & Gail Phillips

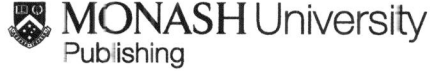

Asbestos in Australia: From Boom to Dust
© Copyright 2019
Copyright of the collection in its entirety is held by Lenore Layman & Gail Phillips.
Copyright of the individual chapters is held by the respective author/s.
All rights reserved. Apart from any uses permitted by Australia's Copyright Act 1968, no part of this book may be reproduced by any process without prior written permission from the copyright owners. Inquiries should be directed to the publisher.

Monash University Publishing
Matheson Library Annexe
40 Exhibition Walk
Monash University
Clayton, Victoria 3800, Australia
www.publishing.monash.edu

Monash University Publishing brings to the world publications which advance the best traditions of humane and enlightened thought.

Monash University Publishing titles pass through a rigorous process of independent peer review.

ISBN: 9781925835618 (paperback)
ISBN: 9781925835595 (pdf)
ISBN: 9781925835601 (epub)

http://www.publishing.monash.edu/books/aa-9781925835618.html

Series: Australian History

Design: Les Thomas

Cover photograph courtesy Mia Lindgren

A catalogue record for this book is available from the National Library of Australia.

Printed in Australia by SOS Print + Media Group (Aust) Pty Ltd.

TABLE OF CONTENTS

Acknowledgements vii
List of Figures ix
About the Contributors xi
Introduction xv
          Lenore Layman & Gail Phillips

Part 1	**The Rise and Fall of the Asbestos Industry** 3	
Chapter 1	The Asbestos Industry in Australia . . . . 5 *Lenore Layman*	
Chapter 2	Asbestos in the Built Environment . . . . 43 *Lenore Layman*	
Chapter 3	Tackling the Dust Hazard: The Response of Public Health . . . 75 *Lenore Layman*	
Chapter 4	Uncovering the Story: Asbestos in the Media . . . . 107 *Chris Smyth*	
Part 2	**Asbestos Related Disease: The Medical Journey** 129	
Chapter 5	Milestones in the Knowledge and Treatment of Asbestos Related Diseases . . . . 131 *A W (Bill) Musk*	
Chapter 6	Asbestos and Mesothelioma—Fifty Years On . . . . 149 *Geoffrey Berry*	
Chapter 7	Health Outcomes of the Women and Children Who Lived at Wittenoom . . . . 167 *Alison Reid*	
Part 3	**Damaged Communities** 183	
Chapter 8	Memories of Wittenoom . . . . 185 *Compiled by Gail Phillips*	
Chapter 9	Working and Living in Baryulgil . . . . 205 *Compiled by Lenore Layman*	

Part 4	Asbestos in the Courts: The Battles for Compensation ...223
Chapter 10	The History of Asbestos Litigation .... 225 *John Gordon*

Part 5	Asbestos Today: The Lingering Legacy 255
Chapter 11	The Ongoing Problem of Asbestos *In Situ*............. 257 *Peter Franklin and Alison Reid*

Part 6	In Their Own Words: The Witness Stories 275
Chapter 12	Wittenoom's Flying Doctor........................ 277 *Dr Eric Saint*
Chapter 13	A Public Health Campaigner's Story .... 281 *Dr Jim McNulty*
Chapter 14	The Story of the Asbestos Diseases Society of Australia... 287 *Robert Vojakovic*
Chapter 15	A Life Recast by Asbestos........................ 297 *Dr Greg Deleuil*
Chapter 16	The Litigator's Story............................ 307 *Peter Gordon*
Chapter 17	The James Hardie Story.......................... 315 *Gideon Haigh*
Chapter 18	The Bernie Banton Story .... 323 *Greg Combet*

Index... 331

ACKNOWLEDGEMENTS

This book is dedicated to the memory of the victims of asbestos who, in telling us their stories, revealed the human cost of an Australian tragedy.

We would like to thank the copyright holders, the State Library of Western Australia and *The Northern Star*, for permission to reproduce photographs in this volume, and Asbestoswise for allowing us to reproduce their graphic of the Asbestos House. We would also like to acknowledge our fellow researchers on the Australian Asbestos Network project: Associate Professor Mia Lindgren of Monash University, whose passion for uncovering the untold asbestos stories led to the creation of the AAN, and Renae Desai of Murdoch University who brought the website into being and nurtured our online community. Many thanks also to Dr Criena Fitzgerald for generously sharing her wide knowledge of health history.

LIST OF FIGURES

Figure 1: Witness Seminar panel: Robert Vojakovic, Greg Deleuil, Rose Marie Vojakovic, Bill Musk, Geoffrey Berry, John Gordon xvi

Figure 1.1: Total asbestos fibre imports to Australia [in short tons] 31

Figure 1.2: Comparison of asbestos fibre prices, Australia 1950-1966 . . . 34

Figure 2.1: A popular attraction at Sydney Royal Easter Show 1949. James Hardie Fibrolite show home. 45

Figure 2.2: "Shangri-la" built of fibro, western Sydney, 1949 46

Figure 2.3: A fibro streetscape, western Sydney, 1946 47

Figure 2.4: Numbers of fibro houses 1921–1971 & as percentage of all occupied private houses 48

Figure 2.5: Distribution of fibro houses, Sydney 1971 52

Figure 2.6: Asbestos insulation blanket on turbine at East Perth Power Station. The turbine's metal casing, which covered the asbestos blanket when the turbine was in operation, has been removed after the station closed in 1980 and during removal of all asbestos from the site. 69

Figure 6.1: Wittenoom workers (men): increases in cases of mesothelioma in male workers up to 2007, and predicted to 2020 164

Figure 6.2: Australian workers (men): predicted annual number of incident mesotheliomas to 2060 165

Figure 8.1: A miner drills in a narrow stope of the Australian Blue Asbestos mine, Wittenoom. 189

Figure 9.1: Workers bag asbestos fibre at Baryulgil mill. 213

Figure 11.1: Asbestos Awareness Healthy House Checklist. A homeowner's guide to identifying asbestos-containing material to manage it safely 259

Figure 11.2: Airborne asbestos fibre concentrations (fibres/mL) measured during selected renovation activities. 264

Figure 13.1: Testing dust levels at Wittenoom's mine and mill, 1966. . . 285

Figure 14.1: Robert and Rose Marie Vojakovic standing outside Parliament House, Perth with some of the widows of Wittenoom. 290

Figure 14.2: Remembering the dead. 295

Figure 15.1: Dr Greg Deleuil 299

Figure 15.2: Alice Deleuil, in the family home in Darwin surrounded by asbestos louvres. 301

ABOUT THE CONTRIBUTORS

Geoffrey Berry is an Emeritus Professor in the School of Public Health at the University of Sydney having retired as Professor in Epidemiology and Biostatistics. He has worked as a biostatistician in medical research for over 45 years; first from 1966 to 1982 at the British Medical Research Council's Pneumoconiosis Unit in Penarth, Wales; then from 1982 to 2001 at the University of Sydney; and since his retirement he has remained active in research on the health effects of asbestos exposure, including working with the University of Western Australia's research group on the Wittenoom workers and residents. He was a Chief Investigator on the NHMRC-funded *Consequences of Asbestos Exposure in WA* and *Dust-related Health Issues in Western Australians* projects. A major part of his work has been in the area of health hazards associated with asbestos, including collaborative research on the epidemiological studies of the Cape and Ferodo factories in the UK set up by Dr Molly Newhouse, the Nottingham women gas mask workers initiated by Dr Stephen Jones, the Wittenoom cohorts of former workers at the mine and mill and residents of the town, and projections of future mesothelioma numbers in Australia. He is co-author of the book *Statistical Methods in Medical Research* (P Armitage, G Berry, JNS Matthews, 4th edn).

Peter Franklin is a Senior Research Fellow and Senior Lecturer in the School of Population and Global Health at the University of Western Australia (UWA), as well as a Senior Scientific Officer at the Western Australian Department of Health. His research and teaching interests are in environmental and occupational health. He has done considerable research in both occupational and community asbestos exposure, and in his government role is responsible for advising on, and reviewing, public health asbestos regulations.

John Gordon is a barrister in Douglas Menzies Chambers, Melbourne. From 1987–1998, he ran the Perth office of Slater & Gordon, including the Wittenoom Asbestos test cases, the CSR asbestos group settlement and James Hardie asbestos claims. From 1994 to 1996 he ran environmental damages claims arising from PNG OK Tedi Gold and Copper Mine. As counsel, he has appeared in important trials for asbestos disease claimants in the WA Supreme Court. He was joint inaugural winner of the Australian Plaintiff Lawyers Association/ Australian Lawyers Alliance Civil Justice Award in 1996 and has been an active and public campaigner on behalf of asbestos disease sufferers and against restrictions of common law rights.

Lenore Layman AM (co-editor) is an Australian historian, currently Adjunct Associate Professor of History at Murdoch University. Her research and publication on Australian asbestos history began in 1983. She was a Chief Investigator on the NHMRC-funded *Consequences of Asbestos Exposure in WA* and *Dust-related Health Issues in Western Australians* projects. She has recently co-authored and co-edited *Powering Perth. A History of the East Perth Power Station and the Electrification of Perth*; *110° in the Waterbag. A History of Life, Work and Leisure in Leonora, Gwalia and the Northern Goldfields*; *Blood Nose Politics: A Centenary History of the WA National Party*; and *Radical Perth, Militant Fremantle*.

A W (Bill) Musk was a respiratory physician at Sir Charles Gairdner Hospital from 1978, and was Clinical Professor of Medicine in the School of Population Health at the University of Western Australia where he is now Emeritus Professor. His research interests are in clinical and epidemiological aspects of lung disease (chiefly occupational and environmental lung diseases) and cancer, particularly related to Wittenoom blue asbestos, Kalgoorlie goldmining and in the Busselton population. He was a lead researcher on the NHMRC-funded *Consequences of Asbestos Exposure in WA* and *Dust-related Health Issues in Western Australians* projects. He is an author on over 320 peer-reviewed scientific articles and numerous reviews and book chapters in the medical literature in these areas of research. In 1992 Dr Musk was awarded Member of the Order of Australia for services to medicine in the areas of asbestos related diseases and smoking control. In 2009 he was awarded the Inaugural Tim Willoughby Medal for Research by the National Centre for Asbestos Related Diseases and in 2011 he was awarded the Thoracic Society of Australia and New Zealand Research Medal. In 2012 he was senior author on the best scientific publication of the year in the *Medical Journal of Australia*.

Gail Phillips (co-editor) is Emerita Associate Professor of Journalism at Murdoch University. She was lead researcher on the Reporting Diversity project funded by the Department of Immigration and Citizenship and a Chief Investigator on the NHMRC-funded *Consequences of Asbestos*

Exposure in WA and *Dust-related Health Issues in Western Australians* projects. She is co-author of *Australian Broadcast Journalism*, published by Oxford University Press (2002, 2006, 2013) and is also co-author of *Journalism Ethics at Work* (Pearson Longman, 2005).

Alison Reid is Associate Professor in Epidemiology and Biostatistics in the School of Public Health at Curtin University. She was a Chief Investigator on the NHMRC-funded *Consequences of Asbestos Exposure in WA* and *Dust-related Health Issues in Western Australians* projects. Her research interests include the occupational health and safety of migrant workers and community exposure to low dose and non-occupational sources of asbestos. She uses both quantitative and qualitative research methods for this work and collaborates widely. She has published extensively in national and international journals.

Chris Smyth is Associate Professor of Journalism at Murdoch University. He has worked in newspapers in Australia and the UK and for 10 years was the state secretary of the Australian Journalists Association (now MEAA). He was a Chief Investigator on the NHMRC-funded *Consequences of Asbestos Exposure in WA* and *Dust-related Health Issues in Western Australians* projects. He is co-author of *Journalism Ethics at Work* (Pearson Longman, 2005) and *Midland Railway Workshops: A History in Pictures 1904–2004* (St George, 2004).

INTRODUCTION

Lenore Layman
&
Gail Phillips

Asbestos has featured in the Australian consciousness from the last decades of the 19th century to the present, initially extolled as a "magic mineral" and after 1977 feared as a deadly dust. For the last 40 years media exposés and stories of asbestos victims together with news of legal battles and accounts of company restructures have run alongside a great number of specialist articles in scholarly journals reporting medical research findings, public policy analyses, and historical and sociological studies of company shortcomings and malfeasance. These writings have provided us with fragments of Australia's asbestos story. A study that overviews, integrates, and completes this story is overdue. It is time for a perspective which spans the 20th century, beginning with the welcome promise of the mineral's versatility and ending with its positioning as a pariah material. We intend this book to provide such a perspective, enabling a better understanding of how and why this health and environmental disaster happened. Our book is a multi-disciplinary collaborative account drawing on specialist knowledges to allow readers the opportunity to see Australia's asbestos history in its entirety.

Australians might assume that asbestos is yesterday's news. After all, mining and manufacturing of asbestos in Australia have long ceased and its import and use have been banned since 2003. However its legacy continues—asbestos remains in our built environment. It remains in our bodies, with the long latency periods resulting in the emergence of asbestos related disease, including the deadly mesothelioma, decades after exposure. And because asbestos products deteriorate over time, a new generation, this time of do-it-yourself renovators, is exposed to the mineral today as they strip away the fences, panels, roofs, carpets, tiles that have remained undisturbed in older houses. A violent storm or a bushfire can result in asbestos being spread around our suburbs, either as broken-off fragments or as airborne particles, putting the entire local population at risk. As well the illegal dumping of asbestos waste is a constant problem around the nation. Even if

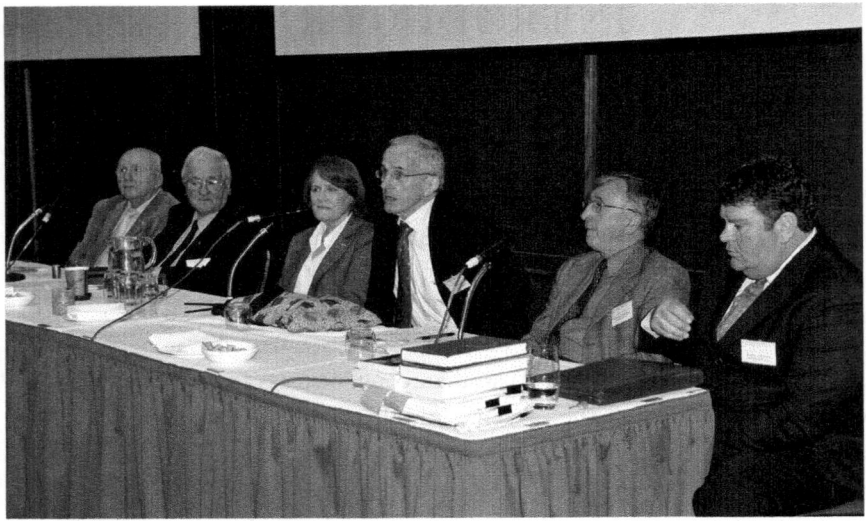

Figure 1: Witness Seminar panel: Robert Vojakovic, Greg Deleuil, Rose Marie Vojakovic, Bill Musk, Geoffrey Berry, John Gordon
SOURCE: Witness Seminar, ANZSHM

asbestos is no longer in use, the need for public vigilance to reduce exposure to the still deadly dust is as important now as it ever was. Asbestos is a problem for today.

This book has its origins in two multi-disciplinary collaborations. The first was a Witness Seminar devoted to asbestos related disease organised as part of the Australian and New Zealand Society of the History of Medicine's biennial conference in 2009. Witness seminars draw together people who have worked in a specific area of biomedicine to share recollections of their involvement and the discoveries, events, and developments they have witnessed and participated in. These individuals have worked on the same topic but often at different points of the process—researchers, clinicians, patients, activists, policymakers, lawyers, historians, journalists, among others. Together they have frequently brought about scientific and social change. This is certainly the case with those working in the arena of asbestos related disease and their testimonies shaped the formation of this book.

The other collaboration which has made this book possible was funded by the National Health and Medical Research Council enabling a cross-institutional team of researchers headed by Professor A W Musk to examine the patterns of exposure and community consequences of asbestos related

Introduction

disease. One of the components of this grant supported the creation of a multimedia website (www.australianasbestosnetwork.org.au), created as an information hub to make scientific research and public health messages accessible to the community, to sketch out a history of asbestos, and to present personal and community experiences of living with asbestos.

This book is therefore the product of a research partnership that has brought together medical and public health researchers, lawyers, historians, journalists, and communication specialists to examine asbestos in Australia from a range of disciplinary perspectives, and to increase public awareness about the ongoing hazard. It covers the history of asbestos in Australia, the progress in the diagnosis and treatment of asbestos related disease, the landmark court cases that sought fair compensation for sufferers, and the public health challenges past, present, and into the future. It also features the voices of many of the key players in the saga, as well as the voices of many victims who have told their stories as a warning to succeeding generations.

In Part 1, *The rise and fall of the asbestos industry*, Lenore Layman charts the growth and demise of mining and manufacturing from 1880 to the present day, the proliferation of asbestos in industry and everyday life, and the role of the regulators who were so tardy in tackling the hazard. Chris Smyth then explores the contribution of dogged investigative journalists in bringing the asbestos tragedy to light via the media. In Part 2, *Asbestos related disease: the medical journey*, the eminent asbestos medical researchers Emeritus Professors Bill Musk and Geoffrey Berry reflect on the path of medical research on asbestos related disease. In Part 3, *Damaged communities*, Gail Phillips and Lenore Layman use oral testimonies supplemented with archival material to convey the lived experience of the residents of the former mining communities of Wittenoom in Western Australia and Baryugil in New South Wales.

Part 4, *Asbestos in the courts: the battles for compensation*, turns to the history of asbestos litigation. Barrister and former Slater & Gordon litigator John Gordon traces the landmark cases that helped to bring justice to at least some of the asbestos industry's many victims. In Part 5, *Asbestos today: the lingering legacy*, public health epidemiologists Dr Peter Franklin and Associate Professor Alison Reid focus on asbestos in the present day, underscoring the need for ongoing public vigilance to limit exposure to asbestos in situ.

In Part 6, *In their own words: the witness stories*, some of the major players in Australia's asbestos history recount their recollections of the momentous events in which they were involved. Dr Eric Saint, Wittenoom's flying doctor, and public health physician Dr Jim McNulty speak of their attempts to alert authorities to the dangers of asbestos exposure at Wittenoom. Robert Vojakovic, founder of the Asbestos Diseases Society of Australia, discusses the role the Society has played in the long battle for compensation for asbestos disease sufferers. Dr Greg Deleuil, a general practitioner who has had a long association with the Asbestos Diseases Society of Australia, tells of the loss of his own mother to mesothelioma. Former Slater & Gordon litigator Peter Gordon took some of the first cases to court and speaks about the challenges facing would-be litigants. Historian Gideon Haigh provides an account of the history of the James Hardie company, responsible for so much of the manufactured asbestos that now provides an ongoing challenge for the community. Finally, former Australian Council of Trade Unions president Greg Combet remembers Bernie Banton, whose landmark court battle in NSW did so much to turn the tide in favour of former asbestos workers.

Everyone associated with this publication hopes that it assists in raising public awareness in order to protect the future wellbeing of the Australian public. We acknowledge Slater & Gordon's assistance at the time of the Witness Seminar. We pay tribute to all those who have struggled to increase knowledge of asbestos related disease, to alert potential victims to their danger, to warn the general public of the looming disaster, to hold the companies to account and fight for legal justice, and to tell their stories of illness and death at difficult and distressing times in their lives. We regret that more was not done earlier. That a seemingly magic mineral turned out to be a deadly dust stands as a warning to us all.

Part 1
The Rise and Fall of the Asbestos Industry

Chapter 1

THE ASBESTOS INDUSTRY IN AUSTRALIA

Lenore Layman

Asbestos stands unique—a world-old rock which is immune to the action of heat, water, weather and wear—a fibrous mineral which can be spun, woven, felted or molded into useful form. So closely does it fit the needs of this new world of steam, electricity and blazing furnaces, that it seems to have been almost purposely designed ... For centuries, Asbestos was but a curiosity—the mystic mineral, the paradox of ages. But today it is a recognised necessity.

Johns Manville, 1923[1]

This statement by Johns Manville Corp., then the US's largest asbestos company, now triggers a strongly negative response—certainly rejection, probably anger. Today, the word asbestos is inextricably associated with danger and disease, a material to avoid and eliminate. It conjures images of deadly dust and terminally ill people. There is fear of the reach of asbestos related disease and anger at the corporate profits made behind a veil of deceit; and there is great concern about the continued presence of asbestos materials in the built environment. But it was not

---

1   Johns Manville Inc., *Johns Manville service to railroads & Johns Manville service to industry* (New York: Johns Manville, 1923), 5–6.

always so. When the above statement was made, asbestos was regarded positively as a material of enormous promise, able to be put to ever more numerous uses that improved modern life. This chapter traces the development of Australia's asbestos industry, the different parts of which it was comprised, and their inter-relations. It examines the business enterprise and government promotion that brought the material into the lives of almost all Australians, and explores a time when asbestos was welcomed to address essential unmet needs in a rapidly developing society.

Introduction

Asbestos became a major Australian industry in the century from the 1880s to the 1970s, built by business and government working together. While the international asbestos companies did not find Australia sufficiently promising to set up either mining or manufacturing ventures themselves, they provided the necessary knowledge about asbestos and its uses for local developers. They shaped the economic and cultural environment in which asbestos was produced and consumed in the capitalist world and therefore they shaped local development. Local capital developed and continued to control the industry in Australia, one company—James Hardie—becoming increasingly powerful by the mid-20th century. As in so many other areas of Australian development, however, the state's role was also crucial. Governments were powerful promoters of the asbestos industry and powerful developers at one remove; certainly far more effective at promoting than at regulating the industry.

Mining and manufacturing of asbestos began in Australia in 1880, around the same time that asbestos products were first imported, and only two years after mining development in Canada marked the commencement of an international asbestos industry. The Australian industry reached its zenith nearly a century later, when fibre imports and consumption peaked in the early to mid-1970s, declining only after 1978.

The illusory promise of "big reefs"

The idea of an asbestos mining eldorado formed the industry's beginnings. Scientific experts voiced their optimism and the search for the "big reefs" began in Australia as soon as mining in Quebec proved a demand for asbestos fibre. Prospectors in the 1880s found numerous scattered deposits and hopes were high for a new colonial mineral industry. "Reports are constantly coming to hand of the discovery of 'big reefs'…. of excellent quality", the Royal Society of Queensland recorded in 1891-92. Like gold that had proved such a bonanza for the Australian colonies, asbestos would be initially a prospectors' mineral. "As it requires no capital but labour", the Royal Society reported, asbestos mining was particularly suited to conditions on Australia's mineral fields.[2] This search indicates the speed with which the idea of asbestos use spread to the colonial antipodes.

The "big reefs" proved illusory, however, and only one discovery was worked in the 1880s. At Jones Creek near Gundagai in New South Wales tremolite asbestos was first mined in 1880 by the Australasian Asbestos Company, and a factory established in Little Collins St, Melbourne, to manufacture "asbestos preparations of various kinds".[3] In total, 26 tons of fibre were produced before the industry failed in 1884. Although hopes were raised by the "long silky white fibres", tremolite had few uses because the fibre was weak and brittle.[4] After 1884 mining at Jones Creek was intermittent before it ceased altogether in 1921. Only 46 tons of fibre were produced in those 37 years.[5] This tonnage, comprising many small parcels, was the work of prospectors who came and went according to movements in fibre prices that alternately fuelled and dashed their dreams of striking it rich. They separated the fibre from its surrounding rock by hand "cobbing", using a hammer.

The pattern of mining established at Jones Creek was repeated at a succession of mining ventures across the continent for the next 80 years: initial prospecting; high hopes and talk of first quality fibre; commencement of commercial mining; failure to maintain mining profitability, most often because the deposit did not prove as rich as anticipated; and finally a reversion to intermittent prospecting. A story of failure, it is a narrative never told in Australia's mining histories.

A second attempt to develop an asbestos mining and manufacturing industry was made in 1899 when the Australasian Asbestos Company began to work the white (chrysotile) asbestos deposits at Anderson's Creek in northern Tasmania in order to manufacture asbestic wall plaster in Melbourne.[6] It was less than three years after asbestic, "The King of Wall

---

2   E Hall, H G Stokes, "Asbestos", *Proceedings of the Royal Society of Queensland for 1891–92*, 8 (4) 1891–92: 114–21.

3   *Gundagai Times and Tumut, Adelong and Murrumbidgee District Advertiser*, 11 August 1882, 2.

4   A Liversidge, "The Minerals of New South Wales", in H Wood, *Mineral Products of New South Wales* (Sydney: NSW Dept of Mines, 1882), 186.

5   A A MacNevin, *Asbestos. The mineral industry of New South Wales*. Geological Survey of New South Wales, 4 (Sydney: NSW Dept of Mines, 1970), 40–41, 47.

6   W H Twelvetrees, *Asbestos at Anderson's Creek. Geological Survey Mineral Resources*, 4 (Hobart: Tasmania Dept of Mines, 1917), 9–10.

Plasters" according to the American industry, was first produced in Canada, utilising short asbestos fibre. In a detailed account of the world industry published in 1897, Robert H Jones concluded that asbestic was "revolutionising the whole industry".[7] Although the conclusion proved incorrect, it testifies to the strong confidence surrounding the new material when the Australasian Asbestos Company prepared to supply colonial markets with Bestic Plaster from its Yarra Bank factory. Fire- and heat-proof, cold-resistant, labour-saving, an effective sound insulator, and inviting decorative embellishments, asbestic would command a significant market, the company and commercial press believed.[8] It did not do so. Adding to the company's problems, the ore body at Anderson's Creek declined steeply in quality. After shipping 374 tons of cobbed fibre, operations ceased in 1901.[9] On-and-off prospecting returned to the field.

Tiny prospecting shows proliferated in the years prior to the 1914–18 war. In Queensland, activity centred on the Rockhampton district, the State Department of Mines in 1904 reporting "the fibres to be finer than the best quality of Italian asbestos", and again in 1916 noting the "encouraging character" of the deposits.[10] A South Australian Geological Survey also described the 1912 workings of an outcrop of blue (crocidolite) asbestos near Hawker as "encouraging" but noted that little work had been done to determine the extent of the deposits.[11] White asbestos was found in Western Australia's Pilbara and several small shows were being worked intermittently by 1912. Canadian mining engineer, author, and world expert on asbestos Fritz Cirkel was sent a large sample of Pilbara fibre and reported that, while it did not have the tensile strength of Quebec fibre, "yet some good crude may be secured".[12] Perhaps the eminent Cirkel's opinion emboldened the Western Australian Geological Survey to report that "there

---

7   R H Jones, *Asbestos and asbestic* (London: Crosby Lockwood & Son, 1897), preface, ch. 10.
8   *Building, Engineering and Mining Journal* (Sydney), 17 December 1900.
9   Twelvetrees, *Asbestos at Anderson's Creek*, 10.
10 B Dunstan, *Notes on asbestos in the Rockhampton District. Geological Survey of Queensland*, 190 (Brisbane: Queensland Dept of Mines, 1904). B Dunstan, Chief Government Geologist, "Queensland mineral deposits. A review of occurrences, production, values, prospects – asbestos", *Queensland Government Mining Journal*, 15, 1916: 372–75.
11 *South Australian asbestos. Geological Survey of South Australia Abstract* Bulletin 11, (South Australia Dept of Mines, Adelaide, 1956).
12 F Cirkel, *Chrysotile-Asbestos. Its occurrence, exploitation, milling and uses.* 2nd Edn (Ottawa: Govt Printing Bureau, 1910), 236–38.

is ... a good margin of profit in working good crude fibre", despite indicating that the fibre seams were narrow, mining costs high, and ore milling untried.[13] Although the lure of the rich find captivated not only prospectors but also government mining experts, nothing materialised. Successful mining development remained a dream, but a powerful one, in the discourse of mining experts.

"Asbestos goods of every description"

Imperial trade links ensured that British asbestos manufactures of all kinds quickly became available to Australian colonists. From the 1880s, British companies advertised their asbestos wares in all colonies, prominent among them Thomas Taylor & Co., United Asbestos Co., Dewrance & Co., India Rubber, Gutta Percha & Telegraph Works Co., Bell's Asbestos, Turner Bros, Imperial Asbestos Co., and Morrison Stanley & Co.[14] As well, enterprising colonial merchants obtained agencies for imported British products made of the new material. The Sydney merchant Leopold Barnett & Co. was unusual in advertising an American manufacture, Danville Asbestic Plaster.[15]

Asbestos product developers promoted the mineral's beneficial new uses. Merchants Wm Adams & Co. of Sydney staged a spectacular demonstration of imported Asbestos Fire-Proof Paint in 1887. Two sheds, one unpainted and the other covered in two coats of the special paint before being shipped from England, were placed on vacant land in Elizabeth Street. Kerosene was poured on both buildings and simultaneously lit.

> The flames spread rapidly, and soon destroyed the unpainted shed; the other, however, with the exception of a certain amount of charring on the wall next to the burning shed, remained intact.[16]

The watching public was invited to wonder at the amazing properties of modernity's magic mineral. Such demonstrations of the wizardry of

---

13 T Blatchford, *Mineral resources of the North-West Division. Investigations in 1912. Western Australia Geological Survey Bulletin*, 52 (Perth: WA Dept of Mines, 1913), 30–54, 120–21.

14 *Victorian Post Office Commercial Directory for Melbourne* 1884/85–1899/1900, H Wise & Co., Melbourne. *NSW Post Office Commercial Directory* 1886/87–1906, H Wise & Co., Sydney. *Tasmania Post Office Directory* 1890–1895, H Wise & Co., Hobart. *Queensland Official Directory* 1389–1907, H Wise & Co., Brisbane. *Western Mail* [Perth], 25 November 1898, 44, 46; 2 December 1898, 45, 46; 9 December 1898, 46.

15 *Building, Engineering and Mining Journal*, 4 January 1902, 5 January 1904.

16 *Australasian Builder and Contractor's News* (Sydney), 25 June 1887, 120.

asbestos became an established marketing ploy proving the paint's "remarkable" qualities, according to Cirkel.[17] Ten years later, the Prince of Wales and other dignitaries watched an identical trial at Millbank in London.[18] This marketing seems quaint today, but at the turn of the 19th century it addressed a growing urban fear. Then the terror of fire in the highly combustible wooden buildings which comprised all rapidly expanding towns and cities was ever present, and most residents had experienced the horror of seeing buildings engulfed in flames and fearing for their lives and property.[19]

There seemed no end to the promise of asbestos:

> It is made into roofing felt, cement, theatre curtains, and various heat-resisting articles, and has been recently spun into a light and fairly strong thread. Even ropes, with or without steel cores, are made from it for firemen. A new and rather surprising application is for army stockings, which have been shown to be less irritating to the feet of soldiers on the march than other stockings.[20]

Another curious new product was asbestos towels which were thought likely to sell well to prospectors: "When dirty it is only necessary to throw them onto a red hot fire, and after a few minutes draw them out fresh and clean".[21] Then there were reports in Sydney's commercial press in 1904 of a wall plaster named Salamanderite that could imitate any form of decoration.[22]

> It may be finished in exact facsimile of quartered oak, mahogany, maple, or any fancy cabinet woods, either plain or in the finest marquetry or bas-relief effects, indistinguishable from the most costly works.[23]

The magic asbestos mineral had been harnessed by modern manufacture to bring facsimiles of expensive goods, which had once belonged exclusively to the elite, within reach of a mass public.

---

17   Cirkel, *Chrysotile–Asbestos. Its occurrence, exploitation, milling and uses*, 278.
18   Jones, *Asbestos and asbestic*, 283–89.
19   R Maines, *Asbestos & fire. Technological trade-offs and the body at risk* (New Brunswick: Rutgers, 2005), ch. 1.
20   *Narandera Argus and Riverina Advertiser*, 8 February 1907, 7.
21   *Mount Leonora Miner*, 24 January 1904.
22   These Salamander decorations were also glowingly described and pictured in Jones, *Asbestos and Asbestic*, 271–74.
23   *Building, Engineering and Mining Journal*, 5 January 1904.

Some of these early asbestos applications were fanciful and short-lived. However most imported asbestos goods which found markets in Australia from the 1880s were used in heavy industry, particularly for steam-driven machinery, and became an indispensable component of industrial growth because of their great superiority to alternatives (mineral wools, felts and cloths, plaster of paris, slag, wood, clay, and such like).[24] In Sydney, merchants Wm Adams & Co., Arthur S Searle, Harrison & Whiffen, and J Blackwood & Son were successful early advertisers of imported asbestos boiler coverings and engine fittings, packings and millboard.[25]

Asbestos coverings, lagging, mattresses, packings, jointings, cloth, rope, and millboard became part of Australian industrial workplaces along with the steam engines for which these asbestos materials provided insulation and fireproofing. The Western Australian Goldfields Water Supply Scheme, completed in 1903 to carry water 351 miles from Mundaring Weir in the Darling Range to Kalgoorlie, provides a major example of this conjunction of asbestos insulation with steam power. Water was pumped the long distance by eight steam-pumping stations that contained, in all, twenty engines and twenty boilers. All were insulated with asbestos coverings and packings, imported as accessories with the pumping engines and boilers.[26]

Asbestos goods on sale in colonial markets by the close of the 19th century were not all imported products. Among the first local manufacturers was the Melbourne-based Australasian Asbestos Co. that advertised its products, including asbestos paint, as early as 1884.[27] Its paint, however, like its Bestic Plaster manufactured from 1899 to 1901, was not a marketing success. Most successful new colonial asbestos manufactures were applications for steam machinery. By the mid-1890s, a group of Melbourne manufacturers advertised a range of such products. In 1893–94, E L Clough developed the "Toope" patent that was a non-conducting fireproof covering for steam pipes, boilers, and cylinders made of asbestos and silicate cotton. One-and-a-half inches in thickness and manufactured in three feet lengths, it was suitable, Clough claimed, "for any hot surface up to 1800 degrees", saving 35 per cent in fuel costs. W H Brewer's "Silex" boiler covering, also

---

24 Maines, *Asbestos & fire*, 34–44.
25 *Australasian Builder and Contractor's News*, 1888–1891. *NSW Post Office Commercial Directory* 1886/87. *Construction and Local Government Journal* (Sydney), 28 January 1913. *Australasian Engineer* (Sydney), 11 January 1915.
26 James Simpson & Co., *Western Australia Coolgardie Water Supply Engines Pumps & Boilers*, Requisition No.1043, 31 October 1899.
27 *Victorian Post Office Commercial Directory for Melbourne*, 1884/85.

an asbestos compound, provided local competition as did both the "asbestos non-conducting boiler and steam pipe coverings and engine packings" made by Wm Adams & Co and Tuck & Co.'s "genuine asbestos goods and engine packing".[28] Protected by Victoria's colonial tariff, these manufacturers were able to develop intercolonial markets prior to federation in 1901.

A modern building material that "lasts for ever"

Enterprising merchants quickly imported asbestos cement sheets and roofing slates, first manufactured successfully in Europe at the turn of the century, the earliest shipment arriving in 1903.[29] Asbestos cement was advertised as an improvement on both nature and older manufactures. "The only building material that constantly grows better with the lapse of time", advised James Hardie & Co., merchant of Melbourne and Sydney and the first importer of asbestos cement products.[30] "They endure not for an age, but for all time", promised merchant F A Spriggs of Newcastle in 1913.[31] Defying the natural cycle of ageing, decay and demise made asbestos cement truly a modern wonder.

First into the building market, James Hardie named its imported asbestos cement sheets and slates Fibro-Cement. Given Hardie's position as industry leader through the entire period in which asbestos cement products were marketed in Australia (1903–1987), it is not surprising that the material was named "fibro" in popular usage. Nevertheless, James Hardie had its competitors virtually from the start, all of whom distinguished their imported products from Fibro-Cement. Spriggs marketed Asbestolite sheets and slates imported from Italy. In 1913–14 the firm was sufficiently established to hold stocks at Sydney, Newcastle, Katoomba, Hobart, and Brisbane, and to produce several catalogues with testimonials extolling the virtues of Asbestolite as compared with other brands.[32] Other competitors included the British asbestos company Bell's Poilite sheets for which

---

28 *Victorian Post Office Commercial Directory for Melbourne*, 1895/96–1899/1900. *NSW Post Office Commercial Directory* 1896/97. *Australian Mining Standard* (Sydney) 1892–1894.

29 James Hardie, *History of James Hardie & Co. Ltd from 1888 to December 1966* (Sydney: James Hardie, 1967), 8.

30 James Hardie & Co., *Fibro-Cement Asbestos Sheets and Slates*. Catalogue 16pp (Sydney: James Hardie & Co., 1911), 1, 13.

31 F A Spriggs, *Spriggs' Asbestolite Sheets and Slates* Catalogue (Newcastle: F A Spriggs, 1913/14), 9.

32 Spriggs, *Spriggs' Asbestolite Sheets and Slates*, 7, 12–16.

Malloch Bros had the Perth agency and Noyes Bros the Sydney one; Speaker's Eternit brand marketed in Sydney by John Sanderson & Co; and other unnamed brands offered by various merchants simply as "Asbestos-Cement Sheets".[33] Buy "Genuine" Fibro-Cement, "The Original Asbestos Sheets and Slates", James Hardie began to advise.[34]

Asbestos cement arrived in Australia in the first years of the 20th century unknown and unproven, and therefore required energetic promotion to break into building markets. The merchants placed advertisements in the daily and commercial press, produced brochures and catalogues explaining and extolling their new products, and published testimonials from satisfied customers and endorsements from architects, builders, and government officials. The messages they chose saw asbestos cement take shape in the minds of Australians. They promoted asbestos cement's suitability for warm climates, its fireproof quality, and its maintenance-free durability.[35] Malloch Bros of Perth listed all the advantages of its Poilite asbestos houses in a 1911 advertisement:

> A cooler house in summer
> A warmer house in winter
> A house that is fireproof
> A house that is weatherproof
> A house that is white ant proof
> A house that looks like a home
> A house that looks one thousand per cent better than a tin house
> A house that is everlasting.[36]

The thermal advantages of asbestos cement were highlighted because the merchants initially concentrated on country markets. Malloch Bros insisted that its asbestos houses were "within the scope of every Farmer" and made better farmhouses than galvanised iron. The South Australian Department of Agriculture agreed, in 1909 publishing the advice of T H Smeaton, builder and politician.

---

33   These included Sydney merchants P C Jones & Co. and Leopold Barnett & Co. See the *Construction and Local Government Journal* 1913–1917 for evidence of the competition in imported asbestos cement products.

34   *Construction and Local Government Journal*, 20 April 1914, 4 January 1915, 19 May 1916, 4 December 1916.

35   *Building, Engineering and Mining Journal*, 5 January 1904. *Construction and Local Government Journal*, 20 April 1914, 12. Spriggs, *Spriggs' Asbestolite Sheets and Slates*, 2.

36   *West Australian*, 8 April 1911, 6.

> Good friend as galvanised-iron has been to our settlers in the back blocks, the best that I can wish is that its glaring unloveliness may soon be banished from the land ... for it bakes its victims in summer and freezes them in winter, and, generally speaking, needlessly increases the burden of the pioneer's lot.[37]

Given this alternative, the advantages of asbestos cement sheeting were undeniable.

Roofing slates in a range of colours (red, purple, blue, black, grey) usually comprised part of import consignments. Marketing rhetoric emphasised their coolness and durability compared with galvanised iron, and their lightness and non-absorbency, compared with clay tiles or quarry slate. James Hardie did early business re-roofing country homesteads and churches. Architect John H Bates from Forbes testified in 1907 to his complete satisfaction with Fibro-Cement slates on such buildings, "being light, cool, and suitable for this western climate".[38]

Being fireproof was another of asbestos cement's advantages, according to the merchants. Spriggs' Asbestolite Sheets and Slates promised "absolute immunity from Bush Fires, and ... a considerable saving in Insurance, viz., 25 per cent".[39] As well as protection from heat, cold, and fire, asbestos cement promised protection from a great number of other threats: white ants and vermin, rust and rot, storm and damp, sagging and shrinking, cracking and crumbling, warping and buckling.[40] It was so hard it was "artificial stone", according to Spriggs.[41] After a severe hailstorm, the churchwardens of St Philip's in south Brisbane testified in 1908, "we consider that you are justified in adding 'hailproof' to its many advantages".[42] Asbestos cement was marketed as resistant to everything, even germs ("the most sanitary of all walls"), and therefore impervious to the passage of time.[43]

The merchants' rhetoric was powerful and the number who chose to try their hand at importing asbestos cement products indicates the building

---

37 T H Smeaton MP, "No.1 Fibro cement", in South Australian Department of Agriculture, *Home-Building in New Districts*. Bulletin 47 (Adelaide: South Australian Dept of Agriculture, 1909), 3–5.
38 James Hardie, "Testimonials", *Fibro-Cement Asbestos Sheets and Slates*.
39 Spriggs, *Spriggs' Asbestolite Sheets and Slates*, 2.
40 Spriggs, *Why Asbestolite? Because!!!* (Sydney: Spriggs' Asbestolite Co., c.1913/14).
41 Spriggs, *Spriggs' Asbestolite sheets and slates*, 1.
42 James Hardie, *Fibro-Cement Asbestos Sheets and Slates*, 9–12 & testimonials.
43 Spriggs, *Spriggs' Asbestolite Sheets and Slates*, 2. James Hardie, *Fibro-Cement Asbestos Sheets and Slates*, 3.

markets' growing interest in the new material. The main disincentive was cost. Imported asbestos cement products were not as cheap as most other slates, clay tiles, weatherboard, or galvanised iron.[44] The merchants could only counter that their imported product would be more economical in the end because it was both cheaper to erect and stronger and therefore more durable than its alternatives. The war, which provided an opportunity for asbestos cement manufacturing in Australia, changed this cost equation and, in so doing, eliminated the merchants from the building materials sector of the asbestos cement market. The legacy of these merchant developers was a pattern of asbestos consumption by Australians on which the new manufacturers could build.

Opportunities of war

As a "material of war", needed chiefly for new naval ships and fire protection, asbestos fibre was in increasing demand after 1914.[45] In the UK, this demand was translated into a search for increased supplies within the Empire. A flurry of correspondence crossed Australia in 1916 as the Australian government sought information on asbestos deposits in order to answer urgent requests from London about the possibility of fibre supply. State government answers were mostly similar and not encouraging: few or no known workable deposits, but considerable prospecting activity because of higher fibre prices.[46] The reply from Western Australia, drafted by the hard-headed State Mining Engineer, sounded a strong note of warning against optimism with regard to the known white asbestos deposits in the Pilbara.

> The narrowness of the vein, hardness of the country, and difficulties of access and transport of the mineral have made working very expensive under existing conditions.[47]

Australia could provide no fibre to ease the wartime shortage and no promise of future exports. An asbestos eldorado had not been found.

---

44 For price comparisons in 1915, see *Construction and Local Government Journal*, 18 December 1916, 7.
45 Twelvetrees, *Asbestos at Anderson's Creek*, 1–2.
46 Commonwealth of Australia. Prime Minister's Dept A2/1 1916/3960. National Archives [ACT].
47 WA Premier's Office to Prime Minister 23 August 1916. Prime Minister's Dept A2/1 1916/3960. NA [ACT].

Only the Tasmanian government reported promising developments.[48] The newly formed Durabestos Co., a subsidiary of Wunderlich Ltd, a well-established Sydney importer and manufacturer of building materials, had begun prospecting at Anderson's Creek where the Australasian Asbestos Co. had mined at the turn of the century. Best known for its manufacture of stamped architectural metalwork and importation of Marseilles roofing tiles, Wunderlich had not imported asbestos cement products prior to the war nor worked with asbestos in any way.[49] Now the company stole a march on its competitors. In August 1916, Durabestos flat asbestos cement sheeting entered the market.[50] In the following year, it began obtaining some of its white asbestos fibre needs for its new manufacturing works, located at Cabarita in Sydney, from Anderson's Creek in Tasmania. Australia's asbestos industry was transformed.

In commencing Australian manufacture of asbestos cement sheeting, Wunderlich took advantage of the virtual cessation of supplies of the imported product caused by wartime shipping disruptions and moved to satisfy unmet domestic demand. James Hardie followed, purchasing a sheet-making machine and accessing expert European advice in 1915, and setting up a subsidiary—The Asbestos Slate and Sheet Manufacturing Company Ltd.—to undertake the business in 1916.[51] Within nine months its Fibrolite flat and corrugated sheeting appeared on the market from its new Sydney factory at Camellia.[52]

The necessity to match prices gradually defeated the merchants. James Hardie's representation of Fibrolite as "the cheapest building material on the market" proved difficult to counter in the low-cost section of the building market.[53] Imported products had to contend not only with a relatively high weight-to-price ratio but also with a protective tariff regime. The British preferential rate, the lowest tariff level, was 15 per cent (of value) for asbestos cement sheets when domestic manufacture began in 1916, and

---

48 Tasmania Geological Survey Office to Prime Minister 3 August 1916. Prime Minister's Dept A2/1 1916/3960. NA [ACT].

49 For a history of Wunderlich Ltd, see S Bures, *The house of Wunderlich* (Sydney: Kangaroo Press, 1987).

50 *Construction and Local Government Journal*, 21 August 1916, 25 September 1916, 13 November 1916.

51 Carroll, *"A very good business": One hundred years of James Hardie Industries Limited, 1888–1988* (Sydney: James Hardie Industries, 1988), ch. 11.

52 *Construction and Local Government Journal*, 18 September 1916, 16 October 1916, 18 June 1917.

53 *Construction and Local Government Journal*, 9 December 1918.

rose to 25 per cent in 1920. Reporting in 1936, the Tariff Board observed that imports of sheeting had been "almost excluded" under this regime.[54] Spriggs continued to offer Asbestolite until 1921–22 but as a smaller and smaller component of its stocks while, in a last hurrah in 1922, Noyes Bros advertised a new line that it named Herculite.[55] Imported asbestos cement building sheets gradually disappeared from the market although the importation of specialised asbestos boards, for insulation and fireproofing, continued. Of the merchants who imported asbestos cement sheeting prior to the war, only James Hardie became an asbestos cement manufacturer. Others also moved into building materials manufacture, but of plywood, gypsum board, and plasterboard.[56] Thus the decisions of Wunderlich and James Hardie to begin the domestic manufacture of sheeting restructured the asbestos cement market.

Wunderlich's 1916 decision to both mine and manufacture asbestos was the first such decision of any commercial consequence since the Australasian Asbestos Co. failed at the turn of the century. Wunderlich began mining at Anderson's Creek in 1917 and erected Australia's first mill to replace hand-cobbing of fibre with mechanical milling. The small plant employed six workers and treated 20 tons of ore a day, producing one grade of fibre, the very fine short fibre being discarded. Mining ceased at Anderson's Creek in 1919, the operators defeated by what the government geologist described as the "irregularity and capriciousness" of the deposit. Mining development encountered low-grade ore in all the quarries, such that 100 tons of rock was required to yield one ton of fibre compared with a Canadian average of 40:1. As a consequence, production costs rose from £20 to £34 per ton and the operation proved uneconomic. In all, 440 tons of white asbestos fibre was supplied to Wunderlich's Cabarita factory.[57]

Although Tasmanian mining failed, asbestos cement manufacturing prospered, James Hardie employing around 100 workers at its Camellia factory by 1919. Fibre supply was the manufacturers' major problem because imported fibre continued in short supply and was highly priced. So, rather than abandon mining, Wunderlich decided to move its mill to Woodsreef

---

54   C/W Tariff Report; *Commonwealth Parliamentary Papers*, 4, 1907–08, paper no.32. C/W Tariff Board's Report on roofing tiles and asbestos cement sheets, etc, 15 October 1936, 6–7; *CPP*, 5. 1937, paper 32.

55   *Construction and Local Government Journal*, 7 February 1921, 7 June 1922.

56   *Construction and Local Government Journal*, 1917–1922.

57   A McIntosh Reid, *Asbestos in the Beaconsfield District. Geological Survey Report* 8 (Hobart: Tasmania Dept of Mines, 1919), 22–27.

near Barraba in northern New South Wales where James Hardie had also opened works.[58] At the same time James Hardie began additional small-scale mining at nearby Baryulgil, employing Bundjalong Aboriginal people, although development of any significance did not begin there until the following wartime period.[59] Imported fibre prices fell after 1920, however, and Barraba's white asbestos deposit proved increasingly uneconomic to mine and mill. In total 2,478 tons of fibre had been extracted by 1923 when both Wunderlich and James Hardie had abandoned mining.[60] These first properly funded ventures into asbestos mining in Australia failed because of circumstances which were to recur throughout the life of this mining: its commencement at a time of exceptional fibre demand; a reliance on asbestos deposits which were relatively expensive to mine and mill; and susceptibility to fluctuations in world fibre prices resulting in ultimately unsustainable mining ventures.

Sharing the interwar asbestos cement market

Asbestos cement manufacturing in Australia grew substantially between 1919 and 1939 with the popularity of the cheap and easily transportable building materials that the industry produced. By the mid-1930s, the annual output of flat sheets totalled 3,700,000 sq. yds and the industry employed 1,200 workers.[61] Numbers of fibro houses in Australia grew from 4,105 in 1921 to 23,125 in 1933 and 107,054 in 1947. All asbestos fibre was imported after 1923, the bulk of it white asbestos purchased from Canadian companies as well as some South African brown amosite asbestos from Cape Asbestos.[62]

Increased demand and higher prices for fibre from 1915 to 1920 had prompted not only the mining developments at Anderson's Creek and

---

58 James Hardie, through its subsidiary Asbestos Mining Co. of Australia, began mining the Barraba deposits in 1918 and Wunderlich in 1919. H Conder, "Asbestos mining in Australia", *Chemical Engineering and Mining Review*, 5 October (1920), 7–10. C Lonsdale Smith, "Asbestos mining in NSW", *Chemical Engineering and Mining Review*, 5 December (1922), 101–02.

59 *The effects of asbestos mining on the Baryulgil community*, Report of House of Representatives Standing Committee on Aboriginal Affairs, October 1984 (Canberra: Commonwealth Parliament, Australian Government Printing Service, 1984), ch. 2.

60 MacNevin, *Asbestos*, 36.

61 C/W Tariff Board's Report, 15 October 1936, 7.

62 White asbestos came from Canada's two major independent producers, Asbestos Corporation Ltd and A F Johnson Company. Evidence of J S Proud, consultant mining engineer to James Hardie, to Tariff Board Inquiry re Asbestos Fibre June 1954, 169.

Barraba but a multitude of tiny workings, many producing experimental parcels of fibre as commercial prospects were tested.[63] Western Australian interests were particularly keen to attempt commercial mining in the northwest but could not match imported fibre prices. They therefore sought tariff protection in order to foster an infant mining industry in a state that felt itself severely disadvantaged by a federal tariff policy which favoured manufacturing. James Hardie and Wunderlich lobbied strenuously against the proposal, which would have increased their costs, making competition more difficult with alternative building materials, chiefly galvanised iron, weatherboard, and plasterboard. In 1922 the Board of Trade refused to impose a tariff on imported fibre.[64] This outcome is unsurprising. While tariff protection was extended very widely to agricultural as well as manufactured products in the 1920s, it did not reach to mine products.[65] Thus the asbestos cement manufacturers were saved, as they were again in 1954, from a fibre-price regime that would have forced them to use uncompetitive Australian fibre.

For most of the interwar period, James Hardie and Wunderlich shared the Australian asbestos cement building materials market. By the mid-1920s the manufacture of Fibrolite flat sheeting and Super-Six corrugated sheeting was the major part of James Hardie's business and its most profitable; in 1926 the company restructured in recognition of this fact. It established new asbestos cement factories in Perth (1921), Melbourne (1927), Brisbane (1934), and Auckland (1938) and manufactured new asbestos cement products: pipes and Tilux decorative board in the 1920s, and moulded brake linings, moulded insulation, and conduit piping for electric cables in the 1930s. The company both undertook its own research, establishing a Laboratory and Research Department in 1933, and purchased the Australian patents for several new pipe-making machines in the 1930s as the manufacture of asbestos cement pipes began to assume commercial importance. That James Hardie had become synonymous with asbestos manufacturing was asserted in the naming of Asbestos House, the company's new twelve-storey Sydney head office occupied in 1929.[66] It was a statement of corporate success, a claim to industry leadership, and a marker of modernity.

---

63 In South Australia, about six such small workings existed in these years. *South Australian Asbestos*. February 1956.

64 "Asbestos Part 1", Prime Minister's Dept A461/1 A325/1/2 Part 1. NA [ACT].

65 Sulphur, which was a by-product of gold treatment, was a partial exception although it was a processed commodity. See C/W Tariff Board Annual Report, June 1923, 8–16.

66 James Hardie & Co., *History*. Carroll, *"A very good business"*. chs 12–14.

Wunderlich's asbestos cement division also expanded with new factories established in Melbourne (1926) and Brisbane (1936). By the mid-1930s Adelaide remained the only mainland capital without either or both a James Hardie and Wunderlich asbestos cement factory and therefore without the ready availability of locally produced asbestos cement building materials. A small South Australian firm, Ausbestos Ltd, endeavoured to fill this gap in the mid-1930s, marketing Ausbestos sheeting, but it did not establish a significant market.[67] Another tiny asbestos cement manufacturer, Asbestos Products Pty Ltd, set up business in Sydney in 1935 marketing Fibrobestos sheets.[68] It also had little commercial success, its historical significance lying in its later acquisition by Colonial Sugar Refining Company (CSR), thereby becoming the vehicle through which CSR entered the asbestos cement industry.

James Hardie attributed the interwar growth in sales of asbestos cement building materials to "intense selling campaigns".[69] Both James Hardie and Wunderlich advertised constantly in the metropolitan and country press, and in building, art, and architecture journals. They reinforced their message by regular mailings of illustrated literature to architects, contractors, and building materials' suppliers. Advertisements for Fibrolite and Durabestos appeared on roadside and railway hoardings. James Hardie built the first of its annual Fibrolite Show Homes for Sydney's 1917 Royal Show, enabling show-goers to inspect a real fibro house.[70] Display homes became an increasingly important component of company advertising. Wunderlich built its first, the Durabestos Demonstration Home, in its Garden Display in Broadway, Sydney, in 1941.[71] It enticed shoppers to "a delightful 'Oasis' in a heavily built-up shopping and industrial area".[72]

James Hardie's and Wunderlich's initial advertising of their new sheeting in the early 1920s portrayed fibro as appropriate for relatively large houses for the well-to-do (often as a holiday house). For instance, Wunderlich suggested that fibro exterior walls could be panelled to achieve "the picturesque half-timber treatments of mediaeval buildings" with "mock [oak] beams" in the interior.[73] In the 1930s and early 1940s, however, advertising shifted to

---

67   C/W Tariff Board's Report, 15 October 1936, 6.
68   Construction and Real Estate Journal [Sydney], 2 January 1936, 17. C/W Tariff Board's Report, 15 October 1936, 6.
69   C/W Tariff Board's Report, 15 October 1936, 6.
70   James Hardie & Co., *History*, 9.
71   Wunderlich Ltd, *Seventy years of Wunderlich Industry* (Sydney: Wunderlich, 1957), 78.
72   Wunderlich Ltd, *Sixty years of Wunderlich Industry 1887–1947* (Sydney: Wunderlich, 1947).
73   Wunderlich Ltd, *Durabestos Asbestos-Cement Sheets and Slates;* catalogue, 1924.

focus on those wanting home-ownership at low cost, "to permit of purchase by a small down payment and regular installments".[74]

Most important of all the companies' marketing strategies were the product catalogues.[75] These booklets, titled "Realising Your Dream of Home" and such like, pictured new, neat, and attractive fibro houses surrounded by colourful gardens and accompanied by house designs. Readers were told how asbestos cement sheeting could be used for walls, ceilings, and roofing to achieve "an attractive and modern home that will combine every desirable feature of comfort, durability and fire safety at a moderate cost".[76] Catalogues reminded country builders that "Durabestos relegates the bush shanty into oblivion. It enables the man of moderate means to own an attractive little home...a home to be proud of".[77]

Fibro's ease of transport was promoted to country people and those wanting a modern seaside cottage.[78] The catalogues told all homebuilders of the advantages of fibro over its major competitor, weatherboard.

> There is no excuse for building a flimsy weatherboard home when Wunderlich Manufacturers enable this bright little cottage to be erected speedily and economically. The weatherboard home is a snare and a delusion. It is cold in winter and hot in summer, invites white ants and should it take fire, becomes a heap of ashes within a few moments.[79]

In emphasising fibro's qualities of maintenance-free durability and protection against fire together with its modern ease-of-use and low cost, the manufacturers reproduced understandings already established by the prewar merchants and spread them more widely among Australians.

Wunderlich and James Hardie catalogues were not simply manuals showing their range of products and detailing specific items. Much more important was the imaginary world which the catalogues created for potential homeowners. It was a world of colour, order, and modest prosperity. Pleasingly painted fibro houses with terracotta roofs were placed against bright blue skies in suburban landscapes of orderly trees, neat lawns, and profusions of flowers, producing images that were visually

---

74 Wunderlich Ltd, *Wunderlich low cost Durabestos homes*; catalogue, 1941.
75 Wunderlich Ltd, *Forty years of Wunderlich Industry 1887–1927* (Sydney, 1927), 188–89.
76 James Hardie & Co., *The way to better homes. Build with Hardie's genuine Fibrolite* (Sydney: James Hardie & Co. Pty Ltd, 1939), 26pp.
77 Wunderlich Ltd, *Durabestos homes*; catalogue, Adelaide, 1920.
78 Wunderlich Ltd, *Seaside cottages*; catalogue, Sydney, 1937.
79 Wunderlich Ltd, *Durabestos homes*; catalogue, Sydney, 1920.

attractive and emotionally enticing. To keep them new and modern, catalogues were regularly re-issued in order to capture changes in design fashions. Wunderlich's asbestos cement catalogues, in particular, were works of art that followed an advertising style the company had developed to promote its elaborate and grand decorative metalwork.[80] These James Hardie and Wunderlich catalogues represent visually and dramatically the industry's message that asbestos embodied material comfort and happiness for all Australian moderns.

Coverings, packings and specialised boards

Unlike the interwar industry in asbestos cement building materials, which consisted of two relatively large domestic manufacturers catering mainly to the house-building market, the markets for asbestos coverings, engine packings, yarn and cord, mattresses for boilers, and specialist boards were diverse and were met by a number of overseas as well as domestic producers. Most of these Australian producers remained very small firms employing a few workers. Beginning in the 1890s in Melbourne, they marketed boiler and steam pipe coverings made of composite material, mainly asbestos, for heat and steam retention. Because these coverings could be a relatively simple product, consisting of loose, packed asbestos fibre bound in cloth, their manufacture attracted small firms.[81] For instance, C J R Le Mesurier, a Perth lawyer and entrepreneur, established the Western Australian Asbestos Manufacturing Company that produced coverings using local asbestos fibre from Bindi Bindi in the Yilgarn in the early 1920s.[82] There is nothing to suggest that the venture was a success.[83] Sydney and Melbourne manufacturers produced engine packings, which were usually composites of asbestos, rubber, and/or cotton.[84] In the interwar years, a British preferential tariff rate of 20 per cent on both coverings and packings assisted local

---

80   Wunderlich Ltd's collection of its catalogues has been archived at the Powerhouse Museum, Sydney, and various Hardie catalogues at the Mitchell Library, Sydney.

81   For a discussion of the distinction between asbestos coverings and packings, see the evidence of F C Wigan; minutes of evidence, Royal Commission on Customs and Excise Tariffs, Division XVI Miscellaneous - Cordage and Twines: Yarns; *CPP*, vol.5, 1906, paper no. 116, 523–25.

82   "Asbestos Part 1", Prime Minister's Dept A461/1 A325/1/2 Part 1. NA [ACT].

83   C J R Le Mesurier, Report of the Royal Commission on the Mining Industry 1925. *WAVP* paper 3, 1925, 167–68.

84   Inter-State Commission of Australia, Tariff Investigation Miscellaneous Group VII Asbestos Manufactures, Report 9 May 1916; *CPP*, 8, 1914–17, paper 266.

manufacturers to some extent, but the market's requirements were too diverse and specialised for domestic production to satisfy it fully. The Tariff Board estimated in 1931 that imports comprised two-thirds of the annual consumption of engine packings.[85]

Most of these asbestos goods were absorbed into industrial workplaces, but some found their way into commercial and public buildings as well as into residences. Where hot-air furnaces heated these buildings, asbestos coverings were used to insulate the furnace and pipes. For instance, in 1921 South Australia's main building journal recommended two or three thicknesses of asbestos paper for insulation of house furnaces. "Furnace men will do the work by contract, but every builder or contractor who has the time can do it as well", the journal advised.[86]

The rise of electricity spread asbestos usage, mostly in the form of special asbestos cement insulating boards. These boards used more asbestos than did the ordinary building board, as well as containing other materials such as bitumen and lacquer. A small South Australian electrical firm, Ellis & Clark Ltd, began production of Zelamite board in 1929 in competition with Sindanyo, one of the many imported products from major British company Turner. By 1930, these two firms divided the Australian market in half. That Ellis & Clark could achieve this market share employing only nine workers indicates the small size of that market. In 1931 the Adelaide firm argued successfully for an increase in the British preferential tariff rate from 25 per cent to 35 per cent.[87] Under this new regime, James Hardie (marketing Dilex) and the small South Australian firm Ausbestos Ltd also began producing electrical insulating boards.[88]

It is not possible to be precise or comprehensive about the range and quantity of goods containing asbestos introduced to Australians as the international asbestos industry expanded. These goods were made of composite materials, and were not necessarily categorised and counted as "asbestos goods". With product diversification, however, we can be sure that there was a great variety of them.

---

85   C/W Tariff Board's Report and Recommendations on cotton packings, asbestos cord, asbestos pipe and boiler covering and greasy packings of jute and hemp, 23 September 1931; *CPP*, 3, 1932–33, paper 114.

86   *Builders' & Contractors' Weekly Gazette* [South Australia], 31 October 1921.

87   C/W Tariff Board's Report and Recommendation on sheets composed of asbestos and cement or of similar materials, 24 April 1931; *CPP*, 3, 1929–31, paper 229.

88   C/W Tariff Board's Report on electrical insulating sheets of asbestos and cement or similar materials, 15 October 1936; *CPP*, 5, 1937, paper 48.

Prospectors continue to come and go

While interwar asbestos manufacturing prospered, no asbestos mining of any commercial significance occurred after 1923. Asbestos remained a prospector's mineral.[89] Prospecting activity increased during the depression as governments encouraged unemployed men out of the cities and into the outback using the lure of striking-it-rich or, at least, achieving subsistence. Rising asbestos fibre prices in the last years of the 1930s further encouraged prospecting. New or previously abandoned leases were worked by hand, the high-grade long fibre extracted by cobbing. In 1936–38, 150 to 200 men joined what the Western Australian Assistant State Mining Engineer described as "the great asbestos rush" to the Hamersley Range in the Pilbara to work the blue asbestos deposits.[90] In July 1938 he reported observing prospectors working at gorge faces on the exposed seams. "It is a day's work for a man to clean from one to two bags (of 100lb) by hand knapping", he reported. Donkeys would then carry the bags out of the gorges where trucks would complete the long journey over rough roads to the coast at Roebourne, itself a tiny northwest town.[91] The isolation, together with the lack of a marketing network, defeated the prospectors.

However, by 1939 two small companies had been formed to mine crocidolite, L G Hancock Asbestos Company, with leases centred on Wittenoom Gorge, and the Asbestos, Molybdenum and Tungsten Company with leases over Yampire Gorge.[92] This renewed mining activity immediately prior to war signalled the beginnings of another period of investment aimed at establishing asbestos mining on a commercial scale. What made it different from previous attempts was the intention to sell fibre overseas rather than primarily on the domestic market. It would prove to be the most expensive and disastrous attempt of all.

Another war, another boost

War in 1939 turned asbestos into a war material again and promoted the industry's rapid growth. James Hardie and Wunderlich were stretched to

---

89 Asbestos prospecting was also a marginal enterprise in New Zealand as is illustrated in Jim Henderson, *The exiles of Asbestos Cottage* (Auckland: Hodder & Stoughton, 1981).
90 J S Foxall, 'The blue asbestos deposits of the Hamersley Ranges and their economic importance', *WA Geological Survey*, Bulletin 100, Part II (Perth: Govt Printer, 1942), 38–39.
91 J S Foxall, report on visit to Hamersley Road Board Asbestos, 19 July 1938. "Asbestos Part 1", Prime Minister's Dept A461/1 A325/1/2 Part 1. NA [ACT].
92 *WA Geological Survey*, Bulletin 100, Part II & Appendices 1, 2.

meet government contracts for sheeting and pipes, Wunderlich's asbestos cement production tripling during the war.[93] Exceptional labour turnover, resulting from enlistments in the defence forces, added to pressures on the companies. They jointly established a new manufacturing plant in Adelaide in 1940 when interstate supply of asbestos cement sheets could not be guaranteed, naming this new sheeting Asbestolite. As war halted the importation of moulded brake linings that normally competed with James Hardie's Hardibestos brake lining, demand for the latter product soared as it did for other asbestos goods normally subject to strong import competition. Hardie's main plant at Camellia moved to three shifts a day and employed approximately 400 workers.[94]

The war increased demand for asbestos products at the same time as it seriously disrupted fibre supplies, especially of South African brown asbestos. World fibre shortages resulted in fibre purchases being managed by the Commonwealth Department of Import Procurement, which further disrupted the Australian industry because it hampered renewal of established contracts and personal contacts with suppliers. As it had done during the 1914–18 war, the Wunderlich company turned to Australian fibre, mining a white asbestos deposit at Baryulgil in north eastern New South Wales from 1942. In 1944 the mine became a joint venture with James Hardie. Despite this venture, Wunderlich still had insufficient fibre. The company therefore decided to introduce some blue asbestos into its asbestos cement mixes and began purchasing Western Australian blue in 1944.[95] This fibre was purchased from a completely new player in the asbestos industry, the Colonial Sugar Refining Company (CSR), one of Australia's largest companies, but not a miner.

Colonial Sugar Refining Company enters the industry

CSR's interest in asbestos followed its 1935 move into the manufacture of building materials with the development of Caneite, an internal wallboard produced from bagasse, a by-product of sugar-refining.[96] This development was quickly followed by another new product named

---

93   Wunderlich Ltd, *Sixty years of Wunderlich Industry 1887–1947* (Sydney: Wunderlich Ltd, 1947).
94   Carroll, *"A very good business"*, ch.18.
95   Evidence of A S P Sangster, Wunderlich Ltd, to Tariff Board Inquiry re Asbestos Fibre 1954, 121–24.
96   C/W Tariff Board's Report on wall and ceiling boards, 26 November 1935; *CPP*, vol.2, 1934–37, paper 215.

Gyprock, a gypsum-based wallboard.[97] The company began investigating asbestos-based external sheeting in 1941, commenced mining and milling white asbestos fibre near Zeehan on Tasmania's west coast in 1942, and took over the small Sydney asbestos cement company, Asbestos Products Pty Ltd, as well as blue asbestos leases[98] and a small mill at Wittenoom Gorge, held by L G Hancock Asbestos Company, in 1943.[99] To undertake this last venture CSR operated through Australian Blue Asbestos Ltd (ABA) that was incorporated in April 1943. Mining ceased at Zeehan in 1945 as CSR's plans for large-scale asbestos mining focused on the Wittenoom deposits.[100] These plans entailed the sale of Australian blue on the international market.[101] Why did a sugar company with no experience in mining or in working with asbestos decide to invest in mining and milling blue asbestos, the least used and most difficult to manufacture and market of the asbestos minerals?

First mined in South Africa in 1893, blue asbestos found no market until the interwar period when it began to be included in some asbestos cement pressure pipe mixes and developed specialist uses in acid-resistant and chemical-resistant packings.[102] South African production—the only commercially significant producer—remained relatively small, between 3,000 to 6,000 short tons yearly, until a boom in 1938–1939 almost doubled total output.[103] Even so, output was small and demand restricted.

CSR investigated Australia's supply of asbestos fibre in 1941–42 and found it inadequate to requirements. Given the company's decision to develop its building materials division and its already considerable investment in the manufacture of Caneite and Gyprock, its move into asbestos cement manufacture and its interest in Australian asbestos fibre is explicable. And certainly political concerns strongly

---

97 Evidence of K O Brown ABA/ CSR, to Tariff Board Inquiry re Asbestos Fibre 1954, 39.
98 Agreement L G Hancock, E A M Wright & others with ABA, 10 April 1943. Plaintiff's Exhibit WV-03951. Motley Rice LLC legal discovery exhibits list, 25 September 2006.
99 WA Mines Dept AU WA S20 cons964 1941/1254. SROWA.
100 CSR operated through the Tasmanian Asbestos Co. Pty Ltd when it mined at the Argent Tunnel near Zeehan. B L Taylor, *Asbestos in Tasmania*. Geological Survey Mineral Resources 9 (Hobart: Tasmania Dept of Mines, 1955).
101 CSR letter to Capital Issues and Building Control, 9 February 1943. Plaintiff's Exhibit WV-03900. Motley Rice exhibits 2006.
102 Great Britain Monopolies Commission, *Asbestos and certain asbestos products*, 5–9. Bowles, *The asbestos industry*, 15.
103 Cape Asbestos and Griqualand Exploration and Finance Company (Gefco) produced almost all this output.

influenced CSR's decision-making; in 1942 it could undertake the development of Wittenoom's deposits only with the strong support of the Commonwealth and Western Australian governments. Both were keen, first, because of the strategic importance of asbestos to national security and Australia's worrying dependence on overseas sources of supply. The Director-General of the Department of War Organisation of Industry wrote to CSR in December 1942 of his government's "complete agreement as to the importance and urgency attached to your projects".[104] Creating "a nucleus of population in the very empty North West of Australia" was the second political goal that Wittenoom's development was intended to achieve.[105]

CSR had a good understanding of the powerful politics of national development, political concerns with which it was already familiar as the Australian sugar-refining company operating chiefly in Queensland, but it failed to gain a similar level of knowledge of the economics and politics of international asbestos. The latter was crucial given CSR's intention to sell its fibre overseas. CSR's growth within the protected world of Australian sugar perhaps explains the blinkers it wore.

James Hardie was highly critical of CSR's Wittenoom decision. The deposits in the Pilbara were well known to the Australian asbestos industry: James Hardie's chairman had examined them in the late 1920s. They were judged uneconomic.[106] In an exchange of letters between chairmen in June–July 1944, James Hardie suggested that "the Colonial Sugar Refining Co.'s knowledge of the asbestos cement industry is of the same order as ours of the sugar refining industry" and questioned the economic viability of CSR's planned investment.[107] CSR ignored the warning.[108]

CSR's operations at Wittenoom from 1943 to 1966 demonstrated conclusively that the company's initial confidence was entirely misplaced. Its ignorance of the complexities of the world asbestos industry—of what was required to operate a profitable fibre export business in the exacting

---

104 Letter, G T Chippindall, Director-General of Department of War Organisation of Industry, 22 December 1942; quoted in evidence of K O Brown, to Tariff Board Inquiry re Asbestos Fibre June 1954, 40.

105 Evidence of K O Brown to Tariff Board Inquiry re Asbestos Fibre June 1954, 40–41.

106 Evidence of J T Adamson, James Hardie & Co., to Tariff Board Inquiry re Asbestos Fibre June 1954, 130.

107 Letter 13 June 1944; Annexure B, James Hardie & Co. submission to Tariff Board Inquiry re Asbestos Fibre June 1954, 136.

108 Letter 21 June 1944; Annexure B, James Hardie & Co. submission to Tariff Board Inquiry re Asbestos Fibre June 1954, 138.

and changeable environment inhabited by large and ruthless international competitors—was palpable from the beginning. Above all, CSR acquired insufficient knowledge to determine what market niche it could reasonably expect to carve out for itself. Undoubtedly, part of the problem was the misleading circumstances of war. In 1942–43, when the company decided to become a blue asbestos miner, it did so knowing that Johns Manville, the largest asbestos company in the US, was searching the world for 2,000 tons of blue every year for gas mask filters; that other US companies wanted it for "various secret processes"; that high grade long fibre—very well-represented in the Hamersley Range deposits—was in strong demand in Britain and the US; and that all asbestos fibres were in short supply everywhere.[109] Even before war's end all these market certainties had evaporated.

CSR moved into mining and milling in 1943 with the intention of producing at least 50 per cent "crudes"; that is, grades 1 & 2 long fibre of spinning lengths. This fibre, CSR believed, would attract high prices on overseas markets and would carry the enterprise. Sales of shorter grades would be a bonus.[110] But, when ABA's managing director visited Europe and the US early in 1945 looking for markets, he found that "the prospects of marketing the top grades are not as bright as we had hoped".[111] In fact, they were very dim indeed: potential for sales of a very small quantity in Britain, and no demand at all in the US which had large war stocks to use up. The company's target therefore shifted to a much greater total output of grade 3 fibre for the domestic market for use in asbestos cement manufacture.[112] CSR planned that part of the output would be absorbed by its subsidiary, Asbestos Products Pty Ltd, and a larger tonnage would be sold to James Hardie and Wunderlich. This changed business plan brought CSR into conflict with James Hardie and Wunderlich, and began a ten-year battle on the issue of how much—if any—blue asbestos fibre Australia's asbestos cement industry wanted to use, was technically able to use, or should be made to use by government direction.

---

109 WA Mines Dept AU WA S20 cons964 1404/41, 1943/0321. SROWA. United States Department of State, *Memorandum of Understanding 6 January 1943, Apportioning of Supplies of African Asbestos, Arrangement between the United States of America and The United Kingdom of Great Britain and Northern Ireland*, Washington, 1943, 2–3.

110 Letter 29 September 1943 C W R Powell CSR to H G Raggatt, Director Mineral Resources Survey, C/W Dept of Supply & Shipping, WA Mines Dept AU WA S20 cons964 1943/0321. SROWA.

111 Letter 22 August 1945 ABA to U/S for Mines, WA Mines Dept AU WA S20 cons964 1943/0413. SROWA.

112 Letters 17 January 1946 & 12 April 1946 C W S Powell, ABA managing director, WA Mines Dept AU WA S20 cons964 1945/0789. SROWA.

The Wittenoom venture was a totally misjudged enterprise. Both company and governments mistakenly trusted each other to be able to rationally assess the likely success of a blue asbestos mining industry. But neither was in a position to do so.[113] CSR's interest in blue asbestos mining originated from L G Hancock Asbestos Company's approach offering sale of its leases, rather than from a systematic analysis of asbestos minerals and asbestos mining.[114] On its side, government advice—particularly that of the Western Australian government—on both the quality of the deposit and the strength of the market was overly optimistic.[115] The Inspector of Mines for Cue district which covered the Hamersley Range deposits was a lone voice warning of dangerous power relations in the international asbestos fibres market: that in the prewar period large overseas combines had absolute control; that the war had halted overseas shipping at the same time as turning asbestos into a strategic material which allowed "the new man" in; and that in a postwar environment the large producers would "indulge in price warfare to squeeze out the new man". He went on to point out that the suitability of blue asbestos in asbestos cement sheets was not established and that what the industry needed, above all, were long-term market contracts.[116] He was correct on all points, but may as well not have written.

Neither company nor government understood the competition South African blue asbestos presented for the Wittenoom venture. The two major South African producers, Cape Asbestos and Gefco, were large mining companies with established places in the international asbestos industry. They held extensive, good quality fibre deposits in both the Cape Province and Transvaal, and access to a plentiful and cheap labour force. South African workings remained highly labour-intensive in the 1940s, still relying heavily on hand-cobbing by large numbers of "native" workers. South Africa's asbestos mines were non-scheduled; that is, not governed by any wage legislation. Wages therefore were low. Generally one "white miner" was employed for every 25 "native miners", the former paid at seven times the rate of the

---

113 Letter 30 September 1943 H G Raggatt to Under-Secretary for Mines; WA Mines Dept AU WA S20 cons964 1943/0321. SROWA. See also the assessment of W H Ifould, former NSW Deputy Director of War Organisation and Industry, in 'Solutions to the Australian housing problem', *The housing problem in Australia*. (Sydney: Angus & Robertson, 1947), 47.

114 Letter 20 September 1942 Peter Wright to U/S for Mines, WA Mines Dept AU WA S20 cons964 1254/41. SROWA.

115 Minute 31 May 1945 U/S for Mines to Minister for Mines; WA Mines Dept AU WA S20 cons964 1943/0413. SROWA.

116 Report 24 October 1945 C F Adams, Inspector of Mines, Cue District; WA Mines Dept AU WA S20 cons964 1945/0352. SROWA.

latter.[117] In the immediate postwar years, Cape Asbestos began a major capital investment to restructure its mining operations in order to increase output and improve fibre quality.[118] It switched from a contract system among its African miners to waged employment.[119] Its production of blue asbestos trebled between 1948 and 1970 while its number of mines was reduced from 22 to 3.[120] When ABA finally sent an engineer to South Africa in 1948 to observe mining and milling practices in order to learn as much as possible from the experienced operators, little was found to be transferable to Wittenoom.[121] And the grim warning about the nature of the price competition Australian blue asbestos faced does not appear to have registered.

Those other companies already experienced in surviving in the asbestos industry proved better judges of the potential of Wittenoom's blue asbestos. In the last months of war the de Bernales-owned West Australian Blue Asbestos Fibres Ltd offered James Hardie the sale of its Yampire Gorge leases, adjacent to those of ABA.[122] James Hardie consulted Wunderlich and advised Turner & Newall of the offer but none was interested, either separately or jointly. ABA subsequently acquired the leases after WA Blue Asbestos Fibres was unable to raise additional capital to continue mining.[123] This lack of interest among those experienced in the industry should have sounded alarm bells within CSR but it did not. The contrast between a tiny, high-cost mining operation in need of government assistance and a booming manufacturing industry was stark and foreboding.

Meeting postwar demand

The postwar years of reconstruction, industrialisation, and economic boom sharply increased demand for asbestos products. Figure 1.1 shows the growth in asbestos fibre imports by a factor of four from the mid-1940s to the mid-1960s.

---

117   Evidence of K O Brown to Tariff Board Inquiry re Asbestos Fibre June 1954, 49–57.
118   Cape Asbestos Co. operated its South African mining interests through three subsidiaries—Egnep Ltd, Amosa Ltd and Cape Blue Mines Ltd.
119   W E Sinclair, "The present status of crocidolite asbestos", *Asbestos*, May 1951, 4–12.
120   Gt Britain Monopolies Commission, *Asbestos and certain asbestos products*, 136.
121   CSR report on inspection of Cape Blue Asbestos Ltd, Union of South Africa. Plaintiff's Exhibit WV-03884. Motley Rice exhibits 2006.
122   West Australian Blue Asbestos Fibres Company, which had taken over the Asbestos Molybdenum and Tungsten Company, was a subsidiary of Austmac Investments Pty Ltd, a de Bernales' family concern.
123   ABA acquired the leases in December 1946. WA Mines Dept AU WA S20 cons964 1946/0180. SROWA.

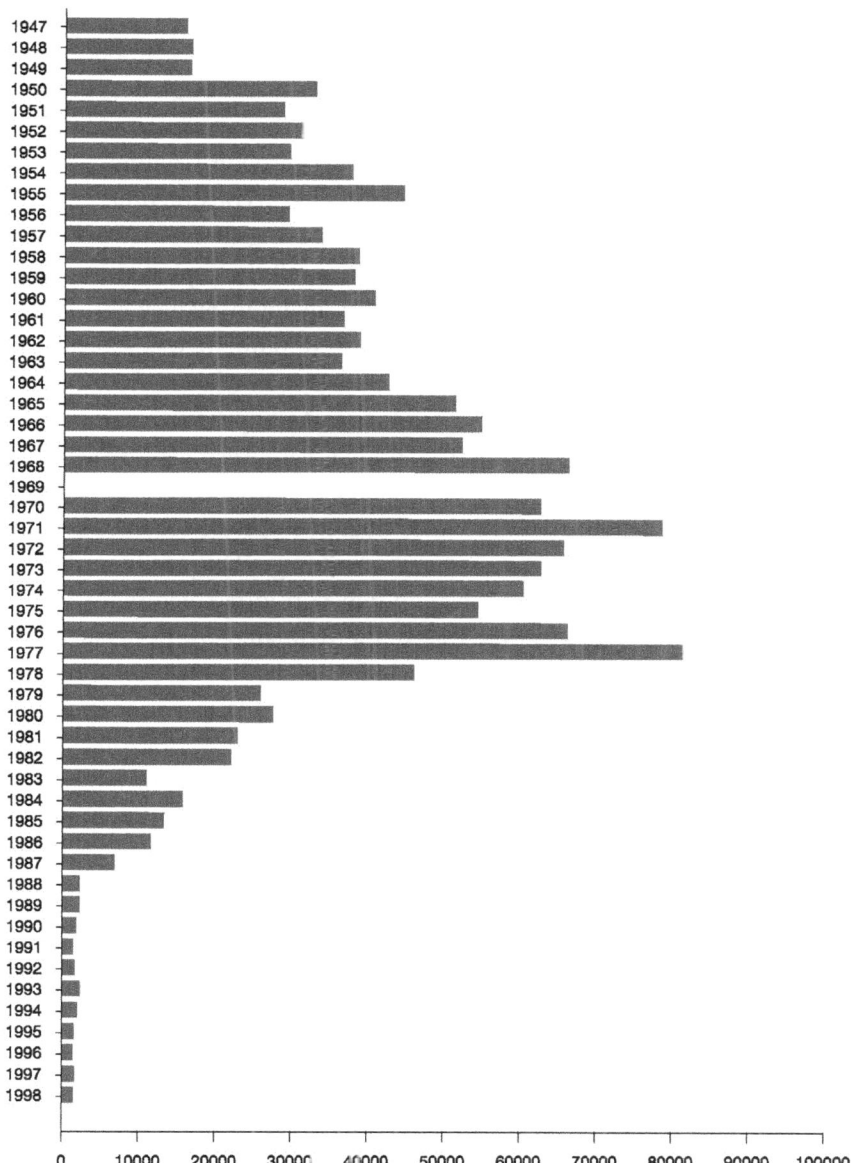

Figure 1.1: Total asbestos fibre imports to Australia [in short tons].
Source: *Australian Mineral Industry Review.* British Geological Survey, *World Mineral Statistics.* Keyworth, Nottingham.

This fibre was mostly white asbestos from Canada with some brown asbestos from South Africa, and almost all of it was absorbed in asbestos cement. Australia consumed more asbestos cement products per head of population than anywhere else in the world in the early 1950s; 19,000kg per head compared with the US figure of 5,261kg in 1951.[124] High demand was caused primarily by a severe housing shortage that was not alleviated in most states until the late 1950s, and later in Sydney. Through Commonwealth/ State Housing Agreements, a key plank of postwar reconstruction, governments combined to fund and build workers' housing in country and city. State housing authorities created new suburbs in all the capital cities, ideal territory for the asbestos cement companies. Chiefly in Sydney and Perth, whole suburbs of asbestos cement housing were built. It was a relatively cheap building material, marketed as modern and maintenance-free, a product that would last a lifetime. This "fibro frontier" was predominantly working class territory, but its use spread into middle class Australia for enclosing verandahs and building extensions, upgrading fences around suburban blocks, and building garages, sheds, and holiday houses. Asbestos cement sheeting was also used extensively in new industrial buildings that proliferated with the postwar growth of manufacturing and transport infrastructure.

Asbestos cement manufacturers used approximately 90 per cent of all asbestos fibre consumed in Australia in mid-century. In 1953, for instance, 89 per cent of all fibre was used in asbestos cement: 60 per cent by James Hardie, 22 per cent by Wunderlich, 5 per cent by CSR's subsidiary, Asbestos Products Ltd, and 2 per cent by the small Tasmanian manufacturer, Goliath Portland Cement Company.[125] A successful cement company, Goliath began manufacturing Tasbestos asbestos cement sheeting in 1947 to cater to the Tasmanian market, given that neither James Hardie nor Wunderlich had established a local plant.[126]

The 10 per cent of imported fibre not used in asbestos cement was incorporated in the small-scale production of a wide range of asbestos goods, James Hardie's brake linings and other friction goods absorbing around 1 per cent.[127] As they had done since the 1890s, many tiny firms manufactured boiler lagging and coverings, engine packings, and jointings. Three somewhat larger firms also manufactured other heat and steam insulation

---

124　Tariff Board Inquiry re Asbestos Fibre June 1954, transcript 134.
125　Evidence of K O Brown to Tariff Board Inquiry re Asbestos Fibre, June 1954, 72.
126　Goliath Portland Cement Co., *The Goliath Works* (Railton: Goliath Portland Cement Co., 1968).
127　L C Noaks, N H Ludbrook, *Asbestos*. Mineral Resources of Australia, Summary Report 17 (Canberra: C/W Bureau of Mineral Resources, Geology & Geophysics, 1945 rev. 1948).

goods—cord, rope, yarn—and fire protection goods—blankets, suits, aprons, and gloves. At least one of these, Tucks Asbestos Ltd, had been in the industry since the 1890s. Locally manufactured asbestos goods for industrial applications, together with continued imports of similar goods, resulted in a substantial accumulation of asbestos in industrial workplaces that was not always visible or recognised. Detailing the many applications of asbestos in 1948, British writer A E Williams observed in relation to asbestos jointing material used in pressure pipelines that "although almost universally used... relatively little is known about it outside the asbestos industry".[128] This was true of many other industrial applications.

Sprayed asbestos insulation, a new product that was heavily promoted from the mid-1950s, proved popular for commercial and public buildings, meeting multiple needs: for fire protection, heat and noise insulation, and condensation absorption. The mixture of asbestos, cement, and water was applied using a spray gun. It set firm only after it had been applied, thus ensuring that it reached into every nook and cranny, giving it an advantage over insulation boards. The British company Turner's Limpet brand was first into the market and most widely used.[129] It was applied by companies licensed to use the process.[130] Similar products were soon competing for the growing market. In 1959 CSR advertised its Silbestos brand, "in many cases, the most inexpensive insulation available".[131] The speed and ease with which the new material could be applied was seen as a significant advance in modern know-how. However asbestos insulation workers quickly experienced a heavy burden of disease, and it was Selikoff, Churg, and Hammond's US paper on asbestosis amongst them, presented at the famous 1964 conference in New York, that was the first effective public exposure of the asbestos health hazard since the US industry silenced opponents in the 1930s.[132] A reckoning was coming, if slowly.

While these were prosperous times for almost all the Australian asbestos industry, tensions existed within the industry relating to the use of local blue asbestos fibre. Conflict erupted in 1954 and was aired publicly in a Tariff Board inquiry.

---

128   A E Williams, *Asbestos. Its preparation and application* (Manchester: Emmott & Co. Ltd, 1948), 20–21.

129   Williams, *Asbestos*, 19–20.

130   See Acoustics (Aust) Pty Ltd's advertisement; *Architecture and Arts*, January 1956, 8–9.

131   *Construction* (Sydney), 16 December 1959, 28–29, 30 December 1959, 10.

132   I J Selikoff, J Churg, E C Hammond, "The occurrence of asbestosis among insulation workers in the United States", *Annals of the New York Academy of Sciences*, 132, 1965, 139–55.

An industry in conflict

CSR's dream of creating an international blue asbestos mining industry at Wittenoom quickly turned to nightmare as the venture proved uneconomic. ABA could not secure its markets because it was not competitive with large-scale, low-cost fibre suppliers like Canada and South Africa. As hopes of overseas markets faded, CSR turned its attention to the domestic market, but this proved out of reach as well. Figure 1.2 compares Wittenoom blue fibre's grade 3 prices with Canadian white grade 4 prices and South African brown prices. These were the grades used in asbestos cement manufacture.

	Canadian white Grade 4/4K Percentage of Wittenoom blue price Perth %	South African brown Percentage of Wittenoom blue price Perth %
1950	44	29
1951	52	30
1952	53	27
1953	67	37
1954	77	41
1955	100	56
1956	99	57
1957	98	60
1958	108	65
1959	109	68
1960	105	68
1961	98	68
1962	92	66
1963	101	73
1964	103	74
1965	94	69
1966	103	74

Figure 1.2: Comparison of asbestos fibre prices, Australia 1950-1966
Source: *Australian Mineral Industry Annual Review*.

The three major companies in the Australian asbestos cement industry—James Hardie, Wunderlich and CSR—did not agree on what fibre, if any,

Wittenoom's blue could replace in asbestos cement mixes. CSR argued that it could replace much of the Canadian white, while James Hardie insisted that it was suitable only to replace brown fibre.[133] The financial implications of the argument can be seen in Figure 1.2 above. Brown fibre was always much cheaper than Wittenoom blue. Canadian white sold at lower prices until 1955 when Wittenoom blue reached parity in Perth, a position which more or less held for the rest of the life of the Wittenoom industry. However another £6 to £10 was added to the Australian blue price by transport costs to the eastern states, making Canadian white always the cheaper fibre in the larger eastern states market. South African blue could always be purchased in Australia more cheaply than Australian blue.

By 1954 ABA had reached crisis point. A stock of 3,000 short tons of blue fibre had built up and the company's accumulated losses had reached £750,000. Assured markets simply had to be found. Wunderlich used some blue in its asbestos cement mixes and had signed a five-year contract with ABA in 1947 to purchase 30 per cent of Wittenoom's output up to 2,000 short tons a year. Between 1947 and 1953 Wunderlich had bought a little over 3,000 short tons of fibre from ABA but complained about the quality of the fibre.[134] The contract was not renewed and, in 1954, Wunderlich turned to cheaper South African fibre. The bigger problem, according to ABA, was James Hardie which used no blue in its asbestos cement mixes. Something had to be done or ABA would have "no course but to shut down at Wittenoom".[135]

For the entire period of Wittenoom's operation ABA argued for, and received, government assistance on the grounds that the venture was serving a political purpose, populating the "empty north", and therefore deserved special treatment. This argument was used in 1954 to demand a protective tariff on imported asbestos fibre. ABA had asked for such a tariff in 1945-46 without success; now it tried again. Supported by the Western Australian government, ABA applied to the Tariff Board for a 40 per cent tariff, with exemption if the imported fibre was included in manufacture that used a minimum of 15 per cent Australian blue. Both James Hardie and Wunderlich opposed the application.

---

133   *C/W Tariff Board report on asbestos fibre*, 24 March 1955, 6–15.
134   ABA letter, 30 September 1949. Plaintiff's Exhibit WV-03887. Motley Rice exhibits 2006.
135   Evidence of K O Brown and M G King, ABA & CSR, to Tariff Board Inquiry re Asbestos Fibre June 1954, 27–96.

James Hardie, which produced 70 per cent of all Australian asbestos cement products in 1955, was the most critical, arguing that

> the development of the remote asbestos deposit in Western Australia was ill-advised and uneconomical, and it is unreasonable to expect asbestos cement manufacturers to pay for such a costly experiment.

Australia ranked fourth in total world consumption of asbestos cement products and first in per capita terms, James Hardie pointed out: between 1950 and 1953, 25 per cent of all new Australian houses and 50 per cent of all those in New South Wales and Western Australia had been built with asbestos cement sheeting. Such success should not, James Hardie argued, be threatened by the burden of a venture that "should never have been started". The cost of Wittenoom "should not be loaded on the working man's low cost asbestos cement home". Wunderlich, which produced 22 per cent of Australian asbestos cement products, gave no more encouragement. It had incorporated blue in its mixes since the war but was in the process of eliminating it and returning to its prewar mix of white and brown. Both companies stressed what Wunderlich described as the "grossly excessive" price of Wittenoom blue.[136]

The Tariff Board ruled that imported asbestos fibre should remain duty free, rejecting the notion that manufacturers should be compelled to absorb Wittenoom blue. It concluded that ABA had "given scant consideration to asbestos cement manufacturers" or to the "cost to the community in general", a reference to the importance of cheap asbestos cement building materials in meeting Australia's postwar housing demand.[137] This decision forced CSR into major compromise with James Hardie. The two companies reached agreement in 1957 that CSR would end its involvement as a manufacturer of Fibrock asbestos cement products and keep out of it in future while, in return, James Hardie agreed to buy Wittenoom blue at prices tied to those of Canadian white. In its last years of operation ABA was selling approximately half its output to James Hardie which was incorporating 18 per cent blue in its products, but considered that it was paying £5 per ton more than the fibre was worth.[138]

---

136 *C/W tariff board report on asbestos fibre*, 1955, 5–16.
137 *C/W tariff board report on asbestos fibre*, 1955, 8–9.
138 Minute, State Shipping Service to Premier 19 October 1965; and CSR Feasibility Study, 29 September 1966; "Wittenoom General", WA Dept of North West, Stack 15 AN 40/5 Acc.1302 A21. SROWA.

This accommodation with James Hardie helped to secure for ABA its most successful years with guaranteed markets. The company had already won a five-year (1955–59) contract with the major US company Johns Manville to supply 7,000 short tons of blue each year.[139] ABA believed it had finally won through to profitability. It was not sustained, however; Johns Manville did not renew its contract and no other significant overseas sales were made despite substantial advertising in the US industry journal Asbestos from 1955 to 1966. In the early 1960s, mining and milling costs rose while fibre prices fell; Wittenoom's blue was again unprofitable.[140] The operation closed in December 1966.

Instead of finding an asbestos eldorado as it had anticipated, CSR joined a long line of defeated asbestos miners. Its failure was the largest of them all and a major corporate misjudgment. That it was also an occupational and environmental health disaster made CSR's culpability of another order altogether, as later chapters will discuss.

The rise and rise of James Hardie

James Hardie had always led the Australian asbestos cement market; by 1977 it held a virtual monopoly. The company took advantage of the opportunities presented by three decades of building and infrastructure construction to strengthen its position as an asbestos cement manufacturer. It undertook a major program of development and modernisation in the 1950s and 1960s, investing in new plants in Perth, Brisbane, and Adelaide, and in new pipe and sheet-making machines at all its plants. Asbestos cement pipes showed greatest growth in demand, by 1962 providing 50 per cent of company profits, compared with 35 per cent from building products and 15 per cent from brake linings and other friction products. The pipes' popularity lay in their cheapness, selling at 25 per cent less than steel pipes and 50 per cent less than concrete.[141] Fibro pipes were used for water reticulation and irrigation, water supply, sewerage and drainage, industrial effluent removal, and conduit for electricity and telephone lines.

Much of the pipes market was dependent on government contracts. Before contracts could be won, authorisation was required from government

---

139   CSR board minutes, 7 December 1955. Plaintiff's Exhibit WV-03891. Motley Rice exhibits 2006. *Asbestos* (Philadelphia), June 1956, 58.
140   ABA letter to WA Minister for Industrial Development, 28 August 1963. Plaintiff's Exhibit WV-03906. Motley Rice exhibits 2006.
141   Carroll, *"A very good business"*, ch. 21.

agencies—for instance, public works departments and water boards—that asbestos cement piping met the specifications for particular usages. These authorisations came piecemeal. For instance, metropolitan water boards responsible for areas where pipes were required to withstand heavy traffic were slower to accept asbestos cement piping than were public works departments responsible for country water supply. Thus government contracts were won first for rural water supply, sewerage, and drainage, and for work in Papua/New Guinea.[142] By 1970 Fibrolite pipe was accepted for sewerage lines in all parts of Australia.[143]

In the 1960s-1970s resource boom, the mining industry—for instance, the Pilbara iron ore ventures—absorbed large quantities of fibro pipes. They were also used extensively in irrigation projects to replace the open channel systems from which water loss by evaporation was severe. In 1956, James Hardie began financial sponsorship of the Water Research Foundation of Australia and added the "Great Thirst" publicity campaign in 1961 to create public awareness of the need for a major water conservation program, an outcome which could not but enhance Fibrolite pipe sales.[144]

James Hardie had the asbestos cement pipe market to itself. Wunderlich attempted to compete by forming a new partnership, Wunderlich Hume Asbestos Pipes Pty Ltd, in 1960 to manufacture pipes. It proved a disastrous decision. The enterprise failed, incurring substantial losses for Wunderlich, and James Hardie acquired the new company cheaply in 1964. Wunderlich was badly damaged and increasingly vulnerable to takeover. The end came in 1969 with CSR's acquisition of the company and its incorporation in CSR's Building Materials Division.[145] James Hardie's competitor for more than fifty years was no more.

The postwar years of prosperity were not without their problems for James Hardie, chief among them being the declining demand for all-fibro houses after the mid-1950s. The company held its share of the building materials market by embarking on a major program of new product design. Instead of a reliance on Fibrolite flat and corrugated sheeting, a plethora of new boards enticed the market: exterior boards of different profiles and colours, some of the most popular simulating wooden boards; interior boards in a great variety of colours; insulation boards; compressed flooring boards; fencing boards; and moulded panelling. With the new product

---

142 James Hardie Asbestos Ltd, *Annual Report* 1968.
143 James Hardie Asbestos Ltd, *Annual Report* 1970.
144 James Hardie Asbestos Ltd, *Annual Reports* 1962, 1963. James Hardie, *History*, 37, 47.
145 Bures, *The house of Wunderlich*, ch. 8.

range James Hardie moved away from an almost total reliance on the housing market into the commercial and public building sector where big buildings absorbed large quantities of asbestos cement, mostly in the form of moulded products. Sales to the housing market revived with the growth of home renovation. These new products and their use in composite constructions increased the quantities of asbestos cement in the built environment while making the material much less visible and identifiable. Wunderlich followed the same strategies but could not match James Hardie in the range of its new products.

A number of takeovers further increased James Hardie's domination of Australian markets. The company acquired Wunderlich's share of their joint South Australian Asbestolite plant in 1956; Asbestos Products Pty Ltd from CSR in 1957 as part of its cessation of hostilities over Wittenoom's crocidolite; Better Brakes Holdings Ltd in 1959 to expand its market in asbestos friction products; and Wunderlich Hume Asbestos Pipes Pty Ltd in 1964. Montpelier Foundry Pty Ltd, a Tasmanian manufacturer of cast iron pipefittings, was acquired in 1969. Turner & Newall combined with James Hardie to form the friction materials company Hardie-Ferodo Pty Ltd in 1961 under James Hardie's management. Expansion into Asia began in 1964 with James Hardie's joint enterprise with Turner & Newall and Eternit to set up an asbestos cement pipe plant in Malaysia, and was followed in 1969 by the establishment of a James Hardie plant in Indonesia.[146] James Hardie's rise culminated in 1977 when it paid CSR £19,000,000 for the former Wunderlich's asbestos cement division (with factories at Rosehill, Sunshine and Gaythorne), thus giving the company a virtual monopoly of Australia's asbestos cement business.[147]

James Hardie Asbestos Ltd had grown into a significant asbestos manufacturer in the world industry. Export markets for its building products and pipes had been developed in east and southeast Asia, and the US.[148] It had cordial relations with Turner & Newall and a shareholding in Cape Asbestos Co., as well as long-established business connections with its Canadian white asbestos fibre suppliers. James Hardie's success was not built on mining activity. While it continued until 1976 to obtain 1-2 per cent of its white fibre from its mine at Baryulgil, no asbestos deposit in

---

146 James Hardie Asbestos Ltd annual reports, 1957–1970. Carroll, *A very good business*, chs 19, 23, 36.

147 "Great profit growth potential in James Hardie", *Rydge's*, 50, August (1977) 33–34. CSR, *Annual Report* 1977.

148 Carroll, *A very good business*, chs 28, 29.

Australia was sufficiently attractive to lead it into establishing a major backward linkage into mining.[149] It was cheaper to import its fibre.

James Hardie's zenith as a major asbestos manufacturer was also the zenith of the Australian asbestos industry, with asbestos fibre imports and consumption peaking in the years from 1968 to 1977. Australian media coverage of the threat of asbestos related disease skyrocketed in 1975 (see below, chapter 4) and the decline of the Australian asbestos industry began soon after. The time of the modern asbestos developer had passed.

Demise

Storm clouds had been building over the asbestos industry in the US since October 1964 when an international conference organised by the New York Academy of Sciences on the biological effects of asbestos marked the end of the long public silence on asbestos related disease.[150] The asbestos companies began placing warning labels on their insulation products in 1964–65, immediately following the conference, but it was already too late. Although the tidal wave of public exposure was delayed in Australia until the mid-1970s James Hardie read the signs and began work on the technology of asbestos-free fibre cement in the early 1970s.[151] Asbestos cement was renamed fibre cement in James Hardie's literature in 1979, although it took a little longer for asbestos to be eliminated from the actual products. Hardiflex II, marketed in 1981, was the company's first asbestos-free fibre cement building material.[152] Asbestos was eliminated from all building boards and mouldings by the end of 1983, fencing sheets (used almost solely in Western Australia) by 1985, and pipes by 1987.[153] Fibre cement prospered; asbestos cement was no more. In 1979, James Hardie Asbestos Ltd became James Hardie Industries Ltd, and the company's head office ceased to be Asbestos House and became James Hardie House.

Over the same period state jurisdictions tightened their asbestos regulations to reduce maximum allowable concentrations of asbestos. Most introduced

---

149 James Hardie sold its Baryulgil mine to Woodsreef Mines Ltd in 1976. MacNevin. *Asbestos*, appendix 1.

150 "Biological effects of asbestos", Proceedings of International Conference on the Biological Effects of Asbestos, New York Academy of Sciences, Waldorf-Astoria, October 1964, *Annals of the New York Academy of Sciences*, 132, 31 December 1965.

151 James Hardie Asbestos Ltd, *Annual Report* 1968.

152 James Hardie Industries Ltd, *The name behind the names*. James Hardie Industries, 1984, 16.

153 James Hardie Asbestos Ltd, *Annual Reports* 1979, 1980, 1985, 1987.

bans on the mining of raw asbestos and the manufacture, import, and installation of products containing blue and brown asbestos from 31 December 1984. The importation of fibre fell precipitately after 1977, as Figure 1.1 above showed (with an initial 86 per cent drop from that peak year to the following one), but through the 1990s the residual import total remained stubbornly at over 1000 short tons per year in order to meet the requirements of friction parts manufacturers for brake pads and linings, and clutch facings. At the end of the century the trade unions took concerted action, the Australian Council of Trade Unions resolving in 2000 to work towards a complete ban on the importation of all asbestos fibre and asbestos products. Finally agreement between the federal, state, and territory governments was reached to ban all asbestos fibre and products containing asbestos from 31 December 2003. The end of the industry in Australia had come.

Conclusion

Asbestos was the 20th century's modern mineral, rising with the new century and turning into a pariah mineral by its end. The small number of transnational corporations which controlled the market in the capitalist world and the companies which dominated the Australian market were technically proficient at developing new usages for the fibres and at creating new commodities. These were promoted as boons to modern life, making life for moderns easier, seemingly safer, and more comfortable thanks to an exploding range of product choices available to more and more people. At the same time, the companies concealed the Faustian bargain that asbestos usage entailed. The "magic mineral" brought with it a hidden curse. The companies arrogantly believed that their technical scientific expertise could eliminate any problem; at the same time, they gambled that they would not be held accountable or financially liable for adverse outcomes. The gamble only partly paid off. It was a peculiarly modern tragedy.

Chapter 2

ASBESTOS IN THE BUILT ENVIRONMENT

Lenore Layman

Houses, cars, trains and planes, home and workplace insulation, household and office appliances, together with electricity, water supply and telephone connections: all of them essential consumer goods and services that by mid-20th century contained asbestos. In industrial workplaces asbestos steam packings, coverings and other insulation were everywhere. Modern buildings—residences, offices and factories—absorbed large quantities of asbestos cement. Asbestos cement pipes found multiple uses. In these many ways asbestos became embedded in all built environments, bringing virtually the entire population into contact with the mineral. However, while asbestos was spread across Australia, that spread was not uniform. There were hotspots—in early postwar housing commission suburbs, particularly in New South Wales, Western Australia and the Northern Territory, in and around asbestos manufacturing works and heavy industrial workplaces, on trade worksites, in office buildings and houses where asbestos insulation was used, in asbestos mining towns, and where asbestos tailings were spread. This chapter discusses this uneven introduction of asbestos into the built environment where much of it remains to this day. The clean up is ongoing.

A modern home in fibro

The asbestos industry promised Australians a home. Fibro houses—that is, timber-framed houses clad in flat asbestos cement sheeting, commonly called fibro—were built in great numbers in suburbs, towns and country areas from the 1930s to the 1960s. At their peak presence in the mid-1960s, nearly half a million fibro houses comprised almost 20 per cent of Australia's housing stock. They were named fibro houses in New South Wales and asbestos houses in Western Australia, the two states that made greatest use of them. The former name has been adopted here. Marketed as new and modern, these houses were more affordable than their alternatives, easy to prefabricate, quick to build when demand was pressing, and relatively simple for owner-builders to construct. For these reasons, asbestos cement building materials became an essential input to the great explosion of house-building from the 1940s to the 1960s.

The single most powerful social promise made to Australians by business and government after the Second World War was the promise of a home. Finding a home of their own was a postwar priority for most married couples, with a national shortfall of over 300,000 houses at war's end.[1] Servicemen and women returned to spouses and children living with parents or sharing accommodation with other families. Couples began married life in garages, sheds or on verandahs. Any potential accommodation, no matter how unsuitable, was pressed into service. In mid-1947, approximately 3.5 per cent of Australians (209,760 people) were sleeping throughout the year on sleepouts or verandahs which were not permanently enclosed; many more slept in similar spaces closed in with louvres, or alternatively with timber or fibro.[2] For both national and state governments, managing the enormous pent-up demand for housing became a major task of postwar reconstruction.

Asbestos cement manufacturing companies targeted these young married couples, urging them to build a Fibrolite home or a Durabestos home or an Asbestolite home (in South Australia) or a Tasbestos home (in Tasmania). Low cost was the major enticement and it remained the cornerstone of advertising.[3] A fibro house would be a modern home, according to the industry.[4] They were modern in that they were starkly simple in shape with clean lines, an absence of ornamentation, low-pitched or skillion roofs, and some interior open planning.[5] The Small Homes Service of the

---

1   *Australian Housing Bulletins* 1–7 (Canberra: Commonwealth Dept of Works & Housing, reprinted 1947).

2   Statistician's Report, *Census of the Commonwealth of Australia* 30 June 1947, 3, 286.

3   *Architecture and Arts*, July 1956, 20. *The Architect*, December 1945, 18; December 1955, 6. *West Australian*, 8 October 1953, 17.

4   James Hardie, *Don't dream—build! Your guide to building beautiful new style homes of Hardie's "Fibrolite"* (Sydney: James Hardie & Co., 1957), 33pp. *Building and Construction Journal*, 18 February 1949, p.4; 1 April 1949, 2; 14 October 1949, 5. *The Architect*, September 1950, 28. *West Australian*, 20 March 1947, 6; 4 February 1948, 4.

5   Wunderlich Ltd, *Designs for small homes*; catalogues, 1955. Powerhouse Museum collection. *Building and Construction Journal*, 14 October 1949, 5. *Architecture and Arts*, September 1956, 20. *The Architect*, December 1956, 40.

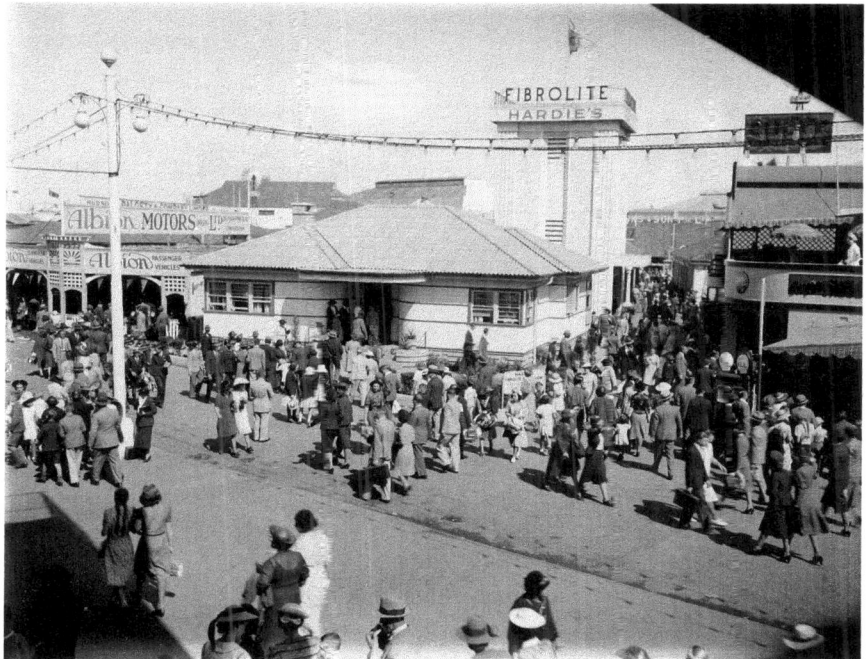

Figure 2.1: A popular attraction at Sydney Royal Easter Show 1949. James Hardie Fibrolite show home.
Courtesy: State Library of New South Wales

Royal Victorian Institute of Architects combined with James Hardie to plan and build just such a demonstration home in the Melbourne suburb of Blackburn in the mid-1950s.[6] It was advertised as "Melbourne's most modern low cost home!"[7] The Fibrolite Show Bungalow on display at the Perth Royal Show in 1955 was another example.[8]

By the mid-1950s, advertisements suggested that family life might happily include home improvements and extensions; after all, "a growing family needs plenty of living space".[9] Using fibro, savings would allow the addition of a sunroom or another bedroom.[10] The new car needed a "modern garage". Or perhaps the family would enjoy "a smart, comfortable weekender—a snug boatshed—a spacious workshop". "Build it yourself", James Hardie

---

6   *The Architect*, June 1956, 14.
7   *Architecture and Arts*, April 1956, 12.
8   *The Architect*, March 1956, cover iii. *West Australian*, 24 September 1955, 28.
9   *West Australian*, 9 May 1959, 16; 21 December 1957, 8.
10 *Architecture and Arts*, September 1956, 20.

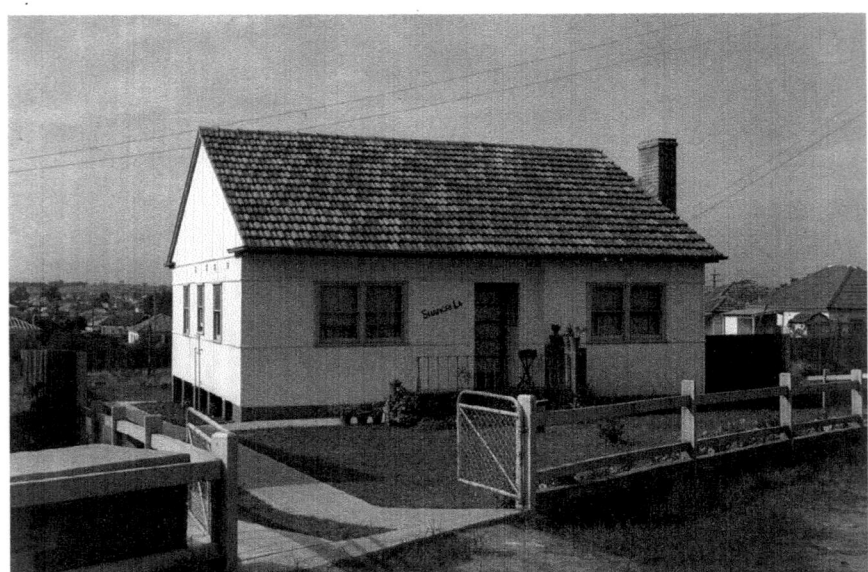

Figure 2.2: "Shangri-la" built of fibro, western Sydney, 1949
Courtesy: State Library of New South Wales

suggested.[11] Or the savings could buy "such expensive extras as a refrigerator, washing machine, hot water service—or even a TV set!"[12] Here was a "blueprint for a Happy Family Life!"[13]

In 1933, there were few more than 23,000 fibro houses in all Australia, an insignificant 1.6 per cent of all housing stock. The take-off in fibro house building occurred in the 1930s; by 1947, their number had increased to over 100,000 and rose rapidly to 495,717 in 1966, which represented the peak of fibro's importance at 18.5 per cent of all houses. The main period of fibro house-building was remarkably short, concentrated in the postwar years of housing shortage between 1947 and 1954, continuing but slowing between 1954 and 1966, and falling away rapidly in the second part of the 1960s.

The fibro house was an embodiment of that period of postwar reconstruction and recovery which saw a gradual transition from the austerity of the 1940s. The period had well and truly passed by the mid-1960s. Between 1966 and 1971 fibro houses fell as a percentage of Australian housing stock from

---

11 *West Australian*, 17 January 1958, 13.
12 James Hardie, *Don't dream—build! Your guide to building beautiful new style homes of Hardie's "Fibrolite"* (Sydney: James Hardie & Co., 1957), 4.
13 *West Australian*, 25 April 1959, 12.

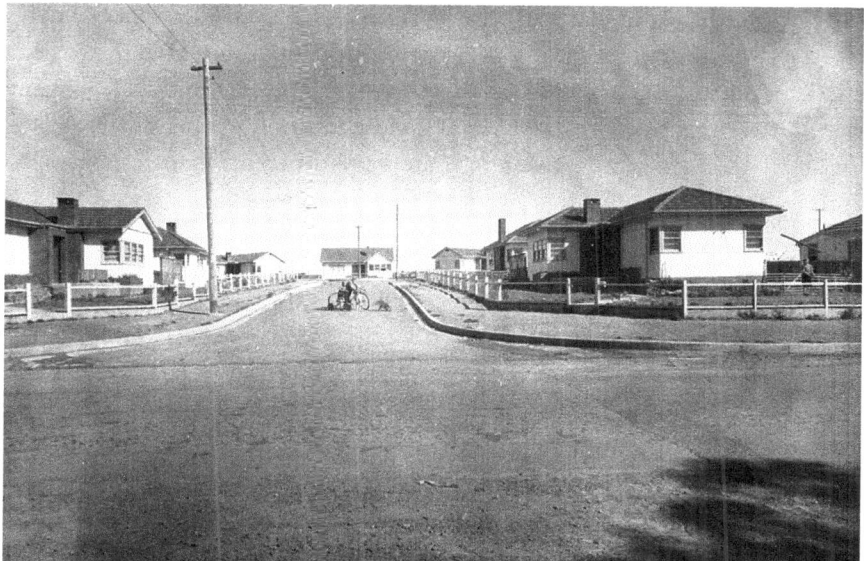

Figure 2.3: A fibro streetscape, western Sydney, 1946
Courtesy: State Library of New South Wales

18.5 per cent to 16.2 per cent. In Victoria, South Australia, Western Australia and the Australian Capital Territory their numbers fell absolutely, a decline probably resulting from some householders reclassifying their houses in census schedules as well as from physical renovations and demolitions.[14] To identify the fibro house with the decades of the 1940s and 1950s is not to suggest that fibro ceased to be widely used in Australian house building after that period. It remained in demand for garages, extensions and interior wall sheeting and, in its corrugated form, for roofing and fencing; but the fibro house itself ceased to be built in great numbers.

State difference in fibro use

While fibro houses proliferated in postwar Australia and became a major component of Australia's housing stock they were not uniformly spread across all states and territories.[15] In 1966, when the proportion of fibro houses peaked Australia-wide, they comprised 30 per cent of all housing

---

14   Where householders named more than one building material in the outer walls of their houses, the Census recorded only the first named material.

15   Census information has been used to identify a fibro house as one with outer walls clad wholly or in large part with asbestos cement wallboard. All census statistics in this period excluded Aboriginal people.

in New South Wales and Western Australia, and over 50 per cent in the Northern Territory; yet only 4 per cent of Tasmanian housing, 7 per cent of Victorian and 8 per cent of South Australian. Queensland's 17 per cent placed it between the two extremes and close to the Australian average (see Figure 2.4). These divergences indicate very different state responses to fibro.

	1921	1933	1947	1954	1961	1966	1971
NSW %	3 063 0.7	16 014 2.9	62 194 10.4	159 339 20.8	244 819 27.5	288 827 30.0	301 002 27.7
VIC %	696 0.2	3 306 0.8	15 357 3.5	34 436 6.0	44 496 6.5	51 668 6.9	43 452 5.1
QLD %	151 0.1	1 334 0.7	14 271 6.0	31 033 10.0	50 070 14.3	63 944 16.7	66 790 15.1
SA %	24 0.02	313 0.2	4 175 3.0	13 787 7.2	20 747 8.5	22 502 8.3	22 253 7.3
WA %	137 0.2	1 968 2.0	9 226 8.5	34 778 24.04	56 097 31.36	61 343 30.5	56 598 22.8
TAS %	27 0.06	134 0.3	1 081 2.0	2 551 3.6	2 804 3.4	3 184 3.6	3 431 3.5
NT %	7 0.7	11 0.9	492 20.2	872 29.1	2 313 52.1	3 252 55.2	4 638 43.5
ACT %	0 0.00	45 2.4	258 8.3	857 13.4	933 8.0	998 5.1	855 2.6
AUST %	4 105 0.4	23 125 1.6	107 054 6.8	277 653 13.5	422 279 17.4	495 717 18.5	499 019 16.2

Figure 2.4: Numbers of fibro houses 1921–1971 and as percentage of all occupied private houses
SOURCE: Census 1921-1971

The variety of house-building practices was shaped by regional differences in the availability and relative cost of building materials, and in differing conventions about what was considered appropriate and good quality housing. The need for effective insulation against the cold limited fibro's use in house building in Victoria, South Australia and Tasmania. In contrast, the Commonwealth Department of Works and Housing which rebuilt Darwin after the war and the Western Australian State Housing Commission which built almost all the postwar houses in the state's north agreed on fibro's value for tropical housing. Fibro's low cost, ease of transport and erection, and the severe postwar shortage of its traditional alternative, galvanised iron, cemented its usefulness in the north.

In New South Wales, where the postwar housing crisis was most severe and prolonged, to build in fibro was the cheapest option. "Thousands of the homes built over the past few years would not have been erected had asbestos cement sheets not been available to the owners concerned at low cost", the New South Wales Association of Co-operative Building Societies insisted in 1954.[16] Comparative costs calculated by the state's Housing Commission quantified the saving achieved by using fibro. The total cost of a three-bedroom fibro house in Sydney in 1963–64 was £2,840 while a brick veneer house of the same size cost £3,655 and a weatherboard house reached £3,790.[17] Yet in Queensland, where it was also significantly cheaper per square foot to build in fibro than in wood, although the price difference was not as great as in Sydney, the majority of new houses continued to be built in weatherboard.[18] Building in timber was a Queensland tradition and one for which local timber was available. In South Australia brick and stone were firmly established as quality local housing products to the extent that, while these materials were regarded as superior housing across all of southern Australia, in South Australia the tradition was so strong as to preclude extensive use of other materials. Brick-only specifications kept fibro (and weatherboard) out of elite suburbs in metropolitan areas, including Canberra.[19] Brick/brick veneer became increasingly important everywhere from the 1960s, although in Queensland it remained relatively insignificant.[20]

The practices of government housing authorities around Australia both reflected and reinforced these state differences in use of fibro. South Australian public housing is a striking instance of state distinctiveness. When the Commonwealth War Workers Housing Trust erected 284 prefabricated fibro "Cabin Homes", each only six squares in area, to house workers for a large munitions plant at the country town of Salisbury, north of Adelaide, in 1942, it challenged South Australian perceptions of proper housing and decent living standards. Most local residents saw "Cabin Homers" as inferior people, as slum-dwellers. Their houses labeled

---

16   Transcript of evidence, Annexure I; Tariff Board Inquiry re Asbestos Fibre, June 1954, 271.

17   Housing Commission of New South Wales, *Annual Report* 30 June 1964, 20. *NSWPP*, 3, 1964–65.

18   *Queensland Year Book*, 28, 1967, 254.

19   Western Australian local governments' "brick area" regulations are noted in the *Building And Construction Journal*; for instance, 19 October 1928, 12 and 30 November 1928, 13.

20   Occupied private houses classified by material of outer walls. Statistician's Reports, *Census of the Commonwealth of Australia* 1933–1971.

and condemned them.[21] Thus, when the South Australian Housing Trust developed a workers' housing estate at Salisbury North in 1949, it built in brick and stone, not in fibro.[22]

On a much larger scale Elizabeth, the model new town developed to the north of Salisbury in the 1950s/1960s by the Trust, was also built in brick. A major satellite town planned and developed as a locality for large-scale new manufacturing industry and therefore with an overwhelming preponderance of workers' housing, and built rapidly from 1954, Elizabeth would have been constructed largely of fibro had it been in New South Wales or Western Australia; as, for instance, was the case with Kwinana New Town built to house workers for the new Kwinana industrial strip south of Fremantle in the early 1950s. In the first two years of building almost all Kwinana's houses (91 per cent) were timber framed with 49 per cent clad completely in fibro and another 23 per cent with composite outer walls.[23] Not so in South Australia. In 1971, 90 per cent of Elizabeth's 8,202 houses were of brick (71 per cent) or brick veneer (19 per cent). Only 349 houses (4 per cent) were of fibro.[24] Planned so carefully by the South Australian Housing Trust as a "city of tomorrow" to attract new secondary industries to the state, the housing stock represented the long-standing South Australian house-building norm.[25]

Similarly, the Housing Commission of Victoria did not turn to fibro.[26] The major developer of suburban housing estates in Melbourne in the first decade after the war, the Commission judged that Victoria's huge housing deficit required the mass production of houses.[27] While Commissioners were aware of the potential of "fibre board" because of its light weight and ease of transport, the prefabricated houses that were trialed were

---

21 M Allen, "Salisbury in the Second World War", *Journal of the Historical Society of South Australia*, 4, 1978, 65–75.

22 M Allen, "Salisbury (S.A.) in transition", MA thesis, University Of Adelaide, 1975.

23 Detail of construction of dwellings taken from SGIO Policy No.HH8853; Insurance of BP Refinery (Kwinana) Ltd Houses. WA State Housing Commission AN150/11 Acc1756 1962/0559. SROWA.

24 *Census* 30 June 1971, Bulletin 7 South Australia.

25 M Peel, *Good times, hard times. The past and the future in Elizabeth* (Melbourne: Melbourne University Press, 1995).

26 R Howe (ed.) *New houses for old. Fifty years of public housing in Victoria 1938–1988* (Melbourne: Ministry of Housing & Construction, 1988).

27 R Howe, "The concrete house frontier: The Victorian Housing Commission and the planning of Melbourne in the 1940s and 1950s", in Davison, Dingle & O'Hanlon (eds) *The cream brick frontier. Histories of Australian suburbia* (Monash University History Dept: Monash Publications in History), ch.8.

built of metal, timber or concrete, not fibro.[28] The prefabricated concrete house was judged to best meet the demands of rapid completion, economical cost, solid and permanent construction, and adequate, comfortable accommodation.[29] Most of the houses that the Commission built in Melbourne in the first decade after the war were of concrete. Houses of brick veneer became more common on Commission estates in the metropolitan area from the mid-1950s.[30]

The Queensland and Tasmanian Housing Commissions built overwhelmingly in weatherboard, using local timber. The Tasmanian Commission experimented a little with concrete housing immediately after the war when seasoned timber was in short supply, while the Queensland Commission imported European pre-cut timber housing in the same period.[31] Both returned fully to local timber as the postwar bottlenecks in supply eased. In contrast, the Housing Commissions of New South Wales and Western Australia built extensively in fibro, both prefabs and conventional constructions.[32]

Nevertheless the brick and tile house was the ideal for most Australians. The fibro house had only a brief florescence in a postwar period marked by a severe shortage of housing and of building materials, the beginnings of an economic boom in which families not previously in a financial position to envisage home ownership were able to do so, and mass migration with newly arrived families seeking an affordable first house as they established themselves in a new country.[33] Once these preconditions eased, fibro's use in new house building declined relative to its alternatives.

---

28 "'Operation Snail'. The Victorian precut housing project" & "The Beaufort home—prefabricated in steel", *Architecture*, October–December 1950, 124–128, 132–134.

29 F Oswald Barnett, W O Burt, F Heath, *We must go on. A study in planned reconstruction and housing* (Melbourne: The Book Depot, 1944), 44–47, 71

30 Howe, "The Concrete house frontier", 79. W Eather, "We only build houses: the Commission 1945–60", in Howe (ed.) *New houses for old. Fifty years of public housing in Victoria 1938–1988*. 75. S O'Hanlon, "Modernism and prefabrication in postwar Melbourne", in R Nile (ed.) *Urban cannibals. romancing the Australian city, Journal of Australian Studies*, 57, 1998, 103–18.

31 *Report of Joint Committee on Home Building 1947. Tasmanian Parliamentary Papers*, 1947 Queensland Housing Commission, *Annual Report* 30 June 1947. *Queensland Parliamentary Papers*, 2, 1947–48.

32 "House out of factory", *Architecture*, October–December 1950, 122–23. CSR advertisement, *The Architect*, September 1947, 26.

33 Housing Commission of NSW, *Annual Report* 30 June 1948, 7–12. *NSWPP*, 1, 1948–49–50.

Landscapes of fibro in Sydney and Perth: a fabric of social difference

The fibro houses that proliferated in Sydney and Perth from the 1940s to the 1960s were not placed uniformly in these metropolitan landscapes. The elite eastern suburbs of Sydney contained almost no fibro houses, in stark contrast to their concentration in the western suburbs. In 1971, less than 1 per cent of houses in the local government areas of Mosman, Waverley, Willoughby and Woollahra were fibro while they comprised more than 50 per cent of houses in Bankstown, Blacktown, Fairfield, Liverpool and Penrith. The elite north shore area of Ku-ring-gai contained few fibro houses and it was only on the outer northern fringes in Warringah and Hornsby that fibro houses were built in any numbers on the north shore (see Figure 2.5 below). Similarly in Perth, the elite riverside and western suburbs of Peppermint Grove, Nedlands, Cottesloe and South Perth had the smallest proportions of fibro houses and the eastern suburban areas of Bassendean, Belmont and Canning the largest.

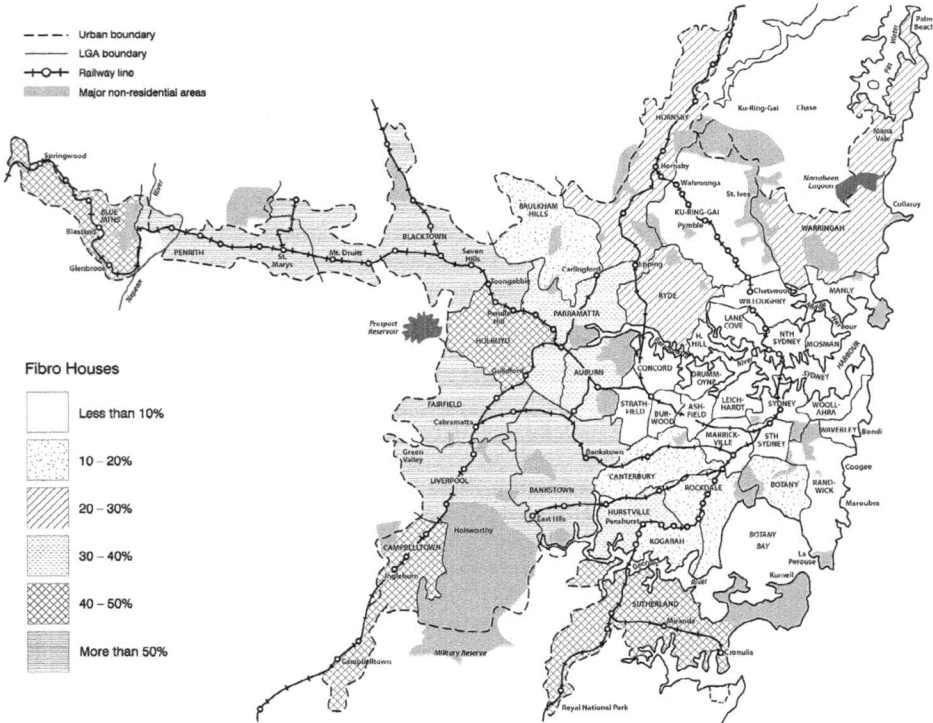

Figure 2.5: Distribution of fibro houses, Sydney 1971
SOURCE: Census 1971, Census of Population & Housing, Bulletin 7, NSW 1971

The Housing Commission of New South Wales reinforced this pattern of difference. It constructed almost 20 per cent of new houses in Sydney in the first decade after the war, more than 35,000 by 1955. Although this percentage declined sharply after 1956 with changes to the Commonwealth State Housing Agreement, the Commission continued building large housing estates in the outer western suburbs. In the ten years from 1945 to 1955, 62 per cent of the houses it built were timber-framed, fibro-clad; in the twenty years from 1945 to 1965 the figure rose to 66 per cent.[34] Building type—brick or timber framed—was chosen according to what was "appropriate to the locality".[35] Thus the Commission built brick houses in suburbs such as Maroubra, Manly, Deewhy, Bexley North and Eastwood, and in areas of inner urban renewal, notably Redfern and Balmain. In its large developments in the outer western suburbs it built overwhelmingly timber-framed, fibro houses; for example, in Granville, Seven Hills and Lalor Park.[36] Two imperatives explain this policy. Ensuring the acceptability of its housing to local government authorities and existing residents necessitated brick housing in already-established brick areas. Otherwise, the Commission built timber-framed dwellings "in the interests of economy".[37] A three-bedroom brick house cost the Commission £2,142 to construct in 1950 compared with £1,764 for a timber-framed, fibro-clad house.[38] This policy intensified the existing patterns of difference in housing types across the metropolitan area and consolidated the perception that fibro was workers' or battlers' housing.

The same pattern was evident on Perth's landscape, concentrations of fibro housing corresponding to the residential areas of industrial workers.[39] The State Housing Commission was Western Australia's major postwar housing developer, building entirely new suburbs around the metropolitan area and completing 20,000 houses by 1955. In the postwar decade,

---

34   The Commission's category from which these percentages are calculated was "timber-framed and other types". I have assumed that "other types" were insignificant in numbers. Housing Commission of NSW, *Annual Reports* 30 June 1955 & 30 June 1965, Annexures "B". *NSWPP*, 1, 1955–56 and 3, 1965–66.
35   Housing Commission of NSW, *Annual Report* 30 June 1947, 6. *NSWPP*, I, 1948–49–50.
36   Housing Commission of NSW, *Annual Reports*.
37   Housing Commission of NSW, *Annual Report* 30 June 1953, 12. *NSWPP*, 2, 1953.
38   Housing Commission of NSW *Annual Report* 30 June 1952, 17. *NSWPP*, 1, 1952–53.
39   "Occupation—tradesmen, labourers or production process workers" in Division of National Mapping & ABS, *Atlas of population and housing, 1976 Census*, 1, Perth, June 1979, 12.

1945–56, the Commission built 41 per cent of all new houses, the great majority timber-framed and fibro-clad.[40] In the mid-1950s, between two-thirds and three-quarters of Commission house completions were timber-framed dwellings.[41] While it is not possible to be exact on the percentage of timber-framed constructions that were fibro-clad as distinct from weatherboard, numbers in particular housing developments indicate the figure at approximately 80 per cent. As was the case in New South Wales, the Western Australian Commission distributed its brick and timber-framed houses unevenly across the metropolitan area. In prestigious riverside suburbs or close to existing brick areas—for example, in Applecross, Mount Pleasant, Manning and Floreat Park—it built in brick. In the old, predominantly working class suburb of Victoria Park, which had a mixture of brick and weatherboard housing, it built almost equally in brick and timber-frame. And in its large new developments close to industrial areas—for example, in Belmont, Ascot, Hilton Park and Willagee—it built almost entirely timber-framed houses.[42]

These government-housing authorities did not see themselves as builders of inferior houses. The New South Wales Commission aimed to build "ideal suburban communities" of "good standard homes" in landscaped surrounds with adequate areas set aside for public use. Each block was to be planted with three shrubs, one small ornamental tree and one large tree to ensure the growth of leafy, pleasant environments. The limits on house size imposed by the 1945 Commonwealth State Housing Agreement resulted in the elimination of entrance halls, the combination of kitchen and dining areas, and the reduction of passage space. Designs were austere with minimum decorations.[43] But these changes were not judged to result in substandard housing. Rather the reverse; housing standards for the mass of Australians were being raised by the program. Reflecting on more than twenty years of activity, the Housing Commission of New South Wales expressed satisfaction at its achievement.

---

40   R Sharp, "A history of public housing in Western Australia. The Workers' Homes Board and State Housing Commission: precursors of Homeswest", History Honours thesis, Murdoch University, 1993, ch.4.

41   In the 1953–54 year, 74 per cent of SHC completed houses were timber-framed; in the 1955–56 year 67 per cent. Western Australia State Housing Commission *Annual Reports* 30 June 1954 and 30 June 1956; *WAPP*, 3, 1954 and 3, 1956.

42   Western Australia State Housing Commission, *Annual Report* 30 June 1954, 32–34. *WAPP*, 3, 1954.

43   Housing Commission of NSW, *Annual Report* 30 June 1946, 9–17. *NSWPP*, 1, 1947–48 & *Annual Report* 30 June 1948, 19–20. *NSWPP*, 1, 1948–49–50.

They are dwellings in which the occupants take pride and in which they can live in contentment, adding the extra amenities they may desire as and when they can afford them.[44]

The fact remained that the Commission built increasingly in fibro as the rest of the New South Wales housing market moved away from fibro houses. Between 1947 and 1954, 59 per cent of all new houses in New South Wales were clad in fibro while, in approximately the same period 1945-1955, fibro constituted 62 per cent of the Commission's new houses.[45] This rough equity persisted until the last years of the 1950s. The austerity or minimal house of the early postwar years—most commonly of fibro—had been a product of building controls, materials shortage and individual endeavours to make a start after the war. As such, it was a housing form shared by the majority of those who built anew in the period.[46] With the passing of austerity in the 1950s this commonality ended. By 1959-60, when the percentage fibro of all new houses had fallen to 48 per cent, the Commission built 70 per cent of its houses in fibro. By 1966-67, the discrepancy had widened to 34 per cent compared to 78 per cent.[47] As late as 1970, the Commission's two major housing developments in the outer west, Green Valley and Mount Druitt, were 70 per cent and 75 per cent fibro respectively.[48]

These very visible fibro estates became stark markers of social difference. Writing in 1970 of his *Ideas for Australian Cities*, Hugh Stretton labeled Green Valley a "ghetto town" of low paid workers together with "a frightening proportion" of "the sick, handicapped, disturbed or deserted fragments of families"; a housing development of multiple disabilities.[49] Used in Commission estates such as Green Valley and Mount Druitt, fibro came to represent social disadvantage. The low-cost fibro house became increasingly identified as government housing at an historical juncture when governments sought to provide mass housing for rent and sale to those in need.

---

44 Housing Commission of NSW, *Annual Report* 30 June 1965, p.11. *NSWPP*, 3, 1965–66.
45 Statistician's Reports, *Census of the Commonwealth of Australia* 1947 & 1954 Housing Commission of NSW, *Annual Report* 30 June 1955, Annexure "B". *NSWPP*, 1, 1955–56.
46 J M Freeland, *Architecture in Australia. A history* (Ringwood Victoria: Penguin, 1972), ch. 13.
47 *New South Wales Official Year Books*, 58 & 60, 1964 & 1969, Tables 332 and 335.
48 Housing Commission of NSW, *Annual Report* 30 June 1970, Annexure "B". *NSWPP*, 4, 1969–70-71.
49 Hugh Stretton, *Ideas for Australian cities* (Melbourne: Georgian House, 1975), 149–55, 259.

A self-help material for the postwar owner-builder

Postwar owner-builders turned to fibro to bypass the long waiting lists for public housing and avoid high building costs in the private sector. Advice books were encouraging: "You can build your own home in your weekends".[50] Most state capitals provided an advice service for the amateur builder, generally in association with the Institute of Architects, where plans and guidance on how to build a small house were easily available. As well, the *Australian Women's Weekly* offered a home plan service with advice centres in major east coast department stores.[51]

Many took up the challenge of owner building.[52] In New South Wales the percentage of completed owner-built houses peaked at 49 per cent in 1953, in Western Australia at 39 per cent in 1953–54.[53] This level of activity gradually fell away through the 1950s and early 1960s as the worst of housing crisis was overcome.[54] The percentage in New South Wales fell to 32 per cent by 1960 and further to 15 per cent by 1965–66 (and just a little more to 14 per cent by 1970–71).[55] Given the relative difficulty of building in brick/brick veneer together with its greater cost, it is not surprising that most owner-builders chose fibro or weatherboard.[56] Almost half the owner-builders in New South Wales chose fibro: 48 per cent in 1957–58 falling slowly to 43 per cent by 1970–71. This continued use of fibro by owner-builders contrasted with the state's contract builders who, by 1970–71, built only 17 per cent of their houses in fibro having moved substantially into brick veneer.[57] Fibro assisted all these people to build family homes in the years immediately after the war.

---

50 The Home Builders' Advisory, Sydney, *You can build your own home*, 6th edn (Sydney, 1954), 5.

51 *Architecture in Australia*, 51, June 1962, 90–92.

52 Spearritt, *Sydney since the twenties*, 103–05. P Cuffley, *Australian houses of the forties and fifties* (Knoxfield Victoria: Five Mile Press, 1993), 75–80.

53 WA State Housing Commission, *Annual Report* 30 June 1955, 19. *WAPP*, 3 1955 *NSW Official Year Book*, 57, 1961, 635

54 For Australian statistics on owner-building from 1951/52 to 1984/85, see Graham Holland, *Emoh ruo. Owner building in Sydney* (Sydney: Hale & Iremonger, 1988), Appendix A.

55 *NSW Official Year Book*, 60, 1969, 436; 62, 1973, 1106.

56 T Dingle, "Necessity the mother of invention, or do-it-yourself", in P Troy (ed.) *A history of European housing in Australia* (Cambridge: Cambridge Uni. Press, 2000), 70.

57 *NSW Official Year Book*, 58, 1964, 409; 60, 1969, 436; 62, 1971, 1106.

Housing for country areas

Proportionately more fibro housing was built in regional than in metropolitan Australia. This was especially so in Western Australia and Queensland where, by 1971, fibro comprised 44 per cent of houses outside Perth and 21 per cent of houses outside Brisbane. In New South Wales, however, fibro houses were as common outside Sydney as within the city.[58] The concentrations of fibro housing in regional areas, and in the Northern Territory, were a product of both government housing practices and the disabilities of distance and isolation, making other building materials expensive to transport and difficult to use without skilled labour. In contrast, fibro cladding was relatively light and cheap to transport and easy to erect by amateur builders. It was even cheaper and easier if fibro was already incorporated in pre-cut housing.[59]

Government housing authorities in New South Wales, Western Australia and the Northern Territory utilised fibro extensively in regional areas. Postwar Darwin, rebuilt after the war by the Commonwealth Department of Works and Housing, was one of Australia's major concentrations of fibro housing, 59 per cent of all housing stock in 1971. The Department built tropical houses in fibro, designed to maximise through-breezes with overhanging eaves for shade and fibro louvres creating "walls that open" to the tropical breezes.[60] In northern Australia, fibro became the modern building material used instead of galvanised iron, more expensive than the latter but not in such short supply in postwar years.[61] The Western Australian State Housing Commission designed special anti-cyclonic houses for the tropical north of the State clad in heavy quarter-inch fibro.[62] The Commonwealth Railways designed arid zone houses of fibro.[63] Even the South Australian government built fibro houses in its remote north.

Government housing for Aboriginal people began to be provided in this era of assimilation although, at a time of shortages, very few resources were directed to Aboriginal families. Most of the small number of houses

---

58 Compared with 14 per cent in Perth Statistical Division and 9 per cent in Brisbane Statistical Division.
59 Western Australia State Housing Commission, "Country housing", in *Home, Western Australia*. State Housing Commission, Perth, 1971, 55.
60 *Architecture*, 36, April 1948, 32–38; 39, July–September 1951, 84.
61 Evidence of J T Adamson, James Hardie & Co. Pty Ltd, to Tariff Board Inquiry re Asbestos Fibre, June 1954, 242–43.
62 WA State Housing Commission, *Annual Report* 30 June 1957, 14. *WAPP*, 4, 1957.
63 *Architecture in Australia*, 52, March 1963, 83–89.

that were specially designed and built in New South Wales and Western Australia were of weatherboard and galvanised iron.[64] However, the Housing Commission in Western Australia in the late 1950s decided that it would provide Aboriginal housing, mostly on the fringes of country towns, as a preliminary step to assimilation into standard Commission rental housing. These transit camp constructions were of fibro, approximately three squares in size, and consisting of one bedroom, living area with open fireplace for cooking, and washing facilities on the back verandah.[65] Put to this use, fibro marked out the most extreme modern housing disadvantage in Australia.

Postwar attempts at decentralisation of industry and population were promoted by the provision of government housing.[66] In New South Wales most activity was directed towards adequately housing coal industry workers in the Newcastle and Wollongong districts. More than 80 per cent of this housing was fibro.[67] In Western Australia in the 1940s and 1950s, Commission houses were built where industry required them: at Wittenoom Gorge for the blue asbestos industry, at Wundowie for the charcoal iron industry, at Boyup Brook to assist the establishment of a flax treatment plant, at Collie for the coal industry, at the major regional ports of Bunbury, Albany and Geraldton, and at numerous tiny south west towns to promote the timber industry.[68] The Commission erected pre-cut fibro houses throughout the southern agricultural region to meet the needs of small country towns and promote rural development. Special housing agreements with new industries, like that with Anglo-Iranian Oil Company at Kwinana, were made in the early 1960s with La Porte Titanium Ltd for workers' housing in Bunbury, with Esperance Fertilisers Pty Ltd for housing in Esperance, and with Broken Hill Proprietary Ltd for mineworkers' housing in Koolyanobbing. In the southern coastal port of Esperance in 1971, for instance, 71 per cent of houses were of fibro. This government

---

64 C Allport, "Nicely furnished cottages: government housing for black and white Australians", in J O'Callaghan (ed.) *The Australian dream. Design of the fifties* (Sydney: Powerhouse Publishing, 1993), ch.7. Sharp, "A history of public housing in Western Australia", ch. 5.

65 K Bell, "The State Housing Commission and aboriginal housing, 1959", in L Layman and T Stannage (eds) *Celebrations in Western Australian history. Studies in Western Australian History*, 10, April 1989, 32–36.

66 Housing Commission of NSW, *Annual Report* 30 June 1948, 26–29. *NSWPP*, 1, 1948–49–50.

67 Housing Commission of NSW, *Annual Reports* 30 June 1952, 21–22. *NSWPP*, 1, 1952–53; and 30 June 1964, Annexure "B". *NSWPP*, 3, 1964–65.

68 WA State Housing Commission, *Annual Report* 30 June 1957, 14–15. *WAPP*, 4, 1957.

housing support for industry was further developed to assist resource development in the North West from the mid-1960s.[69] Government activity placed fibro houses in regional New South Wales and Western Australia where economic development was being fostered. An industrial material itself, fibro became closely identified with the project of transforming Australia into an industrial society.[70]

The fabric of factories and sheds

Fibro also clad and roofed some of the largest of the new factories as well as other large industrial buildings, such as railway sheds, port and aviation facilities, and farm sheds. While many companies continued to build their industrial plants in brick, almost all utilised corrugated fibro for roofing.[71] Where a new plant required a particularly large building and floor area, fibro was a frequent choice for sidings as well as roofing.[72] Automatic Totalisators Ltd's factory at Meadowbank (1948), Hastings Deering's automobile assembly plant at Lidcombe (1950), Thomas Owen & Co.'s paper mill at Burnie (1952), H J Heinz's factory at Dandenong (1954), Westralian Farmers' wool store at Fremantle (1959), Johns & Waygoods plant at Sandringham (1959) and Redmond Inglis & Co.'s printing factory at Notting Hill (1963) were all instances.[73] International Harvesters' new motor truck assembly plant completed in 1953 at Dandenong mapped fibro's place on the industrial landscape unusually sharply: the factory walled and roofed in corrugated fibro, the amenities building covered with fibro roofing, and the administration block constructed of brick with no significant fibro component.[74] Fibro factories fronted by brick office blocks proliferated in all states.

---

69 Sharp, "A history of public housing in Western Australia", ch. 6.
70 "The 'fibrolite' asbestos-cement industry", in *Western Australia - industry, commerce - facts and figures. An account of conditions and opportunities in the western state of the Commonwealth* (Perth: Western Australian Govt, Paterson Brokensha, 1954), 47.
71 Wunderlich Ltd, *Corrugated Durabestos Asbestos-Cement Roofing*; pamphlet, 1938. Powerhouse museum collection. *Architecture*, 36, January 1948, 18; 40, January–March 1950, 38.
72 *Architecture*, 36, July 1948, 24. Wunderlich Ltd, *Wunderlich Deep Corrugated Durabestos for Roofing and Wall Siding*; pamphlets, 1939, 1941.
73 *Architecture*, 36, July 1948, 24; 35, July 1950, 94; 45, April–June 1954, 36–38. *Tasbestos Asbestos-Cement Roofing Sheets and Mouldings* (Railton: Goliath Portland Cement Co. Ltd, 1952). *Architecture and Arts*, 7, January 1960, 12. *Architecture in Australia*, 52, December 1963, 120–21.
74 *Architecture*, 41, October–December 1953, 94.

Holiday places

"Summer Homes for Seaside and Country" were acceptable in fibro even where main, metropolitan residences might not be; for instance, in South Australia. That state's interwar building journals recommended fibro for holiday houses.[75] Wealthy families built their own holiday houses. The majority of families rented accommodation, built by astute locals who recognised the growing demand, or occupied caravan parks and tentlands where new amenities blocks were most often fibro constructions. The new postwar entitlement to three weeks' annual leave for most of Australia's fulltime workforce covered by industrial awards together with the rapid rise in car ownership in the 1950s provided the preconditions for this mass movement of families.

The beach was the most popular place for such holidays. As a result, fibro proliferated around the Australian coast. Queensland's Gold Coast grew from a quiet holiday area for the well-to-do prior to the 1940s into a mass postwar holiday destination built in modern style in boom conditions by investors and speculative builders.[76] In 1971, 32 per cent of the Gold Coast's approximately 14,000 houses were of colourfully painted fibro.[77] No other coastal holiday development experienced the same boom but holiday towns around the country saw much new building. For instance, in Western Australia the popular coastal holiday town of Mandurah, a short distance south of Perth, grew rapidly after the war. In 1971 its housing stock was 56 per cent fibro. The housing in the New South Wales south coastal areas of Bega, Eurobodalla and Imlay was approximately 40 per cent fibro by 1971.[78] The fibro housing which sprang up around the Australian coast varied from substantial standard houses built for the well-to-do to beach shacks, sometimes built illegally by squatters.[79] In this variety of ways, fibro houses and shacks became the place of Australian holidays from the 1930s until holiday culture began to change significantly in the 1970s-1980s.

---

75 *The Builders' and Contractors' Weekly Gazette*, 21 August 1922. *The Builder*, 4 November 1922.

76 P Newell, "Umbigumbi to the Gold Coast", *Architecture in Australia*, January–March 1959, 70–73.

77 *Census of Population & Housing*, Bulletin 7 Queensland, 1971.

78 *Census of Population & Housing*, Bulletin 7 New South Wales, 1971.

79 Most of the illegal squatters' shacks were probably constructed in galvanised iron with a substantial minority in fibro if the Western Australian central west coast is representative. Midwest Heritage Inc., "Squatters of the Midwest Coast of WA", NEGP report 1996.

A changing reputation

The metropolitan fibro house had gained a negative public image by the end of the 1950s, disparagingly labeled "the 'Fibro' box", as James Hardie later acknowledged.[80] Sydney's outer western suburban developments where fibro houses were disproportionately located often lacked essential government services; footpaths, roads, sewerage, streetscaping, health centres and education facilities did not keep pace with the urban sprawl. Shops were distant, bus services meagre and employment a great distance away. When a group of Sydney architects and planners led by Harry Seidler condemned "The Waste of Suburbia" in 1959 and called for urban redevelopment, they labeled the "flimsy" fibro houses, set in their outer suburban "ugliness" with inadequate community services, "the slums of tomorrow".[81] This negative image of fibro housing was compounded by the concentrations of public housing, almost all fibro, which appeared as the Housing Commission built larger and larger housing estates in the outer western areas after completing its early postwar urban infill and renewal projects.

In its cheapness, its sturdy practicality and its grey appearance, fibro had become synonymous with austerity and therefore associated with uniformity, constraints and necessary expedience. As well, it had become identified with working class housing and government housing. These associations made problematic attempts to market asbestos cement building materials as attractive modern products and, consequently, the fibro house as an acceptable consumption choice for families in the 1960s. As the building material for small, relatively uniform rectangular houses, emblems of postwar austerity, fibro became increasingly unacceptable aesthetically and socially. In this market climate the construction of fibro houses fell away and asbestos cement companies had to re-think their marketing strategies.

Transforming asbestos cement sheeting

James Hardie had established its dominance of the industry by providing low-cost housing.[82] By 1959 the company knew that such dependence was not sustainable. If asbestos cement was to hold its share of the building

---

80 James Hardie Asbestos Ltd, *Annual Report* 1977. Jennifer Taylor, *An Australian identity houses for Sydney 1953–63* (Sydney: Dept of Architecture, University of Sydney, 1972), 11.

81 *The Architect*, March 1959, 32.

82 Evidence of J T Adamson, James Hardie & Co. Pty Ltd, to Tariff Board Inquiry re Asbestos Fibre, June 1954, 131–32, 247–52.

materials market, the companies needed to transform both their sheeting products and their marketing to make them modern again. They did both in the five-year period from 1959 to 1964, repositioning their sheeting for another twenty years of good sales. The products were re-designed to meet and encourage the market's changing desires: for colour, choice, decoration, simulation and customisation.

Householders increasingly wanted a colourful home.[83] By the mid-1950s James Hardie had begun to explain that its exterior sheeting could be "painted as colourfully as desired, in keeping with modern trends".[84] And in 1959 the company released New Tilux, its marble-finished bathroom and kitchen wall paneling, in "6 new glorious colours": marbletone, willow green, rose pink, sun gold, sky blue and mist grey.[85] Also new in 1957 was Wunderlich's Duradec for kitchens, bathroom and laundries in five colours—blue, grey, green, black and pink—all with a "distinctive white fleck [which] gives a fresh, modern appearance".[86] James Hardie added Colorbord as "Permanent Colour, Permanent Beauty" in 1960.[87] For exterior as well as interior walls and panels, it came initially in ten colours that increased to seventeen by 1965.[88]

Between 1959 and 1964 James Hardie introduced eleven new exterior boards: Striated and Fluted Fibrolite, New Tilux, Shadowline, Coverline, Colorbord, Asbestolux, Hardiflex, Weatherboard, Ranchline and Log Cabin.[89] Not only were customers given choice but there was also the attraction of new decorative looks. Striated and Fluted Fibrolite, Shadowline and Coverline were vertically ribbed boards; Weatherboard, Ranchline and Log Cabin horizontally ribbed; New Tilux, and Colorbord were variously coloured; Hardiflex had particular flexibility; Asbestolux was a special insulation board. Fibrolite flat sheeting was relegated to advertisements for garages, sheds and holiday houses.[90] Wunderlich's new products paralleled James Hardie's, although the former did not develop as great a range.[91] Durawall, a vertically grooved board, was introduced in 1957 while Log Cabin and

---

83   Cuffley, *Australian houses of the forties and fifties*, ch. 11.
84   *Architecture and Arts*, September 1956, 20.
85   *The Architect*, September 1956, 46 and December 1959, 59.
86   *Architecture and Arts*, 7, June 1960, 86.
87   *Architecture in Australia* 52, 1963: 1.
88   *Architecture and Arts*, 8, 1961, 8. *Architecture in Australia*, 54, 1965, 1.
89   James Hardie Asbestos Ltd, *Annual Reports* 1959–1964.
90   *The Architect*, September 1959, 60; December 1959, 5.
91   *Architecture and Arts*, 6, May 1959, 15.

Ribwall were advertised in the early 1960s.[92] Wunderflex, marketed in 1965, was Wunderlich's new flexible board, its equivalent of Hardiflex.[93] Even in Tasmania's small market Goliath Portland Cement Company diversified from plain Tasbestos wallboard to Flexboard, Shadowall, Fluted Panel and Rustic Sheet.[94]

Fibro's promise of pace-setting, glamorous modernity was achieved by simulation with the boarding assuming more and more disguises. Wunderlich's Ribwall pretended to be board and batten panelling and James Hardie's Weatherboard, Ranchline and Log Cabin all pretended to be timber boards. As marketed, they were better than timber itself. For instance, Weatherboard gave "true weatherboard beauty" but, in addition, offered a "3 in 1 board"; that is, the appearance of three boards in one board, cutting building time, painting costs and, of course, maintenance costs.[95]

This product diversification and simulation of other building materials extended the life of fibro products in the residential market and also spread the material further throughout suburbs which had previously seen few asbestos building products as householders used the cheap and newly attractive materials for extensions and renovations. As well, the companies sought new markets beyond the domestic in the commercial and public sectors.

Customised products for commercial and public buildings

In a final step in product diversification the asbestos companies began manufacturing customised products: moulded panels shaped, coloured and decorated to customers' specifications in order to target businesses and governments. For instance, Wunderlich provided 9,000 specially moulded curved sheets as arched supports on the new Sydney Harbour Bridge roadway in 1959 and similarly customised curved corrugated sheeting for the semi-domed roof of Gilbeys' new factory at Moorabbin in 1961.[96] James Hardie fabricated impressive facade panels for Kogarah's new Civic Centre in 1973 as well as aggregate-faced fabricated balustrades, Colorbord soffits

---

92 Wunderlich Ltd, *Seventy years of Wunderlich Industry 1887–1957* (Sydney: Wunderlich Ltd, 1957), 44. *Architecture in Australia*, 48, January–March 1959, 141; 51, March 1962, 1. *Architecture and Arts*, 10, February 1962, 58.
93 *Architecture and Arts*, 13, June 1965, 12.
94 *Goliath Flexboard* (Hobart: Goliath Portland Cement Co., 1972).
95 *Architecture and Arts*, 10, February 1962, 58.
96 *Architecture in Australia*, 48, June 1959, 105. *Architecture and Arts*, 8, April 1961, 19.

and moulded seating for the new grandstand at Canberra's Race Course.[97] In its custom-made form, asbestos cement could blend chameleon-like into all varieties of composite constructions.

No longer focused primarily on housing, the industry's advertisements prominently featured commercial, industrial and public buildings.[98] Of the new products, James Hardie's Colorbord and Asbestolux (and its successor, Versilux) were intended particularly for offices and public buildings, prestigious markets where asbestos cement had had little success in the past.[99] And corporate sponsorship helped acceptance in these markets. Two sponsorships targeted elite opinion-makers in Victoria, a state where use of its sheeting had been limited. The James Hardie Lecture Theatre was built in the School of Architecture at the University of Melbourne, and James Hardie Project 72 sponsored the Institute of Architects (Victoria) to construct a model for the development of a metropolitan fringe town, specifically the town of Sunbury near Melbourne.[100]

As a result of these changes to company products (the simulation of other materials and customised mouldings) and the manner in which the products were utilised (integrated with other materials and surfaced in materials such as aggregate), asbestos cement became much less visible in the urban landscape from the early 1960s. In his report to shareholders in 1970, James Hardie's chairman described the large decorated moulded panels that the company had made for the facade of a new shopping centre at Indooroopilly in Queensland: "As in many other applications, it is not obvious to the casual observer that the construction is of asbestos cement".[101] Thus more widespread use was accompanied by declining visibility. While the all-fibro houses were no longer being built, the chairman reported in 1969, Hardie's products were "being increasingly used, in some form or other in all buildings".[102] In the mid-1970s, the company claimed that a greater volume of asbestos cement products was being incorporated, per square metre of building construction, than ever before.[103]

---

97 James Hardie Asbestos Ltd, *Annual Report* 1973.
98 *The Architect*, September 1965, 22–23; June 1967, 18.
99 *Architecture in Australia*, 51, June 1962, 1. *The Architect*, March 1965, 15.
100 Royal Australian Institute of Architects (Victorian Chapter), *Sunbury New Town. James Hardie Project 72.* Report prepared for the 21st Australian Architectural Convention. 120pp + Appendices. (Melbourne: RAIA Victorian Chapter, 1972). James Hardie Asbestos Ltd, *Annual Reports* 1969 & 1972.
101 James Hardie Asbestos Ltd, *Annual Report* 1970.
102 James Hardie Asbestos Ltd, *Annual Report* 1969.
103 James Hardie Asbestos Ltd, *Annual Report* 1974.

The new product strategy of the early 1960s continued in the 1970s. More new boards simulated wood (Hardigrain, Hardiplank Woodgrain, Montana Siding) or cement render (Stucco Siding).[104] More colour for external cladding was offered (Shingle Plank).[105] The building materials market was a crowded one and asbestos cement boards had to appear in new guises, promising ever better products combined with up to the minute styles. One section of the market to which James Hardie's extensive range of building board proved well-suited was the rapidly growing area of house renovations; for instance, fibro's light weight made it particularly suitable for second storey extensions.

The fibro home had been relegated to the past. James Hardie's Fibrolite Show Home, which had been an annual fixture at Sydney's Royal Show since 1917, was last seen in 1965.[106]

> Today [1978] we produce textured and decorated products; others are used skilfully in conjunction with a variety of materials so that they are not identified so readily in schools, bus terminals, commercial buildings, hospitals, coal mines, recording studios, railway stations— to name but a few.[107]

Reducing fibro's visibility was important for marketing in the 1960s and 1970s because of the negative image the material had acquired. Especially after 1975 when the threat to health began to become public knowledge in Australia, the asbestos companies had a further reason to encourage a reduction in their products' visibility.

Through this major product transformation one asbestos cement building material—corrugated asbestos cement roof sheeting—remained unambiguously what it had always been. From the 1940s, it had much wider market acceptance than did flat sheeting, its value enhanced because of its suitability for low-pitched and skillion roofs which could not be tiled. In many instances in the 1950s, the only asbestos cement product used in relatively expensive brick houses of modern design was roof sheeting.[108] It was aesthetically acceptable in a way flat sheeting was not. The new Top

---

104 James Hardie Asbestos Ltd, *Annual Reports* 1975, 1977.
105 James Hardie Industries Ltd, *Annual Report* 1980.
106 James Hardie, *History of James Hardie & Co. Ltd from 1888 to December 1966* (Sydney: James Hardie, 1967), 56.
107 James Hardie Asbestos Ltd, *Annual Report* 1978, 8.
108 *Architecture and Arts*, December 1956, 20–23. *The Architect*, March 1957, 36. *Architecture*, 39, October–December 1951, 108–09 & 112–13. *Architecture in Australia*, 46, January–March 1957, 55; 51, March 1962, 88–89.

Dog Men's Wear Production Centre at Dee Why, roofed in corrugated fibro, won a Sulman Award for architecture in 1950.[109] And the winning designs of the main stadium and the swimming and diving pools for the 1956 Melbourne Olympics featured corrugated fibro roofing.[110] As early as the mid-1940s James Hardie advertised that "Many thousands of factories, industrial works, wharves, government and commercial buildings have been roofed with this durable material".[111] In the mid-1970s, Hardie's Super Six was marketed as "the great Australian roof".[112] The fibro roofing market remained strong from the 1940s to the 1970s, with additional sales of corrugated fibro for fencing, chiefly in Western Australia, in the 1970s.

Reducing this sea of asbestos cement

While the less visible customised asbestos building products are most often a corporate or public sector responsibility increasingly subject to auditing, monitoring and planning for their eventual removal, the fibro houses are proving more difficult to identify and monitor. Most of this housing stock remains *in situ* although not in Darwin where Cyclone Tracy swept it all away in 1974, a story Dr Greg Deleuil tells in chapter 15 of this book. He points to the disease and death caused by a clean up of fibro building materials carried out without protection from airborne fibres and without adequate planning for the disposal of the building materials and contaminated rubble. This natural disaster and its follow-up serve as a warning of the potential danger in the process of asbestos removal.

Around Australia some fibro houses have been demolished but many more have been renovated—most often painted and sometimes the fibro panels encapsulated. Asbestos roofing that has become dirty and friable, with fibres being washed into gutters and into the ground with every rain, has frequently been replaced or sometimes painted. Where the original roofing remains in a friable state it poses an immediate health danger. Workplace Health and Safety Queensland has instituted a program to stop the use of high-pressure water cleaners on fibro roofs by a combination of community education and manufacturers' labelling.[113] But clearly the problem grows as the roofs age.

---

109 *Architecture*, 8, January–March 1950, 28–29.
110 *Architecture*, 41, January–March 1953, 16–17; 41, July–September 1953, 74.
111 *The Golden West. Western Australia's Illustrated Annual*, 1945–46, 1946–47, 1947–48. *Architecture*, 35, October 1947, 2.
112 *Architecture in Australia*, 64, February 1975, 19.
113 *National Strategic Plan for Asbestos Management and Awareness Progress Report 2015–16* (Canberra: Australian Government Asbestos Safety and Eradication Agency), 54.

Otherwise the asbestos embedded in these houses is safe until disturbed, but at this point the problem of lack of knowledge arises: is asbestos material present in the building? Most often no one is sure and sometimes the question is not asked, posing a major safety risk to both occupiers and tradespeople. A government taskforce on asbestos in the Australian Capital Territory in 2005 estimated that four in every five residential properties in the Territory contained the material in some form, although in many cases this presence will be slight. Professional assessments are necessary, and one of the recommendations of the Australian government's 2012 Asbestos Management Review was that local councils should systematically identify the presence of asbestos materials within their localities and maintain databases of the information for public consultation.[114] For instance, the Barkly, Central Desert and MacDonnell Regional Councils in Central Australia, where the extent of the fibro problem is not known, have set up such community asbestos mapping programs. The health risk for remote communities is particularly sharp where harsh physical environments are often coupled with inadequate or no building maintenance and the dumping of broken materials on the outskirts of communities. The Regional Councils' program includes the establishment of asbestos registers, remediation planning, and asbestos education and training.[115] There is a very long way to go in the removal of asbestos cement building materials from Australia's residential environments and, in the meantime, a third wave of asbestos related disease is catching the home renovators and weekend handy-people.

Particularly sensitive has been the ongoing presence of asbestos in school buildings. Most of this is fibro used for school roofing and also for the construction of "relocatable" or "demountable" classrooms that could be moved to schools with overflow enrolments at times when school populations grew rapidly. Once set in place many have remained. State governments have responded to community concerns and much of the fibro roofing has been replaced. The Victorian Government has committed to the removal of all dangerous asbestos-containing materials from its schools by 2020. Much of this material is located in 780 relocatable classrooms.[116] Whether this goal will be achieved is not yet clear. Elsewhere throughout Australia's residential areas the asbestos legacy remains a massive challenge.

---

114 *Asbestos Management Review Report* (Canberra: Department of Education, Employment and Workplace Relations, 2012), 7, 23–24.
115 *National Strategic Plan for Asbestos Management and Awareness Progress Report 2015–16*, 34–37.
116 *National Strategic Plan for Asbestos Management and Awareness Progress Report 2015–16*, 50.

Asbestos insulation and its removal

Insulation products add to the asbestos load that accumulated in Australia's built environment through the 20th century. This insulation came in three forms—as covers for boilers and pipes (containing more than 50 per cent asbestos); as sprayed loose coatings (up to 85 per cent asbestos); and as board for fire protection, heat and sound insulation, circuit boards, electrical panels, ceiling tiles, wall linings, and partitions (20–45 per cent asbestos). Given that asbestos cement products generally contained 10–15 per cent asbestos, it is evident that asbestos insulation products are potentially the more deadly.[117]

All heavy industrial worksites where heat protection was essential became laden with asbestos insulation. The rising number of steam driven, coal fired power stations were prime examples. Most commonly white asbestos was mixed on site with plaster into liquefied pugging which was trowelled on steam pipes as lagging. It set hard, coating the pipes and needing to be chipped away and then re-applied when repairs to joints, valves or flanges were necessary. Asbestos rope was wound around the boilers and asbestos cylindrical batts were strapped on to pipes. Bricklayers used high concentrations of asbestos in their mortar mixes when re-bricking boilers. Boiler houses were full of asbestos lagging, approximately 50 per cent of which was asbestos fibre.[118] Turbines were covered in asbestos blankets. Asbestos mouldings were poured in blacksmiths' shops. Electrical circuitry boards also contained asbestos as did gaskets for water and steam valves. Asbestos blankets were placed over hot surfaces while welding or fitting jobs were done.[119]

As well as bringing disease to generations of power station workers, this heavy asbestos burden left workplaces requiring extensive remediation. Much of this has had to await decommissioning and demolition, as was the case with the Munmorah Power Station on the New South Wales central coast, which was built in 1967 and decommissioned in 2012. It was a 1400 MW coal-fired station and its demolition included four steam-driven

---

117 A *Literature Review of asbestos fibre release from building materials following weathering and/or corrosion* (Canberra: Australian Safety and Compensation Council, 2008) 7.
118 Analysis of asbestos content in boiler lagging at East Perth Power Station. Workers' Compensation Miscellaneous Correspondence, file 16/21/2 vol.1, box WP16125. Western Power records. Western Power archive.
119 L Layman, "Health, safety and welfare: remembering 'the way it was'", in L. Layman (ed.) *Powering Perth: A history of the East Perth Power Station* (Perth: Black Swan Press, 2012), ch. 7.

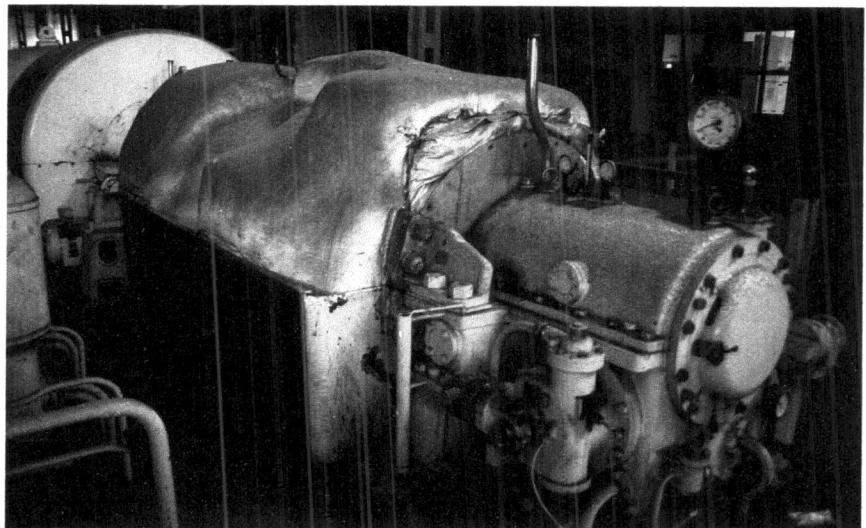

Figure 2.6: Asbestos insulation blanket on turbine at East Perth Power Station. The turbine's metal casing, which covered the asbestos blanket when the turbine was in operation, has been removed after the station closed in 1980 and during removal of all asbestos from the site.

Courtesy: Ian Fieldgate

turbo-alternators, two chimney stacks, boiler house, coal handling plant and conveyors, and extensive ash lines, making it the largest such project carried out in Australia up to 2017. The most time-consuming aspect was the removal of all the asbestos, bonded and friable, from the structures, approximately 30,000 square metres in total, and its safe disposal.[120]

The widespread use of sprayed asbestos insulation carried friable asbestos beyond industrial environments into commercial and community ones. It was developed in the 1930s, particularly for acoustic insulation and fireproofing, was extensively used in wartime naval shipping and advertised after the war as a boon to major building projects, given that the coating would bond to undersides and curved surfaces.[121] Its reach extended even into suburban houses; for instance, the Home of the Week in the *Australian Women's Weekly* in January 1973 was an expensive modern, two-storey family home in Brisbane with the ceilings of the living-room, kitchen, and children's bedrooms of sprayed asbestos fibres.[122]

---

120   Liberty Industrial, "Munmorah Power Station". http://libertyindustrial.com.au/projects/munmorah-power-station/. Accessed 11 October 2018.
121   *Sydney Morning Herald*, 7 December 1954, 10.
122   *Australian Women's Weekly*, 10 January 1973, 20–23.

Turner & Newall's limpet asbestos, a mix of 60 per cent asbestos fibre with cement, advertised in its name that it attached firmly to any surface. When *The Advertiser* newspaper office in central Adelaide, built in 1960, was demolished in 2006, more than 800 cubic metres of friable limpet asbestos was removed from the 14-storey building. The sprayed asbestos fireproofing had covered the structural steel columns and beams on all 14 levels.[123] When Shell's Clyde Refinery in Sydney was demolished in 2015 after operating from 1925 to 2013, 500 tonnes of hard-set limpet asbestos was removed.[124] Auditing and regularly monitoring the asbestos-containing materials in major CBD business premises and public buildings has become an important component of corporate responsibility and public sector accountability.

Between 1968 and 1979, one Canberra business D Jansen & Co. Pty Ltd made the disastrous decision to market a product it named Asbestosfluf as ceiling insulation for Canberra houses. It was loose-fill asbestos composed entirely of brown asbestos (or less frequently of blue asbestos). In 1972 the product was rebranded Amoswool (avoiding any mention of its asbestos content).[125] The company went by the name of Mr Fluffy and installed the material in the ceilings of 1022 houses in the ACT and an unknown number in NSW, mostly in nearby Queanbeyan.[126] The asbestos was "fluffed" up by hand on the back of a truck and then blown by hose and fan into the ceiling cavity. Each ceiling absorbed 113kg of asbestos. Expert NSW occupational health officer Gersh Major (who took the only reliable readings of dust levels at Wittenoom in 1966) was asked for his advice on the new business in 1968. He recommended that the company be "dissuaded or even prevented" from proceeding with the dangerous enterprise. Despite wearing respirators, the workmen were certainly in danger while, in the then-current state of medical knowledge, "there is some evidence that community exposure ... is undesirable", Major argued. Air currents would carry the fibres from the ceiling cavity into the living spaces of the house. The ACT Health Services Branch supported Major's report but no government action was taken and the business went ahead.[127] This cheap insulation

---

123 *Advertiser Building Asbestos Removal & Demolition Report*, McMahon Services.
124 http://dert.com.au/portfolio-item/clyde-refinery-removal/ Accessed 17 October 2018.
125 A Dunn, "Mr Fluffy: acquiring a toxic legacy", *Canberra Law Review*, 13,1, 2015, 41.
126 *NSW Taskforce Report: Loose-Fill asbestos insulation in NSW homes* (Gosford: Work-Cover NSW, 2015).
127 G Major, "Asbestos hazard", July 1968 in "Asbestosfluff Insulation", ACT Health Services Branch report to Dept of Interior, December 1968. ABC Background Briefing documents, 2014.

spread more widely when some Canberra residents bought bags of asbestos and installed it themselves in their houses and beach houses. As well, a small NSW company, Bowers Asphalt Pty Ltd, used loose-fill asbestos for home insulation in Sydney.[128]

In the face of householders' concerns,[129] the Commonwealth government in 1988 began a publicly funded program to identify and remove the insulation from Canberra houses, the ACT government joining the effort in 1991. The program ended in 1993 without the clean up being complete. Asbestos residue remained even in the houses previously cleaned and, when the public crisis revived in 2013, the ACT government decided that the only "enduring solution" was the demolition of affected residences.[130] This has proceeded. The NSW government eventually came to a similar decision and has decided to voluntarily purchase and demolish the estimated 511 houses with similar loose fill in ceilings.[131]

Fear of continuing exposure to asbestos because of inadequate clean up of asbestos contamination, or none at all, now exists throughout the community and is quickly aroused. Former asbestos manufacturing and waste disposal sites trigger recurrent alarms.

Clean ups at asbestos factory and mine sites

Factories and workshops that manufactured asbestos cement and other asbestos products closed from the early 1980s onwards with the industry's precipitate decline after 1978. Site remediation involving the removal of asbestos materials as well as contaminated soil was carried out under state government statutory management. As well, asbestos disposal or dump sites, which existed alongside all manufacturing sites, were identified and contained, buried or capped to prevent the release of asbestos fibres. Enforcing remediation to the required standard followed by regular monitoring of these sites are state responsibilities. Nevertheless community concerns are not easily allayed, given the risk of mesothelioma from low fibre exposure and its inevitably fatal outcome.

---

128 Dunn, "Mr Fluffy: acquiring a toxic legacy", 42.
129 Editorial, *Canberra Times*, 9 October 1987, 2.
130 *Long term management of loose fill asbestos insulation in Canberra homes* (Canberra: Asbestos Response Taskforce, ACT Govt, 2014).
131 Voluntary Purchase and Demolition Program. NSW Government Fair Trading. https://www.fairtrading.nsw.gov.au/housing-and-property/loose-fill-asbestos-insulation/about-the-program. Accessed 12 October 2018.

In 2014, community alarm was raised at Sunshine North in Melbourne that there was risk of mesothelioma from elevated dust levels in the roof cavities of houses close to the site of a former Wunderlich asbestos cement factory. Tests found that dust levels in houses were not elevated but that there was evidence of illegally dumped asbestos waste in surrounding areas.[132] Later that month, communities living around Wunderlich's Gaythorne site and James Hardie's site at Newstead, both in Brisbane, also raised the alarm. The Queensland Government's investigation arrived at almost identical conclusions to those in Victoria a few months earlier—no dangerous dust levels in the houses but evidence of more illegal dumping.[133] This dumping was not from the era of asbestos manufacturing and is symptomatic of ongoing Australia-wide illegal dumping of old asbestos waste.

In some instances ground contamination spread far beyond the factory gates. At Camellia in Sydney asbestos tailings (residue from milling) were used to infill low-lying areas and as street cover around James Hardie's first asbestos cement manufacturing plant.[134] In Perth James Hardie allowed tailings to be spread at Castledare Boys' Home at Wilson as infill for a miniature railway track, exposing a generation of young boys and visitors to the danger of mesothelioma in later life.[135] The most reckless and indefensible of all such instances was the spread of tailings all over the townships of Wittenoom and Baryulgil. Coloured blue from Wittenoom's blue asbestos, it covered roads, road verges and footpaths, driveways, school playgrounds and the surrounds of all town buildings and amenities. It was better than the red dust, residents thought, and softer for children to play in. Many of these children have died of mesothelioma in early adulthood.[136]

The former asbestos mining and milling sites together with their workers' housing and tailings dumps in the surrounding bush have proved most challenging of all the asbestos clean ups. At Wittenoom the clean up started earliest and still continues. The state government began phasing out the townsite and encouraging residents to relocate from 1978. Some houses and town buildings were demolished and amenities withdrawn – school, nursing

---

132   *Update: Mesothelioma and asbestos in the Sunshine area - 1 April 2015* (updated from 24 October 2014) (Melbourne: Dept of Heath & Human Services Victoria, 2015).

133   *Queensland Health report on the investigation into asbestos related concerns due to former asbestos manufacturing factories at Gaythorne and Newstead* (Brisbane: Queensland Health, 2015).

134   *Camellia Precinct: Contamination study, Part 1: High level contamination review for New South Wales Dept of Planning* (Sydney: Golder Associates, 2015), 13.

135   *West Australian*, 1 September 2009.

136   *Sunday Times*, 19 August 2018, 35.

post, police. The airport closed in 1993. In 1994 a renewed effort was made to phase out the town, although the 15 remaining residents refused to leave. Mine buildings were demolished and the rubble buried onsite in the gorges.[137] Then in 2006, the town's official status was removed, the power grid shut off, and in June 2007 the townsite was officially degazetted. The area was declared a contaminated site in 2008. Wittenoom's name was removed from official maps and road signs: the town is no more. But it has not been fully cleaned up; this would be a very costly and difficult task, and the government has opted for de-listing with warning signs throughout the district. The Ashburton Shire, which includes the town and mine site, requires its employees to wear full protective clothing with breathing apparatus should they need to visit.[138] Unfortunately some casual tourism continues.

Woodsreef near Barraba in northern New South Wales was Australia's last asbestos mine, commencing operations in 1970 and closing in 1983.[139] Its clean up was long delayed, a delay criticised by the New South Wales Ombudsman in a 2010 report on successive governments' failures to adequately deal with the state's asbestos legacy.[140] Only limited site fencing and water erosion controls had been put in place, and Barraba residents, 20 km distant, treated the mine site as a tourist attraction, the Ombudsman reported. A public awareness campaign was needed to inform the community of the risks of asbestos exposure and the wisdom of avoiding the site.[141] In the following year the government undertook a major rehabilitation project involving demolition of all mine buildings and infrastructure, closure of Crow Mountain Road which ran through the site, and the burial and capping of all processed friable asbestos and waste onsite. Of course it was impossible to cover and cap the surrounding tailing dumps that total approximately 25 million tonnes of asbestos milling residue.[142]

---

137 Occupational Health & Safety Practitioner, *Demolishing and removing buildings in Wittenoom* (West Perth: Worksafe, 2007).

138 EMP02 Prohibited Areas-Wittenoom and Yampire Gorge, Ashburton Shire minute 12-07–1045, 13 March 2013. https://www.ashburton.wa.gov.au/library/file/council_policies/EMP02. Accessed 12 October 2018.

139 Commonwealth Bureau of Mineral Resources, Geology and Geophysics, *Record*, 15, 1985, 50.

140 NSW Ombudsman, *Responding to the asbestos problem: The need for significant reform in NSW* (Sydney: NSW Ombudsman, November 2010), ch. 6.

141 NSW Ombudsman's Report 2010, 12.

142 D Blackmore, "Woodsreef Mine major rehabilitation project", 2016 International Summit on Derelict Mines (Sydney: NSW Dept of Industry, 2016). https://www.crccare.com/files/dmfile/2016DerelictMinesConferenceWoodsreefMine-David-Blackmore.pdf. Accessed 11 October 2018.

Conclusion

Today asbestos-containing materials are a blight on Australia's built environment. Government requirements for registers, audits and monitoring have begun to reveal the extent of the challenge facing eradication efforts. The clean up is in progress and, in the meantime, community awareness and education programs seek to lessen people's interactions with the material. While legal action has forced the asbestos companies to answer to their workers and product users, providing some compensation to those affected by asbestos related diseases, the wider public and private toll has been left to be borne by all Australians.

Chapter 3

TACKLING THE DUST HAZARD: THE RESPONSE OF PUBLIC HEALTH

Lenore Layman

"The worker is entitled to breath an atmosphere free of dust."

Dr Charles Badham, 1938[1]

That employers owe a legal duty of care to their workers was hammered home in the 1980s in a series of high profile cases where courts found against Australia's asbestos companies and awarded damages to plaintiffs with asbestos related diseases. The prime responsibility to avoid foreseeable workplace dangers is the employer's, and Australia's asbestos industry did not meet that obligation. However, in the operation of mines, factories, and other industrial workplaces, networks of statutory regulation devised by state governments were also imposed to protect workers' health and safety. Government departments overseeing factories, labour and industry, and mines all operated inspectorates to ensure compliance with a myriad of occupational health and safety regulations. Although the systems devised by state jurisdictions varied in detail, in all cases they sought to balance advisory assistance to industry with enforcement of the rules. These regulatory regimes involved a number of government departments and agencies. The least influential among them were the public health departments where physicians, those with the clearest understanding of potential health hazards, strove

---

1   International Labour Office, *Silicosis. Proceedings of the International Conference held in Geneva, 29 August–9 September 1938* (London: PS King & Son, 1938), 82.

to convey to engineers, managers, administrators, and workers the lethal dangers that dealing with asbestos fibre generated. These fractured regulatory regimes proved ineffective despite the best efforts of many of those involved in them.

Delay in public health's initial responses

The year was 1935. Charlie W had been employed in asbestos cement manufacture for ten years and had felt unwell for five of those years.[2] He had worked for six years in the blending and grinding mill of an asbestos cement factory where he shovelled asbestos fibre into a grinding pan and then shovelled the finely ground fibre out and rubbed it through a sieve from where it was blown into settling rooms. His workplace had no mechanical system of dust control. He complained of tightness of the chest, coughing, frequent colds, and a lack of appetite, and looked "drawn and haggard". He often had to visit his local doctor who advised him to drink large quantities of milk and take concentrated cod liver oil. When his usual doctor was absent on one occasion, another told him that his ill health was probably caused by his job and advised him to leave the industry. For reasons that are not indicated in the surviving records, he remained at his job. Like Charlie W, Eric K worked in the grinding mill during his five years' employment at the same asbestos cement factory. He left because his health "completely broke down". He described the same symptoms as Charlie and attributed them to the heavy manual work and heavy dust. Ern M worked with raw asbestos fibre for 11 years in the mixing and blending room before leaving the factory because of increasing illness. Ern had the same symptoms as Charlie and Eric but did not see a doctor because he began to feel better as soon as he left the asbestos cement works. His only continuing problem was a husky voice. George E also worked in the mixing and blending room. He remained employed in the factory after ten years. He was first reported to have needed time off work because of sickness caused by workplace dust, but later insisted that he had never needed to consult a doctor and had never been forced to stop work through illness. As a precaution, he drank a bottle of milk each day at work and took olive oil "freely" at home. He would not discuss his health in detail.[3]

---

2   People experiencing ill health who have been named in this chapter have been given pseudonyms to respect their privacy.

3   Reports of Factory Inspector Mooney, 8 March 1935, 21 May 1935; WA Dept of Labour AN25/1 Acc 749 1935/0178. SROWA.

All these men had been employed at James Hardie's asbestos cement sheet and pipe factory in the Perth suburb of Rivervale. They had worked in the dustiest parts of the manufacturing process where asbestos fibre was emptied out of bags, blended, and ground finely before being fed to the wet asbestos cement process. Their workplaces had no mechanical systems of dust control. They came to official notice in 1935 because the factory inspectorate of the Western Australian Department of Labour decided to investigate workplace dust levels and the state of health of the factory's 68 workers. Armed with a worrying report which detailed the illnesses outlined above, the Chief Inspector asked the Western Australian Public Health Department to conduct medical examinations to decide whether the men's ill-health was symptomatic of asbestosis. The Public Health Department, however, declined to investigate, the workers were not examined, their condition was not diagnosed, and they were left to pursue their existing health regimes of milk and cod liver oil. Another 23 years passed before a diagnosis of asbestosis was publicly recorded in Western Australia.

The first recorded diagnosis of asbestosis in Australia was made in 1933 in New South Wales in an asbestos millhand. Clinical examination found bronchitis along with evidence of asbestos fibres in his sputum; X-ray of his lungs led to a definite diagnosis of asbestosis.[4] This item in the New South Wales Department of Health's annual report announced the existence of asbestosis in Australia. Not until the 1950s, however, did asbestosis begin to be diagnosed in any numbers, with Dr D L Gordon Thomas' 1952-57 survey of Victorian industry.[5] Even then, between 1942 and 1968 only two NSW asbestos manufacturing workers received workers' compensation, indicating just how invisible asbestos related disease remained for another 30 years or more after 1933.[6] Australia's asbestos industry had been in existence for half a century before the first recorded case of asbestosis, and operated for more than 70 years before asbestosis began to become a public health concern in the 1950s.

Perceiving and naming the fibrosis of the lungs caused by exposure to asbestos dust was delayed throughout the industrial world. In 1928, however, as the medical profession was naming and forming its understanding

---

4   "Report of the Medical Officer of Industrial Hygiene for the year ended 31 December 1933", *NSW Department of Public Health Annual Report*, 1933, 63.

5   D L Gordon Thomas, "Pneumonokoniosis in Victorian industry", *Medical Journal of Australia*, 19 January 1957, 75-77.

6   *Report of the NSW Workers' Compensation (Dust Diseases) Board*, 30 June 1968, Appendix 10.

of asbestosis,[7] the UK's factory inspectorate instituted an investigation into the health conditions of the asbestos industry. E R A Merewether, a medical inspector of factories, and C W Price, an engineering inspector, produced a *Report on Effects of Asbestos Dust on the Lungs and Dust Suppression in the Asbestos Industry* in 1930.[8] In the same year in the UK, legislation was amended to include asbestosis as a compensable occupational dust disease.[9]

The Merewether and Price report became a benchmark, alerting government labour and public health officials around the English-speaking world to the threat of asbestosis, as can be seen in these mid-1930s events in Western Australia and New South Wales. Factory Inspector Mooney, who investigated James Hardie's Perth asbestos cement plant in 1935, cited the report extensively. As well as recommending the introduction of exhaust ventilation at the factory, Mooney identified all workers who had been employed for five years or more, guided by Merewether's finding that the incidence of asbestosis among workers rose rapidly after five years' exposure. He reported that, although the factory had been operating for 14 years, few employees had worked there long; only four of a manufacturing workforce of 62 had been employed for more than five years.[10] In declining to examine the workers, Western Australia's Public Health Commissioner recommended that they consult their general practitioners and, if diagnosed with pneumoconiosis, seek workers' compensation.[11]

The Western Australian Public Health Department had no occupational health division until 1959 and no evident interest in industrial medicine;

---

7   W E Cooke, "Fibrosis of the lungs due to the inhalation of asbestos dust", *British Medical Journal*, 26 July 1924, 140–42,147. W E Cooke, "Pulmonary asbestosis", *British Medical Journal*, 3 December 1927, 1022–25. Sir Thomas Oliver, "Clinical aspects of pulmonary asbestosis", *British Medical Journal*, 3 December 1927, 1026–27. F W Simson, "Pulmonary asbestosis in South Africa", *British Medical* Journal, 26 May 1928, 885–87. H E Seiler, "A case of pneumoconiosis. Result of the inhalation of asbestos dust", *British Medical Journal*, 1 December 1928, 982. A C Haddow, "Clinical aspects of pulmonary asbestosis", *British Medical Journal*, 28 September 1929, 580–81. W Burton Wood, "Pulmonary asbestosis. Radiographic appearances in skiagrams of the chests of workers in asbestos", *Tubercle*, 10, May 1929, 353–63. W Burton Wood and S Roodhouse Gloyne, "Pulmonary asbestosis", *Lancet*, 1 March 1930, 445–48.

8   E R A Merewether and C W Price, *Report on effects of asbestos dust on the lungs and dust suppression in the asbestos industry* (London: Great Britain Home Office, 1930), 9–14.

9   Sir John Collie, *Workmen's compensation. Its medical aspect* (London: Edward Arnold & Co., 1933), ch. xiii.

10 Report of Factory Inspector Mooney, 8 March 1935, WA Dept of Labour AU WA S321 cons749 1935/0178. SROWA.

11 Commissioner of Public Health to Chief Inspector of Factories, 30 July 1935, WA Dept of Labour AU WA S321 cons749 1935/0178. SROWA.

rather, it was narrowly preoccupied with the traditional public health concerns of sanitation and control of acute infectious diseases.[12] At first sight, the neglect of industrial medicine seems unbelievable, given the importance of the goldmining industry to the state's economy and the prevalence of silicosis among miners.[13] The Department, however, played virtually no part in the public health controls which were established to attempt to reduce the incidence of silicosis and tuberculosis among miners. The Federal Government was responsible for the establishment (in 1925) and operation of the Kalgoorlie Laboratory which compulsorily X-rayed miners periodically for lung disease until 1954 when the State took over responsibility. The Western Australian Department of Mines was responsible for inspection of dust levels in the mines and for occupational health practices in the mining industry. Asbestosis, like other pneumoconioses, fell well and truly between the large gaps in this fragmented regulatory regime.

The Division of Industrial Hygiene in the Commonwealth Department of Health, established in 1921, was active until 1932 promoting research into occupational hazards and diseases, more effective regulation of industry by greater uniformity in state legislation and regulatory practices, and the establishment of industrial medical services by employers. But staff worked within a paradigm of public health rather than of industrial medicine, concentrating on industrial diseases rather than industrial workplaces and on the elimination of sick workers from those workplaces, rather than on improving workplace conditions. At Kalgoorlie, as at Bendigo and Port Pirie, this approach guided the operations of the Commonwealth Laboratory.[14] Then the closure of the Commonwealth Division in 1932 as a budgetary economy during the Depression left industrial medicine even weaker than it had been. The Division of Industrial Hygiene in the New South Wales Department of Public Health became the only significant government authority in Australia dedicated to medical investigation of workplace health hazards and diagnosis of occupational disease. It is therefore not surprising that Australia's first diagnosis of asbestosis, in 1933, should have been made by that Division.

---

12   Western Australia Public Health Department [PHD], *Annual Report* 1943.

13   C Fitzgerald, *Turning men into stone. A social and medical history of silicosis in Western Australia 1890–1970* (Perth: Hesperian, 2016).

14   R Gillespie, "The limits of industrial hygiene: Commonwealth government initiatives in occupational health, 1921-1948", in *Reflections on medical history and health in Australia. Third national conference on medical history and health in Australia 1986*, eds H Attwood and G Kenny (Melbourne: Medical History Unit, University of Melbourne & Medical History Society, 1987), 101-20.

New South Wales starts investigating but not enforcing

Unlike its Commonwealth counterpart, the New South Wales Division did have statutory authority to inspect workplaces, direct managements, and penalise employers in the interests of industrial health. Unlike the other state public health departments without such a division, New South Wales had the appropriate medical expertise on occupational ill health within government. However, the Division was tiny, consisting until 1938 of just one medical officer with two assistants, a physicist, and an engineer. Dr Charles Badham, medical officer in charge from the Division's inception in 1923 until his death in 1943, was an internationally recognised researcher on pneumoconiosis.[15] He aimed to advance medical knowledge of dust diseases by scientific investigation: clinical and X-ray examinations, pathology and chemical analysis, and animal studies. This work drew him into industrial workplaces, but it was the sample of workers, not their workplaces, on which his concentration focused. Laboratory examination of deceased workers' lung tissue became an increasingly important aspect of his research.

Badham began his research on dust disease by investigating the hazard of sandstone dust for tunnellers, quarrymen, miners, and stonemasons,[16] and from 1928 researched dust fibroses other than silicosis, particularly fibrosis in coal-miners, chiefly because of the rising tide of workers' compensation claims in the New South Wales coal industry.[17] His 1936 study of the pathology of 76 lungs of workers from a variety of dusty occupations demonstrated scientifically the existence of coal dust fibrosis at a time when international medical opinion tended to discount it as a disease separate from silicosis. Not one of the lungs he analysed, however, came from an asbestos worker.[18] Perhaps he could not obtain one; more likely he did not

---

15 B Gandevia, "The Australian contribution to the history of the pneumoconiosis", *Medical History*, 17, 4 1973: 377. See Badham's contributions to the International Labour Office (ILO) conference, *Silicosis. Records of the international conference held at Johannesburg, 13–27 August 1930* (Geneva: ILO, 1930).

16 Studies in Industrial Hygiene, 2, 4, 5, 12; NSW Department of Public Health, *Annual Report* 1924, 1927.

17 NSW Department of Public Health, *Annual Report*, 1929, 55; 1930, 67–68; 1931/32, 62.

18 C Badham and H B Taylor, "The lungs of coal, metalliferous and sandstone miners and other workers in New South Wales, chemical analysis and pathology", *Studies in Industrial Hygiene*, 19; NSW Dept of Public Health, *Annual Report* 1936. Also "The lungs of coal miners in New South Wales, chemical analysis and pathology", *Studies in Industrial Hygiene*, 20; NSW Dept of Public Health, *Annual Report* 1939.

seek one out. It was a missed opportunity, but not a surprising one. In most Australian minds, dust disease was associated with mining and quarrying, and asbestos mining, beyond prospecting, had ceased in Australia in 1923, not to resume until the early 1940s. Almost all asbestos manufacturing plants were small at that time and therefore unlikely to come to the factory inspectorate's notice. Consequently, they were rarely drawn to the NSW Division of Industrial Hygiene's attention. Not until 1938 did the Division investigate the dust hazard in an asbestos manufacturing workplace.

The Division began to assess the extent of that hazard in 1938 because it was given a standard on which to base its judgment. In 1938 the United States Public Health Service published a proposed threshold limit value (which became known in Australia as a maximum allowable concentration) for dust exposure in the asbestos industry of five million particles per cubic foot (5mppcf) which converted to 176 particles per cubic centimetre (176ppcc).[19] This proposal, subsequently known as the Dreesen standard, remained in place until the late 1960s. It was a dust count (that is, including non-asbestos particles), not an asbestos fibre count. The technologies for fibre counting were not given practical application until the late 1950s, although Badham's work to refine dust counting with an Owen's Dust Jet Counter did enable his Division to assess approximately what percentage of dust was asbestos. Even in 1938, US evidence existed to show the 5mppcf level to be too high to prevent asbestosis developing in long-time asbestos workers. The level was, however, achievable by asbestos companies; in fact already achieved in many large US textile mills, and therefore relatively acceptable to the US industry.[20]

The dust levels recorded in 1938 at James Hardie's Sydney factory manufacturing insulation sheeting, which combined asbestos and magnesite, were far in excess of the new standard; this result in spite of the fact that the very dusty process of cutting the sheeting into its required shapes was not in operation during the testing. While dust in the centre of the room measured 532ppcc, approximately three times the standard, the work area where asbestos and other ingredients were hand-mixed to form the sheeting recorded 1,710ppcc, almost ten times the standard, and almost all of it asbestos dust. The Division described this latter exposure as "gross". When the dust counts were repeated six months later, the labour process of hand-mixing had permanently ceased but a reading of 10,000ppcc was recorded

---

19 Division of Industrial Hygiene, "The dust hazard during the manufacture of insulating packing and fibro-cement", NSW Dept of Public Health, *Annual Report* 1938, 105.

20 Castleman, *Asbestos: medical and legal aspects*, ch. 4.

at the circular saw cutting the sheeting. Only 2 to 3 per cent of this dust was asbestos, the Division estimated, but even that percentage exceeded the standard and should be reduced. The company acted to end the dustiest work in its production process only after it had been exposed by government investigation. Similarly, the dustiest parts of fibro sheeting production, although initially far less dusty than insulation sheeting production, had also become less dusty again when the Division revisited after six months.[21] There were no disincentives on employers to ensure that dust control measures were put in place before direction to do so came from government regulators; certainly employers were not self-motivated to make dust control a priority for managements.

While the manufacture of asbestos cement was carried out by a relatively small number of large companies, the manufacture of asbestos coverings, packings, and similar insulation products for industrial machinery was carried out in a large number of very small workplaces. The New South Wales Division of Industrial Hygiene took dust samples in such a workplace for the first time in 1940. A factory manufacturing asbestos rope carried out the dangerously dusty processes of winnowing, tearing, and carding asbestos fibre, preliminary steps in rope-making, without mechanical ventilation. Dust counts measured 560ppcc, three times the standard. Exhaust ventilation should be installed, the Division directed.[22]

Ten years passed before these initial fragmentary investigations began to be systematised. In 1950 dust samples were taken at a factory producing asbestos lagging (most often used as covering for boilers). It was typical of the tiny workplaces in this section of the industry. Merewether and Price in 1930 described the "unsatisfactory" character of the small works which manufactured boiler compositions in Britain.[23] Poorly designed buildings and plant also characterised most of these Australian workplaces. The asbestos lagging factory investigated by the New South Wales Division in 1950 had no mechanical ventilation for dust control. Its premises and plant were "unsuitable" and "crude". It employed two to three workers who came and left quickly. Dust counts measured an astonishing 500mppcf, 100 times the standard. The Division was moved to an unusual comment on the entire labour process: "the only remedy appears to be a completely new plant and

---

21   NSW Dept of Public Health, *Annual Report* 1938, 104–05.
22   Division of Industrial Hygiene, "Asbestos", NSW Dept of Public Health, *Annual Report* 1940, 5.
23   Merewether and Price, *Report on effects of asbestos dust on the lungs and dust suppression in the asbestos industry*, 20.

premises". The solution, however, was not to shut the factory down in the meantime because, the Division explained, "this material is of the utmost priority in industry, including power stations now under construction". Consequently, it was decided to require the installation of exhaust ventilation and frequent medical inspection of employees.[24] Allowing the existing plant to continue operating in the interest of industrial development illustrates the presence of influences other than industrial health in a government regulator's decision-making.

While the Division argued that high labour turnover protected most workers from disease, asbestosis was diagnosed in increasing numbers of NSW asbestos workers from 1950.[25] It "suspected" dust levels throughout the asbestos industry to be in excess of the Dreesen standard and pneumoconiosis to be "widespread throughout industries handling or manufacturing asbestos products"; systematic investigation of the dust hazard was indicated, the Division decided.[26] Major surveys were carried out in those sections of the asbestos industry where workplaces were large—in asbestos cement production and at James Hardie's Sydney plant which manufactured a range of asbestos products. However the numerous small plants producing industrial insulation (coverings, engine packings, and so on) were not surveyed. It would have been a time-consuming and laborious task; too much for the resources of the tiny Division.

The asbestos cement section of the industry comprising three plants, those of James Hardie, Wunderlich, and Asbestos Products, was surveyed in 1952–53. Dust levels at all stages in the production process were tested. The dustiest jobs were found to be among workers who emptied bags of chrysotile and amosite or crocidolite asbestos, blended it by shovel, and then shovelled the blend into pulverisers, generating dust levels of 15.7mppcf, more than three times the standard. At other stages later in the production process, dust levels ranged from 2.6mppcf to 0.3mppcf, well within the standard. The report recommended the introduction of exhaust ventilation where the labour of unbagging and blending occurred.[27] Yet again, companies failed to invest in dust-reduction equipment until directed to do so.

---

24   Division of Industrial Hygiene, "Asbestos. Manufacture of asbestos lagging", NSW Dept of Public Health, *Annual Report* 1950, 67–68.

25   NSW Dept of Public Health, *Annual Report* 1950, 68.

26   NSW Dept of Public Health, *Annual Report* 1950, 68 and 1951, 68.

27   C G Roberts and H M Whaite, "A survey of dust exposure and lung disease in the asbestos cement industry in New South Wales", *Studies in Industrial Hygiene* 24 (NSW Division of Industrial Hygiene, Sydney, c.1954).

Despite this intervention the dust hazard continued unabated, as was demonstrated when the Division carried out another survey of all production components at James Hardie's large Sydney plant at Camellia in 1957. The dustiest workplaces in the plant were those where insulation sheeting was manufactured. Of 56 dust counts carried out on this production process, 29 (52 per cent) exceeded 5mppcf and of these 4 (25 per cent) exceeded 20mppcf, four times the standard. The standard was, in fact, breached in almost all major sections of the factory: in 9 (27 per cent) of the 33 counts taken in asbestos cement production; in 5 (23 per cent) of the 22 counts in the production of brake-linings; in 6 (30 per cent) of the 20 counts where asbestos gangs manhandled bags of asbestos in the first stages of all the production processes; and in 5 (62 per cent) of the 8 counts taken during scrap reclamation.[28]

The Division carried out these dust counts with scientific precision to a high standard; however the unsatisfactorily high levels of workplace dust which they recorded do not appear to have been conveyed to plant managers with force or urgency. Neil Gilbert, deputy and then factory manager at James Hardie's Camellia plant in these years, commented on the communications: "What they told us was always in passing like: 'It's very dusty down there. You should have a look'. And we usually did".[29] Not until a meeting with Dr Alan Bell in 1966 was stronger pressure exerted.[30] Even allowing for some misremembering here, evidence suggests that the asbestos companies could afford to make only cursory attempts to lower dust levels. They faced no effective compliance pressure to ensure their production processes met the Dreesen standard. The 5mppcf standard did not have the legal status of a maximum allowable concentration; it remained only the measure by which the New South Wales Division of Industrial Hygiene judged the dust hazard of the asbestos processes it was called to investigate. In this restricted role, it appears to have had little effect on dust levels in the industry.

These dust levels produced asbestosis. Of a total workforce of 960 at the three Sydney asbestos cement plants, 175 men were clinically examined and X-rayed in the 1952–53 survey. Nine of them (5 per cent) were diagnosed with asbestosis.[31] In the 1957 investigation of James Hardie's plant, 99 workers of a workforce of 919 were selected for examination because they

---

28 NSW Dept of Public Health, *Annual Report* 1953–1957, 93.
29 G Haigh, *Asbestos House. The secret history of James Hardie Industries* (Melbourne: Scribe, 2006), 74–77.
30 Haigh, *Asbestos House*, 93–94.
31 Roberts and Whaite, "A survey of dust exposure and lung disease in the asbestos-cement industry in New South Wales", 8–10.

worked on dusty processes. Among these 99 workers, 14 cases of asbestosis were diagnosed which represented 14 per cent of the men in dusty jobs and 1.5 per cent of the entire workforce.

Shiels takes action in Victoria

New South Wales did not adopt the Dreesen standard as a maximum allowable concentration until 1964, and then only for mines.[32] In the meantime Victoria had moved ahead, employing Dr Douglas Shiels to take responsibility for industrial hygiene in 1937 and establishing a Division of Industrial Hygiene under his control in 1939. Shiels, fresh from employment at Mt Isa Mines, followed Badham in researching occupational dust diseases; and in 1939 his first factory inspections, which included asbestos manufacturing plants, found excessive dust counts.[33] He promised to be an energetic regulator and so he proved to be. It was Shiels who secured Victoria's adoption of the Dreesen standard as the maximum allowable concentration for all handling of asbestos in 1945.[34] And, under Shiels, Dr D L Gordon Thomas undertook a major investigation of Victorian industry for pneumoconioses. His 1952–1957 survey found asbestos workers to be among the worst affected of the "dusty trades" with 15 per cent of the 300 workers tested showing lung damage. The incidence of asbestosis "is far too high", Thomas concluded.[35] Unfortunately the impact of his article was greatly weakened by criticism of his X-ray readings by experts from other jurisdictions.[36] As a result, Thomas' findings became an outlier, rediscovered as significant only recently with the benefit of hindsight.[37]

Shiels made a final effort to tackle the hazard before retirement by overseeing the drafting of specific regulations for the handling of asbestos; however after he retired in April 1956 these new regulations, although accepted, were never gazetted. There seem to have been a number of reasons for this administrative failure, but at least one was the departure of an

---

32   *The effects of asbestos mining on the Baryulgil community*, Report of House of Representatives Standing Committee on Aboriginal Affairs, October 1984 (Canberra: Commonwealth Parliament, Australian Government Printing Service, 1984), 37.
33   *Age*, 8 April 1938, 7. P E de Silva, *Science at work. A history of occupational health in Victoria* (Blackburn: PenFolk Publishing, 2000), 58–60.
34   *Victoria Government Gazette*, 21, 7 February 1945, 637–39. C Hunter, "Perceiving a dust hazard in ordinary conditions of work", *Health and History*, 13, 2011, 8.
35   Thomas, "Pneumonokoniosis in Victorian industry", 77.
36   de Silva, *Science at work*, 77–78.
37   Haigh, *Asbestos House*, 78–79.

effective regulator who actively focused on the asbestos hazard in the workplaces for which he was responsible.[38] Certainly the attention of Victoria's Industrial Hygiene Division shifted to other workplace hazards and subsequently adopted a more cautious and strictly scientific stance, for which it was criticised when the extent of the asbestos hazard became public and a union priority in the later 1970s.[39]

While the focus and drive of individual regulators were factors in explaining the effectiveness or otherwise of regulation of the asbestos industry, employers' resistance to hearing about and acting on the findings of regulators was equally important. Shiels noted as early as 1938 that it was difficult to obtain the cooperation of employers for his work,[40] and it is evident that this was true of both private and public sector employers, not only the asbestos companies themselves. The attitude of Victoria's State Electricity Commission is a good example.

Heavy industry absorbed large quantities of asbestos, much of it in the form of lagging for heat insulation, and nowhere was this more so than in the Latrobe Valley's power stations, as a former power station mechanical fitter George Wragg has vividly detailed.[41] The constant high levels of workplace dust inside the stations resulted in the Valley producing the highest incidence of asbestos related disease in the state. Shiels' focus on dust hazards, together with the concerns of the Federated Engine Drivers and Firemen's Association, led him to examine conditions in the Yallourn power station in 1944. His recommendations to reduce boiler cleaners' dust exposure were not accepted by the State Electricity Commission's engineers who ran the station, leading Cecily Hunter to conclude in her case study of dust hazards in that industry in the 1940s and 1950s that "his [Shiels'] expertise was not taken seriously by the senior engineers".[42] This attitude did not change. George Wragg recalled the offence taken by State Electricity Commission managers at union action which called the Division of Industrial Hygiene back in to carry out testing at Yallourn in 1965–66. The workers' air quality concerns were a "family matter" which should not have been taken "outside", according to managers.[43] Such paternalism served the interests of the managers themselves, not the workers.

---

38   de Silva, *Science at work*, 77–86.
39   de Silva, *Science at work*, 155–79.
40   *Age*, 25 March 1938, 18.
41   G Wragg, *The asbestos time bomb* (Melbourne: Catalyst, 1995), ch. 3.
42   Hunter, "Perceiving a dust hazard in ordinary conditions of work", 1–25.
43   Wragg, *The asbestos time bomb*, 32–35.

Victoria's State Electricity Commission's engineers were confident that they were best able to identify and manage dust hazards in power generation, their confidence stemming both from their high regard for the expertise of their own profession as well as from their belief that external investigators without technical workplace knowledge or experience (for instance, medical scientists) were unlikely to contribute any useful or practical advice. It was not until the public scandal generated by the industrial dispute at Vic Rail concerning workers' exposure to crocidolite (blue asbestos) during the refurbishment of Melbourne's Harris ("blue") trains in 1977–78 that management culture began to shift.[44]

Mine regulation fails: the Wittenoom disaster

In Australia's asbestos mining industry worksites, suffused with mine and mill dust, the over-confidence of engineers employed in both mining companies and departments of mines proved even more obstructive to effective dust control. This complacency began early and continued for the life of the country's asbestos mining. Australia's first mill, run by Wunderlich at Anderson's Creek in northern Tasmania, operated from 1917 to 1919 with no system of dust control. Dust "in great volume" escaped and bleached the surrounding country a vivid white.[45] In an explanation which was to be repeated in various ways by government mining officials around Australia for the next half-century, Hartwell Condor, the consulting engineer and former State Mining Engineer, advised that the problem was "being dealt with" by the introduction of fans and machine covers.[46] Luckily for those workers, that mill soon closed. Baryulgil's largely Aboriginal workforce was not so lucky, its old mill operating until 1958 without any system of dust control. The "dense cloud of dust" inside the mill that made it "impossible to see anywhere" generated diagnoses of early asbestosis by 1952.[47]

---

44   Peacock, *Asbestos. Work as a health hazard*; Broadband ABC radio transcripts (Sydney: Australian Broadcasting Commission, 1978), ch.7. John Benson, "Union involvement in health issues: The VIC RAIL asbestos dispute", *New Zealand Journal of Industrial Relations*, 6, 1981, 57–65.

45   A McIntosh Reid, *Asbestos in the Beaconsfield District*. Geological Survey Report No.8, Tasmania Department of Mines (Tasmania Govt Printer, 1919), 20–21.

46   H Conder, Consulting Engineer & former Tasmanian State Mining Engineer, "Asbestos mining in Tasmania", *Australian Industrial and Mining Standard*, 6 December 1917, 358–59.

47   *The effects of asbestos mining on the Baryulgil community*, 44. For more on Baryulgil, see chapter 9.

At Wittenoom in Western Australia's northwest the dust hazard in mine and mill reached its Australian zenith. Colonial Sugar Refining Company (CSR), of which Australian Blue Asbestos (ABA)—Wittenoom's management company—was a subsidiary, had almost no mining experience. It was a sugar company and its only other mining venture was at Zeehan in Tasmania producing small quantities of chrysotile (white asbestos). There were no Australian precedents for mining and milling crocidolite except for some tiny prospecting shows scattered around Western Australia.[48] The process at Wittenoom would be one of trial and error and depend for its success on the expertise and innovative practice of management. Australian Blue Asbestos did not prove equal to the task; for the most part it was not even competent.

From the establishment of Australian Blue Asbestos in 1944 Western Australia's Mines Department commented on its inexperience and labelled its management "amateurs".[49] The Department was used to competent, trained managers in the state's large goldmines and expected this level of professionalism from CSR; instead management practices had more in common with the traditional "ad hocery" of small outback mining ventures than they did with the effective operation of a large corporate enterprise. It was only in 1943 with its purchase of the Wittenoom leases that CSR added basic mine engineering and technical books to its corporate library in Sydney;[50] the company's directors and managers truly were mining amateurs. Stories illustrating management's low standards have been a common element in workers' recall of their time in Wittenoom, whether they worked there in the 1940s or the 1960s (see chapter 8 below).

The state's Mines Department was responsible for overseeing the industry. It was a powerful institution because of the importance of minerals to the state's economy and because it forcefully promoted state development which reflected the views of Western Australian governments of all political persuasions.[51] The Mines Department both fostered and regulated the state's mining enterprises and shared with the mining industry a belief in the value of resource development and a confidence that workplace

---

48   WA Mines Dept AU WA S20 cons964 1943/0321, 1945/0789 SROWA.
49   WA Mines Dept AU WA S20 cons964 1943/0413, 1945/0352. SROWA.
50   CSR memo, 3 June 1943. Plaintiff's exhibit WV-03867. Motley Rice LLC Motley Rice LLC legal discovery exhibits list, 25 September 2006.
51   L Layman, "Development ideology in Western Australia 1933–1965", *Historical Studies*, 20, 79, 1982. L Layman, "Changing resource development policy in Western Australia, 1930s–1960s", in *State, capital and resources in the North and West of Australia*, eds E J Harman and B W Head (Nedlands, 1982), ch.8.

problems could be solved with engineering and technical know-how. The Department, while without medical expertise, did not lack concern for the health hazards of mining, but this concern was tempered by a strong desire to encourage new mining ventures and a pragmatic view of what could reasonably be expected of new, geographically isolated, financially marginal or small-scale mining ventures. And its officers knew that a certain measure of dust and dust disease had always been associated with the industry.

Wittenoom appeared to be a promising mining venture owned by one of Australia's largest companies; all the signs augured success. The Department was confident that it had the expertise to advise on and regulate not only Wittenoom's underground mining but also the milling of crocidolite, a technical process it had seen before, but only in the milling of tiny quantities of the fibre. The District Inspector's report in 1945 concluded sanguinely:

> The problem to be faced in the future development of the asbestos industry in this State is purely a mining one. The metallurgical requirements of the undertaking are comparatively simple, since the separation of the fibre is an entirely mechanical process, and since the deposits are so large and regular the geological aspect is also relatively simple.[52]

Such optimism proved entirely misplaced as satisfactory dust control (by the standards of the times) and fibre quality in milling were never achieved, and unexpected variations in the length and quality of fibre revealed the deficiency of geological knowledge.[53] Failure to control the dust created Wittenoom's epidemic of asbestos related disease, now an internationally infamous case study of an industrial disaster.

Over the period of Wittenoom's operation (1943–1966) the Mines Department's confident optimism did not flag. Year after year its inspectors ruled that dust control was unsatisfactory but that conditions were *about* to improve because of some planned change. In 1945 the Inspector reported that

> The plant is equipped with a carefully designed dust collection system. Dust escapes at certain points, but these are minor matters and can be corrected. The collection of dust at the final discharge is not satisfactory. This is to receive further attention.[54]

---

52   Report, Inspector of Mines Cue C F Adams, 25 October 1945, WA Mines Dept AU WA S20 cons964 1945/0352. SROWA.
53   CSR's Feasability Study, 29 September 1966, WA Dept of North West, "Wittenoom General", Stack 15 AN40/5 Acc1302. SROWA.
54   Report, Assistant State Mining Engineer, E E Brisbane, 6 August 1945, WA Mines Dept AU WA S20 cons964 1945/0523. SROWA.

The 1946 inspection recommended "a slow current of air distributed over a large area" to solve the continuing problem and that "when this is carried out, and it can be done easily and cheaply, the dust nuisance will disappear".[55] In 1949 the erection of a new milling plant was noted with the addendum that "dust nuisance and similar defects will now be overcome".[56] The installation of dust extractors in the mill resulted in "a general improvement all round", the District Inspector reported in 1950.[57] In 1952 mill extensions caused renewed concern but the Inspector advised that "at my request the mill building is being totally enclosed and a great improvement can already be seen in dust control". By the close of the year he was satisfied that "the dust is now controlled by extractor fans and cyclones placed in the roof".[58] Yet a tour of inspection in the following year by the Assistant State Mining Engineer found conditions less than satisfactory.

> Mill operation, at the time of our visit, was very dusty being brought about by the installation of new plant and the removal of dust curtains. The mill staff advises that the dust will only be a temporary nuisance and should be well under control within a week or two.[59]

Despite the reassurance, the 1954 inspection found the mill in a "disgraceful" condition with dust polluting the entire plant. This inspector had yet another solution: "the most effective remedy would be to exhaust large volumes of air through the roof of the mill building".[60] Both the underground workings and mill were included in the annual three-day inspections, but one inspector's work diaries for 1954–1961 show that two of those days were regularly spent underground where the workplace and work process were more familiar than that of the mill with its apparently simple mechanical process.[61] His report to the company in 1956 showed

---

55 Report, Inspector of Mines Cue, C F Adams, 17 September 1946. WA Mines Dept AU WA S20 cons964 1945/0789. SROWA.

56 Report, Inspector of Mines Cue, J Boyland, 1949, WA Mines Dept AU WA S20 cons964 1949/0037. SROWA.

57 Report, Inspector of Mines Cue, J Boyland, 1950, WA Mines Dept AU WA S20 cons964 1950/0037. SROWA.

58 Report, Inspector of Mines Cue, J Boyland, 31 December 1952, WA Mines Dept AU WA S20 cons964 1952/0031. SROWA.

59 Report, Assistant State Mining Engineer, K Lloyd, 8 December 1953, WA Mines Dept AU WA S20 cons964 1953/1238. SROWA.

60 Report, Inspector of Mines Cue, A W Ibbotson, 31 December 1954. WA Mines Dept AU WA S20 cons964 1954/0031. SROWA.

61 J Faichney, "Diary 1950–1958, 1958–1966"; 2 vols in possession of C Fitzgerald.

the same imbalance, despite his observation of the mill's " very high dust hazard".[62]

After more than ten years of milling dust levels had not been brought under control. What had seemed to the mines inspector in 1945 a minor matter proved an intractable problem. Given that a new mill was being designed perhaps, CSR reflected, it was time to get advice from a company experienced with the control of dust emissions in a dry processing plant; or perhaps dust from enclosures around mill machinery could be blown into the upper part of the old mine workings?[63] Trial and error continued.

The Mines Inspectorate was never satisfied with Wittenoom dust counts and constantly negotiated with management on the matter, but common to all its responses to the high dust levels was a professional confidence that the problem had a simple technical solution which the Department could competently identify, combined with a professional optimism that the problem was about to be solved. The NSW industrial hygienist Gersh Major, who took dust readings in the plant in 1966 just prior to its closure, concluded that the task of dust control required the determined and skilled attention of an industrial hygienist over some period of time. It should not, he concluded, "have been the responsibility of busy mines inspectors".[64] Nevertheless the Mines Department believed it had the time, experience, and expertise to handle the problem and resisted any suggestions otherwise. Like the State Electricity Commission's engineers in Victoria, the Western Australian Mines Department did not believe the Public Health Department's physicians held useful knowledge.

Until the mid-1950s that Mines Department's judgment of the Public Health Department's expertise was an accurate one; the latter department had little knowledge of or interest in industrial medicine. It played no part in the Commonwealth Health Department's Health Laboratory at Kalgoorlie which ran the miners' compulsory X-ray program from 1925.[65] A Commonwealth mobile X-ray unit was responsible for X-ray examinations of miners beyond the Golden Mile, the unit travelling by rail and ship as well as road to reach isolated mining centres, either biennially or annually depending

---

62   J Faichney, Assistant Mines Inspector to ABA, 6 December 1956. Plaintiff's Exhibit WV-03964. Motley Rice exhibits 2006.

63   CSR letter to ABA, 20 April 1956. Plaintiff's Exhibit WV-03931. Motley Rice exhibits 2006.

64   G Major, "Asbestos dust exposure", in *Proceedings of the First Australian Pneumoconiosis Conference*, 12-14 February (Sydney, 1968), 474.

65   J H L Cumpston, *Health and disease in Australia. A history* (Canberra: Commonwealth of Australia, 1989), 166-68.

on the remoteness of the location and the size of the workforce. In 1947 and again in the early 1960s a more up-to-date unit replaced the older equipment.[66] In the 1940s the mobile X-ray unit made the Marble Bar–Yilgarn–Wittenoom trip bienially.[67] This unit also carried out initial medical checks and issued certificates prior to 1948.[68] Medical acceptance of radiological examination as sufficient evidence for a diagnosis of silicosis (although not for assessing the degree of disability which people with silicosis experienced) made this Commonwealth public health initiative viable. The State Health Department did not take over this X-ray screening role until 1954, combining it with mass tuberculosis screening of the whole population from 1956.[69] It did not establish an Occupational Health Division until 1959, and added a second physician, Dr Jim McNulty, to join Dr Don Letham in 1963.[70] A pneumoconiosis section within the Division in 1964 signalled the Public Health Department's increased activity in the area.[71] In other words, the Public Health Department came late to industrial medicine.

Dr Saint issues warnings in vain

The medical practitioner who first realised the extent of Wittenoom's asbestos dust danger was Dr Eric Saint (see chapter 12 below). One among a group of general practitioners recruited in the UK by the Public Health Department in the postwar period to ease the medical shortage in remote areas of the state, he was appointed to the northwest coastal town of Port Hedland and serviced Wittenoom as a Flying Doctor between 1948 and 1951. What made him unusual (probably unique) in Western Australia at this time was his doctorate in industrial health from England's Newcastle University. His extensive knowledge of industrial disease included a specific understanding of the danger of asbestos dust from his experience of asbestos manufacturing near Newcastle.[72] Consequently he was horrified by what he saw on his first visit to Wittenoom and wrote immediately to his superiors in Perth stating that

---

66 D A Darroch, *The origin and a history of the mobile x-ray unit for the mining industry in Western Australia* (D A Darroch, 1993), 1–24.
67 WA Dept of Labour AN 25/1 Acc 749 1949/ 0479. SROWA.
68 WA Mines Dept AU WA S20 cons964 1945/0523, 1945/0352. SROWA.
69 WA PHD *Annual Report* 1957, 10, 32, 33.
70 Discussion with Dr D D Letham, 15 May 1984. Interview with Dr J C McNulty, 10 May 1984.
71 WA PHD *Annual Report* 1963, 8.
72 Interview with Dr E Saint, 27 April 1984.

in a year or two ABA [Australian Blue Asbestos] will produce the richest and most lethal crop of cases of asbestosis in the world's literature... Naturally I think some of these chests should be looked into.[73]

The Commissioner of Health responded positively to Saint's concerns, acknowledging that "these workers could easily incur a greater hazard than do workers in our gold mines". He tried to reassure Saint by advising him that X-rays in Perth would be required of all workers before they commenced employment at Wittenoom, and that his department was endeavouring to arrange for the Commonwealth's mobile X-ray unit to make annual (rather than biennial) visits to Wittenoom.[74] Annual visits began in the mid-1950s. Given the transience of Wittenoom's workforce, however, with 60 per cent of a total workforce staying for six months or less, this timeframe remained inadequate.

Saint also tackled Wittenoom's employer, Australian Blue Asbestos, in 1948.

> I said "Look, you've got problems"...They pooh-poohed me and in fact they labelled me as a troublemaker...They didn't listen. I was just a young man, a Flying Doctor...I'd only just come out from England and they thought "Who's this jumped-up fellow?" That was the attitude.[75]

And yet Wittenoom's management had first-hand knowledge that the mill produced asbestosis because their dependable mill superintendent had "shown signs of asbestosis" when X-rayed by the travelling laboratory in 1946 and had been advised to "get away from the dust" which he did.[76] This early case of asbestosis at Wittenoom appears to have escaped medical records but clearly not the company's.

Nevertheless management ignored Saint and both the Public Health and Mines departments seemed to him uncomprehending of the scope of the potential disaster.

> It was the local experience. They'd never encountered asbestos. They'd never had occasion to look it up in the literature. It wasn't in the

---

73 Letter, E G Saint to Commissioner of Public Health C E Cook, 6 June 1948; WA Dept of Labour 1949/0479.
74 Letter, Commissioner of Public Health C E Cook to E G Saint, 16 June 1948, WA Dept of Labour 1949/0479.
75 Interview with Dr E Saint, 27 April 1984.
76 ABA internal letter, 6 September 1946. Plaintiff's Exhibit WV-03974. Motley Rice exhibits 2006.

front of their consciousness. All they were thinking was what they knew, that there was a certain amount of silicosis among the miners in Kalgoorlie ... The mining people were looking at the morbidity amongst miners; what interested them was silicosis.[77]

Wittenoom's crocidolite works were deemed a mine and therefore came under the provisions of the *Mining Act*, which did not touch on health at all, and of the *Mines Regulation Act*, which vested in the Mines Department the powers of inspection and supervision and of framing regulations relating to sanitation, safety and health.[78] The latter Act defined "mine" widely to include not only the place of extraction of a mineral/metal but also "a place ... where the products of any such place are being treated or dealt with".[79] Thus Wittenoom's mill was a mine for the purposes of the Act.

Although Dr Saint was not aware of it, his letter in 1948 warning of the asbestosis danger at Wittenoom spurred the Public Health Department to try to change this legal situation. In 1949 the Department proposed that an area within five miles of Wittenoom's mill be excised from the jurisdiction of the *Mines Regulation Act* and be brought within that of the *Shops and Factories Act* so that factory inspectors could inspect the works and "enforce improvements".[80] The attempt was blocked when the Solicitor General, on advice from the Mines Department, ruled that Wittenoom was a mine and therefore not a factory.[81]

The Public Health Department tried again on a broader front in 1953, this time in response to Kwinana's industrial growth, calling for co-ordination to replace the piecemeal approach of the past.[82] The response was again negative, a parliamentary draftsman advising that such legislation would cut across at least ten Acts as well as industrial awards. And it was unnecessary as "ample legislative power already exists to bring about what is desired without further expense to the State".[83] The Commissioner of Public Health

---

77   Interview with Dr E Saint, 27 April 1984.
78   Mining Act, 1904–1957, Mines Regulation Act, 1946–1957. *The Reprinted Acts of the Parliament of Western Australia*, 12, 10.
79   Mines Regulation Act, 1946–1957. *The Reprinted Acts of the Parliament of Western Australia*, 10, 3.
80   Minute, Acting Commissioner of Public Health to Minister for Public Health, 14 November 1949. WA Dept of Labour AU WA S321 cons749 1949/0479. SROWA.
81   Minute, Secretary of WA Department of Labour to Chief Inspector of Factories, 15 December, 1949. WA Dept of Labour AU WA S321 cons749 1949/0479.
82   Report 1953. WA Dept of Health AU WA S268 cons1003 1964/0473.
83   Response of Assistant Parliamentary Draftsman and Chief Conveyancer, 5 May 1953, WA Dept of Health AU WA S268 cons1003 1964/0473.

protested that it was not possible under existing legislation for his Department to maintain adequate medical supervision of other authorities who were "without the medical knowledge required to appreciate the problems involved".[84] However nothing changed.

Dr McNulty stirs public health action

Despite the lack of an immediate government response Saint's intervention had raised awareness in the Public Health Department and attitudes began to change. By 1954 the Department saw the mining industry as "a blight on its [the state's] public health".[85] Then the appointment of Dr Jim McNulty as Kalgoorlie Chest Physician and Mines Medical Officer in early 1957 introduced a young doctor who had clinical experience with dust diseases. This included both silicosis, because of work in the potteries in Stoke on Trent, and also coalminers' pneumoconiosis which he had seen in many dusted miners when he worked at the Thoracic Surgery Centre in Sully, South Wales. McNulty was determined to extend the Public Health Department's influence with the aim of reducing occupational dust disease among the state's hard rock miners. For too long the prevention of industrial disease had been "entirely the prerogative of engineers".[86]

The Public Health Department voiced its growing concern that dust control at Wittenoom was "unsatisfactory" and criticised the Mines Department's inadequate dust counting equipment—the Watson Vector Konimeter—which was used to count asbestos fibres as though they were dust particles.[87] No maximum allowable dust concentrations were in place, with the mines inspectors aiming to achieve what was reasonable and practical in particular mine circumstances.[88] The Public Health Department, on the other hand, believed the asbestos dust limit to be that set by the Dreesen standard—176 particles per cubic centimetre (176ppcc). Wittenoom's mine and mill dust breached that standard; but no one knew by exactly how much until 1966 when the Public Health Department

---

84   Minute, Commissioner of Public Health, 28 May, 1953. WA Dept of Health AU WA S268 cons1003 1964/0473.
85   WA Public Health Dept, *Annual Report* 1954, 8.
86   Committee on Pneumoconiosis, 24. For more on Dr McNulty's role see chapter 13, below.
87   WA Public Health Dept, *Annual Report*, 1959, 47 and 1962, 32. Cumpston, *Health hazard at Wittenoom*, 1.
88   Committee on Pneumoconiosis, 23–24.

finally persuaded the Mines Department to allow a dust-testing expert to be brought in from New South Wales (on condition the Public Health Department pay all costs) to take samples.[89] The results were alarming: samples reached 1,500ppcc in the stopes (more than eight times the Dreesen standard) and 3,000ppcc in the bagging section of the mill (seventeen times the standard).[90]

The Mines Department knew that Wittenoom's dust was excessive, but this mine was just one of many dusty mining workplaces around the state. Inspectors regularly reported dust counts (mostly in gold mines) of more than 1,000ppcc, former mines inspector Jack Faichney recalling that "sometimes in the very dusty places you got a very crowded dust sample and you couldn't distinguish them; you'd generally place them as 1000+".[91] In 1962, for instance, there were 111 such samples of 1,938 samples taken around the state, with an average count of 308ppcc.[92] It is not difficult to see why a parliamentary committee appointed in 1963 to inquire into pneumoconiosis should conclude that "the methods, extent and apparent lack of system in dust count testing were disturbing".[93]

McNulty commented wryly:

> When Cassandras ... advised that dust was a problem [at Wittenoom] and predicted the development of disease it didn't ring any alarm bells in the people concerned in the mining industry because they were used to it; they expected it.[94]

For the Mines Department, dust remained an inevitable part of mining; "they were fatalistic about it".[95]

A medical practitioner stationed at the northwest coastal town of Roebourne and serving Wittenoom as a Flying Doctor in the period 1952–53 also recalled that

> At this stage they were not concerned about lung disease caused by asbestos. They were more talking about dust on the lung which a

---

89 J C McNulty, interview with C Fitzgerald, 15 November 2002, 59.
90 Major, "Asbestos dust exposure", in *Proceedings of the First Australian Pneumoconiosis Conference*, 12–14 February 1968 (Sydney, 1968), 467–518.
91 J Faichney, interview with C Fitzgerald, 6 August 2008, 72.
92 WA Mines Dept A/R 1962, 25.
93 Committee on Pneumoconiosis, 23.
94 McNulty interview, 57.
95 McNulty interview, 58.

miner usually gets. They were concerned about the miner that worked directly in the mine.[96]

Experience suggested to Mines Department officers that men with a history of mining behind them, exposed for long periods to the silica in quartz rock, were in danger of developing silicosis. The greater danger of asbestos dust, and particularly to Wittenoom's mill workers, in a workplace laden with asbestos dust, but who were almost all newcomers to and transient in the mining industry, was not fully recognised.

Indeed the threat of asbestosis at Wittenoom was subsumed in the ongoing prevalence of silicosis. In 1959 the Public Health Department calculated that one worker in every 30 who entered the mining industry developed silicosis with an annual incidence of ten per thousand.[97] As far as the state's mining industry was concerned asbestos generated a dust danger more or less equivalent to that of silica. This misperception is evident in Arbitration Court hearings in 1949 when union advocates challenged Wittenoom management's argument that "merely because there are clouds of dust it does not mean that that dust is dangerous".[98] While the unions firmly rejected this notion of the dust as just a nuisance, an inevitable part of manual work like heat and noise, it was silicosis—not asbestosis—that concerned them. The Australian Workers' Union advocate, despite quoting medical advice about asbestosis as well as silicosis, urged that Wittenoom must not be allowed to develop into "a silicosis-producing mine".[99] He focused on the underground mine not the mill because he shared the Mines Department's concern about long-term mine workers, especially underground workers, those who spent their working lifetime in the mines. Only in 1959 when, on the basis of its first asbestosis diagnoses, the Public Health Department calculated that 12 per cent of Wittenoom workers developed asbestosis on average after four years' exposure and that mill workers were most at risk, did perceptions begin slowly to shift.

The first publicly recorded asbestosis diagnosis was made unexpectedly in 1958 during surgery at Wooroloo tuberculosis sanatorium. The patient was found to have asbestosis. Dr McNulty in Kalgoorlie was advised and read up on the literature, while the mobile X-ray unit sent Wittenoom's most recent X-rays to him. From those he diagnosed five more cases of asbestosis. Dr Letham, who was setting up the Occupational Health Division at the

---

96 Interview with Dr Kowal, 30 August 1983.
97 WA Public Health Dept, *Annual Report* 1959, 47.
98 Employer advocate, Arbitration Court of WA, 15 July 1949; Awards 41/48, 12/49, 22/49; transcript of evidence, SROWA.
99 Australian Workers Union advocate 3 June 1949, 21–22.

time, immediately travelled to Wittenoom to examine the workforce and McNulty followed him in the following year.[100] By the close of 1960 these examinations had identified 19 cases of asbestosis, silicosis or a combination of the two,[101] figures which were "something of a shock" to the State Mining Engineer.[102] They were also a shock to Wittenoom's more experienced miners, the District Inspector of Mines reporting "an exodus of skilled miners" confronted by evidence of the asbestosis risk.[103] Searches of medical records from 1958 to 1961 increased the number of diagnoses to 25 while further searches took the number to 34.[104] In December 1962 the number had reached 42.[105]

Empowered by this evidence, public health physicians demanded immediate action to reduce the dust, pressuring government, company and Mines Department. One physician wrote to Sydney specialist Dr H M Rennie, consultant physician to CSR, concerning a former Wittenoom worker then dying in "very considerable distress": "if the officers of the CSR…were to be compelled…to hear his struggling for breath they would be a little less satisfied 'that they had gone as far as they can with the present knowledge'." He quoted another public health physician who described Wittenoom as "a festering sore".[106]

The shock of the diagnoses reverberated and action followed. The Mines Department began to listen to the public health physicians; it increased its ventilation staff, organised more frequent and detailed Wittenoom ventilation inspections and became less tolerant of management shortcomings. ABA appointed a full time ventilation officer and engaged two companies with expertise in dust control to visit and advise on dust reduction in the mill.[107] Despite these efforts, however, the Senior Inspector of Mines

---

100 McNulty interview, 92–94.
101 Wittenoom chest X-ray survey 1960. Plaintiff's Exhibit WV-04157. Motley Rice exhibits 2006.
102 Memo State Mining Engineer to Unser Secretary for Mines, 17 November 1960. Plaintiff's Exhibit WV-04158. Motley Rice exhibits 2006.
103 District Inspector of Mines to Senior Inspector of Mines, 12 December 1960. Plaintiff's Exhibit WV-04164. Motley Rice exhibits 2006.
104 Dr J McNulty to Dr H M Rennie, 25 October 1961. Plaintiff's Exhibit WV-04098. Motley Rice exhibits 2006.
105 Dr J McNulty to Dr H M Rennie, 10 December 1962. Plaintiff's Exhibit WV-04105. Motley Rice exhibits 2006.
106 Dr B Hunt to Dr H M Rennie, 25 September 1961. Plaintiff's Exhibit WV-04090. Motley Rice exhibits 2006.
107 Plaintiff's Exhibits WV-04187, WV-04186, WV-04191. Motley Rice exhibits 2006. Motley Rice exhibits 2006.

concluded at the end of 1961 that "the dust menace has not declined".[108] Tensions, threats and complaints rose among the parties. These continued until Wittenoom's closure in December 1966, CSR eventually conceding that it was not possible to satisfy rising concerns.[109]

From 1959 until the mine's closure in 1966 public physicians targeted Wittenoom with regular visits to undertake clinical examinations alongside the annual X-ray examinations.[110] The X-ray changes in asbestosis had been found to be subtle and therefore difficult to detect, and it was hoped that additional clinical examination would enable earlier diagnosis.[111] During these yearly clinical examinations Dr McNulty found that the wisest advice he could give was not wanted.

> Perhaps the only medical advice one could have given, in view of the dusty conditions and history was "If you are thinking of going—don't!" and "If you are there—leave!" but this was not the advice they wanted ... If there were no signs of clinical disease, one could not advise them to leave.[112]

At the end of his life Jim McNulty grappled with the thought that he should have done more, but also remembered the hard reality of the time.

> I talked to everybody I could find and I stood in a pub having a drink talking to people ... and I visited people and people invited me home for meals ... and I spoke to individual miners that I examined and, short of hiring a hall and having a public meeting, which could never have happened ... they didn't do things like that in those days ... Subsequently they would have [been] interviewed [by] *Today Tonight* ... but in those days you didn't do it ... it just wasn't seen as a role ... You would talk to them and persuade them to leave but that was their decision if they wanted to stay. It was their lives to lead ... If they had TB, of course, that was different; that was a danger to other people, so they had to be removed, whether they liked it or not.[113]

---

108   Senior Inspector Mines to ABA, 6 November 1961. Plaintiff's Exhibit WV-04195. Motley Rice exhibits 2006.
109   CSR Director K O Brown speech, 20 September 1966. Plaintiff's Exhibit WV-04541. Motley Rice exhibits 2006.
110   J C McNulty, "Asbestos mining—Wittenoom, Western Australia", in *Proceedings of the First Australian Pneumoconiosis Conference*, 12–14 February (Sydney, 1968), 449.
111   J L Elder, "Asbestosis in Western Australia", *Medical Journal of Australia*, 2, 1967, 583.
112   McNulty, "Asbestos mining—Wittenoom, Western Australia", 453–54.
113   McNulty interview, 99.

New asbestosis cases were diagnosed each year from 1958.[114] By 1967, immediately after the mine had closed, 60 former Wittenoom workers had been certified with asbestosis by the Pneumoconiosis Board.[115]

Wittenoom increases understandings of asbestosis

Medical understandings about the disease asbestosis had been changed by the Wittenoom experience. First, the average period of exposure required to produce the disease was found to be shorter than had been reported in the medical literature. For instance, the New South Wales Division of Industrial Hygiene staff who carried out the 1950s surveys in Sydney framed their interpretation of their results in the context of both the Merewether and Dreesen studies when they wrote:

> Asbestosis has only been found to occur after prolonged exposure and even with work in very high dust concentrations, the disease is rare in workers with less than five years' exposure.[116]

In asbestos cement manufacture, more than half the workers (57 per cent) were employed for less than five years. They therefore were seen to have escaped asbestosis. Even at exposures of 500mppcf, experienced in asbestos-lagging manufacture, workers were protected by transience, the Division had argued in 1950.[117] Examining the Wittenoom statistics, however, Dr Janet Elder in 1967 found asbestosis occurring in a 1.5–12 year range with an average of less than 7 years; McNulty in 1968 found a 1–14 year range with an average of 5.25 years among mill workers and a range of 3–12 years with an average of 6.6 years in mine workers.[118] Exposure for less than 5 years did not protect workers, as previously assumed.

Second, the rapidity of onset of the disease at Wittenoom was also surprising, NcNulty reporting:

> A man with two years exposure in the mill might have a normal chest X-ray and no symptoms one year, but have dyspnoea, finger

---

114 WA Mines Department Annual Reports 1959–1966.
115 Elder, "Asbestosis in Western Australia": 579. These 60 workers were diagnosed with either asbestosis or asbestosis and silicosis.
116 NSW Dept of Public Health, *Annual Report* 1950, 68.
117 NSW Dept of Public Health, *Annual Report* 1950, 68.
118 Elder, "Asbestosis in Western Australia", 582. McNulty, "Asbestos mining—Wittenoom, Western Australia", 456.

clubbing, basal crepitations and an abnormal chest X-ray the following year.[119]

Third, the chest X-ray, which worked so well in the diagnosis of silicosis, was not adequate for asbestosis both because radiological change was not the earliest sign of disease and because the X-ray was difficult to interpret, with considerable variation among readers. Sadly the limitations of X-ray diagnosis had already seriously damaged the impact of Dr Gordon Thomas' 1957 findings set out in the *Medical Journal of Australia* that 15 per cent of all the Victorian asbestos workers he examined showed signs of asbestosis. Experienced X-ray readers in New South Wales and the United Kingdom did not diagnose the disease in the same X-rays and Thomas' conclusions were somewhat discredited and, as a result, discounted.[120]

Added to the growing load of asbestosis cases came the lethal threat of a newly diagnosed and named disease, mesothelioma. Following immediately on Wagner, Sleggs and Marchand's groundbreaking South African findings published in 1959,[121] McNulty diagnosed the disease in a former Wittenoom mill worker in 1960.[122] It was a shocking development. Dr Janet Elder, respiratory physician at the Perth Chest Hospital (later Sir Charles Gairdner Hospital), saw many of the early cases of both asbestosis and mesothelioma and established lists of both cohorts which she pinned to the wall of her office. So Western Australia's Mesothelioma Register began from McNulty's first diagnosis. Dr Elder explained:

> We realised that this problem of mesothelioma in particular was going to be much more of a problem in the future because of the long latent period ... of course it has been almost an epidemic since.[123]

Wittenoom's closure in December 1966 ended any significant asbestos mining in the state to the relief of all health staff involved in the saga. Then in the mid-1970s Dr McNulty's carefully cultivated courteous relations with the parent company CSR resulted in an extraordinary breakthrough.

---

119 McNulty, "Asbestos mining—Wittenoom, Western Australia", 451.
120 de Silva, *Science at work*, 76-77.
121 J C Wagner, C A Sleggs and P Marchand, "Diffuse pleural mesothelioma and asbestos exposure in the North Western Cape Province", *British Journal of Industrial Medicine*, 17, 1960, 260-71.
122 J C McNulty, "Malignant pleural mesothelioma in an asbestos worker", *Medical Journal of Australia*, 2, 1962, 953-54.
123 Dr J Elder, interview with C Fitzgerald, 20 April 1995.

He arranged a meeting between CSR representatives (regional manager Russell Leith and several Sydney staff) and researchers from the Public Health Department at the University of Western Australia led by Professor Michael Hobbs at which CSR agreed that Wittenoom's personnel records would be made available for medical research.[124] This welcome and surprising decision came at a time when CSR was first facing adverse publicity in relation to its involvement with asbestos. The *Bulletin* magazine's cover story in July 1974 warning of "Blue Asbestos: Is there a killer your house?" led the way in alerting Australians to Wittenoom as "a tragic chapter in our mining history".[125] How was CSR to respond, secure as it thought it was at the time behind the corporate veil? In June 1978 the company set up the Wittenoom Trust to expend $2,000,000 over ten years in order to relieve personal hardship among former Wittenoom workers. Perhaps its decision to facilitate medical research was an earlier example of a similar effort to display philanthropy while projecting a positive company image. Whatever the motivation, access to the records was the essential prerequisite for the major epidemiological project which established Wittenoom as a "modern industrial disaster" of international proportions.[126]

1970s: a changing environment

In 1978 asbestos fibre imports to Australia began to fall from their all-time high in 1977. Although James Hardie first produced fibre cement boarding containing a reduced percentage of asbestos in 1963 and seriously committed to research on asbestos-free fibre cement in 1972, usage of asbestos fibre continued to climb in the first half of the 1970s.[127] Woodsreef chrysotile mine at Barraba in New South Wales began production in 1972 with James Hardie its major customer. When Matt Peacock visited the mine for his ABC documentary in 1977 he saw "vast quantities" of tailings dust "blowing into the mill", and the New South Wales Mines Minister's response to his challenge on the matter indicated that the failure of mine regulators across state jurisdictions stretched to the end of asbestos mining in Australia:

---

124 Emeritus Professor M S T Hobbs, interview with L Layman, 1 October 2008, 35.
125 T Hall, "Blue asbestos: Is there a killer in your house?", *Bulletin*, 6 July 1974, 30–33.
126 A W Musk, N H de Klerk, J L Eccles, M S Hobbs, B K Armstrong, L Layman and J C McNulty, "Wittenoom, Western Australia: a modern industrial disaster", *American Journal of Industrial Medicine*, 21, 5, 1992, 735–47.
127 James Hardie Asbestos Ltd, *Annual Report* 1968.

> ... we want some immediate action because undertakings have been given by the Company before and ... the position did improve but now they've deteriorated and the position is back as bad as it was eighteen months ago.[128]

The pattern of dashed hopes was starkly reminiscent of the Wittenoom experience.

Efforts at the national level to reduce workers' exposure to airborne asbestos began in the late 1960s with the 1969 recommendation of the National Health and Medical Research Council (NHMRC) for the adoption of a maximum allowable concentration of asbestos fibres of 4 fibres per cubic centimetre (4fpcc). Subsequent NHMRC recommendations in 1978 and 1983 reduced that maximum further. Implementation required each state to embed the recommendations in statutory regulations, and the individual jurisdictions began to do so at various times through the 1970s: Queensland in 1971; South Australia in 1976; New South Wales, Victoria, and Western Australia in 1978; and Tasmania in 1979.[129] As asbestos regulations were finally being gazetted, the tide of public opinion was turning against the asbestos industry. From the mid–1970s a flood of sensational and heart-rending media exposés of the asbestos hazard shifted public perceptions sharply (see chapter 4). Knowledge grew and fear surged.[130]

Workers in all parts of the asbestos industry mostly learnt of the extent of the asbestos hazard they faced at work from the same sources as the public and at around the same time. The government regulatory model examined in this chapter had neither a component for informing and educating workers nor a specified industrial health role for workers' trade unions. Companies were under no regulatory obligation to inform workers of the hazard of workplace dust levels nor even provide a full accounting of workers' own test results. And indeed the asbestos companies failed to fully inform and educate their workers. CSR conceded as late as 1974 that in all its factories that handled asbestos there was an "apparent lack of effective communication of the hazards of asbestos to all personnel".[131] This failure was industry-wide and workers had to find out about the asbestos hazard in their workplaces elsewhere.

---

128 Mines Minister Pat Hills quoted in Peacock, *Asbestos. Work as a health hazard*, 70.
129 Report, *The effects of asbestos mining on the Baryulgil community*, ch. 4.
130 For Wittenoom's transformation in the public mind, see "Wittenoom: Public memory reframed", *Public History Review*, 4, 1995, 2–24.
131 CSR memo, "Review of precautions taken throughout CSR on handling of asbestos", 12 July 1974. Plaintiff's exhibit WV-03573. Motley Rice exhibits 2006.

For the most part trade unions did not take up the issue of workplace health hazards until the 1970s. The response of the Australian Workers' Union to Wittenoom's dust levels is a case in point. The union began well in 1948 by protesting twice to the State Mining Engineer about the "heavy clouds of dust...drifting through the plant" and the "thick covering of dust" surrounding the mill, following up these complaints with press and radio publicity.[132] This challenge was not pursued however, the union (together with other unions whose members worked at Wittenoom) opting instead for increases in dust money to compensate workers for their unsatisfactory working conditions.[133] They continued to see the dust as a "nuisance", their members "breathing and eating dirt".[134]

It was not until the 1970s that most trade unions developed research and education sections and became better informed about less obvious workplace hazards. Strikes and other direct actions around occupational health and safety issues increased. Melbourne's Harris ("blue") trains strike at Vic Rail in 1977–78 had the most extensive media coverage at the time and is best remembered, but there were other actions, including a successful strike in 1978 at Western Australia's Midland Railway Workshops to secure similar protection for workers removing asbestos insulation from old railcars.[135] As well, from the early 1970s the Builders Labourers' Federation (BLF) in the ACT, Queensland, and South Australia organised direct actions when members were exposed to asbestos on the job. "Asbestos Kills" became a popular union rallying cry.[136] And some unionists proved particularly adept at spreading the message; South Australian BLF organiser Jack Watkins was among the most passionate. In the early 1970s he placed bright yellow stickers carrying a black death's head and a "Danger" warning on the front doors of Adelaide business premises to force owners to begin asbestos removal programs. Even more dramatically on 16 September 1982 he disrupted parliament by throwing two sealed bags of asbestos fibre at South Australian cabinet ministers, shouting "You're killers, all of you", to protest

---

132 *Kalgoorlie Miner*, 13 May 1948, 1. Plaintiff's Exhibits WV-03998, WV-03890, WV-03893. Motley Rice exhibits 2006.

133 WA Employers' Federation to ABA, 14 December 1956. Plaintiff's Exhibits WV-04024, WV-04031. Motley Rice exhibits 2006.

134 AWU to Workmen's Inspector, 5 March 1958. Plaintiff's Exhibit WV-04033. Motley Rice exhibits 2006.

135 P Bertola, "Occupational health at the workshops", in *The Workshops*, eds P Bertola, B Oliver (Perth: University of Western Australia Press, 2006), 158–71.

136 H McQueen, *Framework of flesh. Builders labourers battle for health and safety* (Port Adelaide: Ginninderra Press, 2009), 134–40.

their inaction on the removal of crocidolite from the ceilings of public hospitals.[137] For the asbestos industry this sort of publicity was lethal: with its growth well and truly ended and its reputation increasingly laid waste, the long process of asbestos removal began.

Conclusion

Control of workplace dust in the Australian asbestos industry across the 20th century failed. The asbestos companies have been forced to acknowledge their failure and their ongoing responsibility and culpability for the harm they have caused. And what of those regulators on whom this chapter has focused—the public health component of the statutory framework? They worked within a regulatory model that was judged a failure and replaced at this time (1970s–1980s) by a new model based on the Robens principle of tripartite responsibility of employers, unions, and governments. The old model was condemned as a maze of complex, intertwined and, in some instances, conflicting legislation resulting in overlapping and confused regulatory responsibilities, made worse in Australia's federal system by six divergent state jurisdictions. As well, for all its complexity, there remained gaps in coverage and ineffective processes for recognising and preventing occupational diseases with long latency periods. The framework did not have a systematic review process and did not involve trade unions or other workers' representation. Inspectorates were underfunded and too small to carry out their monitoring responsibilities fully. They almost never prosecuted employers for breaches, preferring to advise and educate rather than enforce compliance; and this practice continued despite its repeated failure to eliminate or even reduce ongoing workplace hazards.[138] Financial constraints, the hierarchical administrative cultures fostered within individual inspectorates, and the social expectations of governments and industry provide the wider context which hamstrung the operation of the state regimes.

All these weaknesses can be seen at play in this account of failed attempts to regulate the asbestos hazard in Australian workplaces. Most striking was the incapacity of the model to move beyond scientific measurements of dust levels and evidence of dust disease to effective implementation of workplace improvements. In some jurisdictions public health did not have the necessary

---

137 McQueen, *Framework of flesh*, ch. 6. Senator A McEwen, *Commonwealth Parliamentary Debates Senate*, 13 February 2008.

138 M Quinlan, P Bohle, *Managing occupational health and safety in Australia. A multidisciplinary approach* (Melbourne, Sydney: Macmillan, 1991), 194–206.

authority; in others there were no effective implementation processes to persuade or enforce improvements; in yet other instances changes of personnel changed inspectorates' practices. There are no heroes in this history, but some public health practitioners stand out as crusaders, if ultimately failed ones: Dr Douglas Shiels and Dr Gordon Thomas in Victoria, and Dr Eric Saint and Dr Jim McNulty in Western Australia. All of them pushed as hard as they could to lessen the asbestos hazard for the workers they examined; all strained (and sometimes railed) against the circumstances of the time. That they continued to try is to their personal credit; that they failed was a product of the regime in which they operated.

Chapter 4

UNCOVERING THE STORY: ASBESTOS IN THE MEDIA

Chris Smyth

The danger of asbestos and the effects it has wrought in Australia are common knowledge today. It wasn't always so. The story of asbestos as we now know it—one of industrial disease, personal tragedy, and corporate malfeasance—was concealed for much of the 20th century. Key media stories in different countries, published decades apart, helped reveal the atrocious scandal. This chapter identifies the news stories and programs that lifted the lid on that scandal. There are similarities and common themes in how these came about. There are reasons why the details in these stories lay unrevealed for as long as they did. Among the common themes are first, the lengths to which the big asbestos firms and their affiliated entities kept information from their employees and the community, including their tactic of creating doubt in discussion about hazard and their use of public relations professionals to hone their message. Second there was the often complicated language of disease and the conundrum of establishing scientific certainty. And lastly, the revelations were often as the result of key protagonists without whose courageous persistence the story may never have seen the light of day. The story of uncovering the story also offers insights into the way journalists work and think, the news culture itself, and the pressures exerted by commercial and official interests in the news process. This chapter reviews the work of reporters and also draws on interviews with some of the participants as well as material from the Australian Asbestos Network project, which documented the story of asbestos in Australia.[1]

Early news reporting of asbestos: 1920s to 1950s

What would the average early–20th century reader of the press have known about the dangers of asbestos?

---

1   www.australianasbestosnetwork.org.au

Barry Castleman, who has chronicled the scientific and legal knowledge of asbestos, and given testimony on who knew what and when, notes a few early stories in the US press that mention the risk of disease. In 1932 the Chico (CA) *Enterprise* said asbestos caused "'serious if not fatal condition' in the lungs" and the *Chicago Tribune* in 1933 cites asbestos work as "among the 'most harmful trades'" in an article on dust hazards.²

A search of the online archive of the *New York Times* shows that the newspaper first mentions asbestos in relation to industrial disease in a 1935 two-page review of a book about American workers written by the leftist reporter and author John L Spivak. The reviewer Robert Luther Duffus relates Spivak's observations about the Blue Heaven neighbourhood of Charlotte, North Carolina:

> The Blue Heaven is inhabited by Negro workers in the asbestos mills. White men working in those mills, Mr. Spivak reports, may live as long as seven years. Negroes, more susceptible to tuberculosis, don't live so long.³

Later that year Spivak takes up a public spat through the pages of the *Philadelphia Record* with the president of the Southern Asbestos Company Mills in Charlotte over a report by Spivak about the company's worker compensation practices and its dominance of the town.⁴

Previous to 1935, the *New York Times* mentioned asbestos and disease only incidentally in news stories. In the 1800s asbestos is mentioned in trade notices and industry gossip. By the 1900s asbestos is reported in terms of its special qualities in the making of theatre curtains, subway cars, and protective suits. The first general-news story in the *New York Times* linking asbestos to disease appears in 1937 with a page 4 story about lung-function tests to determine compensation claims for silicosis, "a disease to which an estimated million industrial workers are potentially exposed". The story goes on to say:

> Dr. McCann, authority on pneumoconiosis, believes that state compensation laws should require objective tests to determine when actual disability begins in the diseases resulting from such mineral dusts as sand, granite and asbestos.⁵

---

2 B Castleman, *Asbestos: medical and legal aspects*, 5th Edition (New York: Aspen, 2005), 723.

3 R L Duffus, "The American worker today", *New York Times*, 28 July, Book Review, 1, 1935.

4 Castleman, *Asbestos: medical and legal aspects*, 723.

5 "Rochester pushes tests in silicosis", *New York Times*, 5 December 1937, 4.

Throughout the 1950s and into the 1960s the newspaper covered asbestos disease in 16 stories—typically in articles about medical research on cancers and about industrial safety. No asbestos stories are given prominent positions in the newspaper.

Readers of Australian newspapers, too, would have been made aware generally of the industrial hazard posed by asbestos, along with other dusts. For example, the *Newcastle Morning Herald and Miners' Advocate* covered the International Labour Organisation meeting in Sydney in March 1950 at which pneumoconiosis experts called for a scheme to classify X-rays of workers in dusty industries. Asbestos is mentioned as one of the dangerous materials. The report summarises the recommendations of the meeting, including the need for more research on how the size of particles affects health, on the efficacy of treatment using aluminium dust, on methods to suppress dust, and a recommendation that "a worker suffering from pneumoconiosis should be entitled to receive compensation, regardless of the time which has elapsed since he was exposed to dust".[5]

However, the asbestos media message was mixed. Within a month of that story running in Newcastle across the country on the west coast the Perth afternoon newspaper the *Daily News* reports, under the headline "Asbestos used to treat heart complaint", the following:

> Reports have reached the Australian Blue Asbestos management at Wittenoom Gorge of experiments being undertaken in the United States in the treatment of heart complaints with asbestos.
>
> The treatment was described to a conference of top heart surgeons by Dr. B. N. Carter, of the University of Cincinnati. It involves injecting powdered asbestos into afflicted parts of the heart and then encasing it with the same material.
>
> The operation is designed to increase the blood supply to the diseased heart by virtually glueing the patient's healthy lung to his heart by means of asbestos "painted" on to the surface of each. The paste is made by putting powdered asbestos in a salt solution.
>
> Dr. Carter told the conference that the function of the asbestos was to serve as an 'irritant' that would cause nature to form new tissues at the point of attachment and provide tiny blood channels between the lung and heart.[7]

---

6   "X-rays of dusted lungs: uniform plan for world", *Newcastle Morning Herald and Miners' Advocate*, 11 March 1950, 3.

7   "Asbestos used to treat heart complaints", *Daily News*, 3 June 1950, 4.

The leading paragraph betrays the source of the story.

Avid newspaper readers of that city would have read on the same day in their morning daily the *West Australian* a page 2 report on the Australian Medical Congress meeting in Brisbane, which warns that process workers should wear respirators and have periodic medical examinations for dust on the lung caused by "the more dangerous dusts", including asbestos.[8]

While these stories of the 1950s and 1960s reported the danger of asbestos, they were sparse and not prominent. The informed reader of the day would have concluded asbestos affected only workers in occupations that were dirty and dangerous, and in particular those workers with heavy or prolonged exposure. These stories also pointed out that industrial injuries and complaints were matters of concern for industry (if for nothing else than productivity), the medical profession, government regulators, and boards established for compensation. But it was not news that affected the community at large.

1960s: Mesothelioma in the news

In 1964 a key news story raises a new spectre—mesothelioma—and a broader threat. For the first time, in a *New York Times* story of October 7 entitled "A rare carcinoma believed on rise: Study of asbestos workers shows a high incidence", readers are introduced to the cancer mesothelioma, which was rare in the general populace but "far more common" among African asbestos miners and New York builders exposed to asbestos dust. The story, covering a report to the American Public Health Association annual meeting by New York asbestos researcher Dr Irving Selikoff, goes on to say:

> the specialists... expressed worry that the danger might not be entirely restricted to a limited occupational group, but that it might be more general and possibly of considerable importance. There is no direct evidence to substantiate this, they said, but some of the available findings hint that this may be the case.

It further warns that "even a single heavy exposure could conceivably produce cancer after a latent period of 20 years or more".[9]

---

8   "An unshapely nose no bar to beauty", *West Australian*, 3 June 1950, 2.
9   "A rare carcinoma believed on rise; study of asbestos workers shows a high incidence", *New York Times*, 7 October 1964, 24.

Mesothelioma had been linked to asbestos exposure both in miners and those living around asbestos mines in South Africa. This had been published in a landmark article in the *British Journal of Industrial Medicine* in 1960[10] (Wagner 1960), but it had not been publicised widely by the press. The *New York Times* article does mention this South African study as it cites Selikoff and his colleague Dr E Cuyler Hammond, who spoke "at a news conference before their talk". Certainly from this point in the American asbestos story Selikoff becomes the go-to expert on asbestos and disease. As we will see, he plays a significant—international—role in public awareness-raising of asbestos diseases from the mid-60s.

Among asbestos disease researchers, the conference in October 1964 of the New York Academy of Sciences on the topic of "Biological Effects of Asbestos" became a watershed, not just because it gathered leading researchers from around the world, but also because it became a clarion call for greater awareness and action over the asbestos hazard. However, it did not receive the press that in retrospect it deserved. Did the media miss the moment? According to Barry Castleman,

> One reason for limited coverage was the protests of the asbestos companies over the press releases Selikoff was planning to hand out, but evidently did not . . . (calling) attention to a cancer hazard to the public from asbestos air pollution. [11]

One publication, the *Science News Letter*, did report from the NYAS conference. Under the punchy heading "Asbestos Workers Live Longer But Get Cancer", the eight-paragraph article cites two researchers from Wales, one of them J C Wagner, who told the gathering that animals injected with any of the three types of asbestos developed mesotheliomas.[12]

Asbestos becomes a front page story

It was across the Atlantic in the following year that the next big story broke. London's *Sunday Times* of October 31, 1965 carried a front page story about a study in London that confirmed the wider public hazard of asbestos.

---

10   J C Wagner, C A Sleggs and P Marchand, "Diffuse pleural mesothelioma and asbestos exposure in the North-Western Cape Province", *British Journal of Industrial Medicine*, 17, 1960, 260–271.
11   B Castleman, email to the author, 20 January 2015.
12   "Asbestos workers live longer but get cancer", *Science News Letter*, 7 November 1964, 297.

A disquieting "new" occupational disease capable of killing not only the exposed workman but also perhaps his womenfolk and even people living near his place of work is the subject of intensive behind-the-scenes activity by British scientists, experts on industrial health and representatives of at least two Government Ministries.[13]

In the authoritative and revelatory voice of the Fleet Street weekly, medical correspondent Dr Alfred Byrne tells of the "remarkable report" by the two researchers who have "brought this whole matter to the surface" with their epidemiological work on the medical, working, and living circumstances of 76 patients who died of mesothelioma.

The reporter tells how the two scientists, Dr Muriel Newhouse and Mrs Hilda Thompson, pored over patients' case notes and asbestos company records, and interviewed family doctors and relatives. As well, the reader learns of experiments on rats in Wales and research from the US and South Africa. It concludes rather coolly—with a pun and a certain reserve about the hazard: "Asbestos is therefore very much in the air. Whether these particles could possibly cause other unwelcome changes in the lungs is one of the vital questions that remains to be answered by research". Unwelcome changes, indeed.

The *Sunday Times* is considered to have pioneered modern investigative journalism in the UK when it established its *Insight* team in 1963. The team went on to uncover the Philby spy ring and the thalidomide compensation scandal, the latter presenting issues not dissimilar to those that chilled media disclosure about asbestos for so long during the 20th century. The paper had a well-honed sense of smell when it came to injustice wrought by corporate and bureaucratic power. It is for this reason that the story about asbestos has impact and departs from previous coverage. The newspaper recognises the importance of the story and brings the paper's authority to the matter—this is the first front-page story about asbestos in a major newspaper. It is international in its scope. It goes beyond medical research to point out that industrial disease compensation does not extend to workers' spouses and dependants. And, tellingly, it angles the reader's perspective somewhat away from the factory and the laboratory and places the "workman" and his "womenfolk" (archaic as it is reads today) in the centre of the story. In doing this, the *Sunday Times* story presages later media reporting of asbestos diseases, which goes further to personalise the subject as the scale of the asbestos problem becomes greater and more broadly recognised.

---

13 A Byrne, "Scientists track down a killer disease", *Sunday Times*, 31 October 1965, 1.

Byrne continued to write stories about asbestos into the 1970s, including on regulatory recognition of diseases, new treatments, and legal cases. Indeed the *Sunday Times* upped the ante when it devoted a feature by a staff writer and an industrial lawyer in its April 2, 1972 magazine. The hook of the feature is a recent High Court compensation case and the problems of industrial inspection, but the focus of the piece is a London asbestos worker, Bob Smith, one of a group of plaintiffs. The paper quotes Smith whose fingers have swollen so he can't grip a cup of tea and gets "out of breath with the slightest exertion". The magazine uses a haunting picture of him, prematurely aged by the ravages of asbestosis.[14]

Brodeur and *The New Yorker*

While an asbestos story had made the front page in London, American journalists and editors had confined stories to the inside pages. Indeed it was not until 1971 that the subject appears in an editorial—a comment on a national health survey, under the heading "Health of Americans".[15] And it wasn't until September 1974 that the *New York Times* ran a front page story—on a study of 933 New Jersey asbestos plant workers and their families from the 1940s, some of whom were suffering from mesothelioma from "their peripheral and often brief exposure to this insidious mineral".[16]

However, the looming catastrophe of asbestos had been writ large in 1968 by a compelling piece of journalism in *The New Yorker* by Paul Brodeur. It was entitled, innocuously enough, "The Magic Mineral", but it blew open the issues confronting medicine, industry, the environment, and public policy.[17]

Originally a short-story writer for *The New Yorker*, Brodeur said the magazine's editor William Shawn had encouraged him to write about the environmental and health impacts of American industry. This field came to define his award-winning journalistic career. Through his many series of magazine stories and books on asbestos and other environmental hazards, Brodeur came to "discover that the manufacturing sector of the vaunted private enterprise system ...was squandering the lives of thousands upon

---

14   P Gillman and A Woolf, "The dangerous dust", *Sunday Times*, 2 April 1972, 91–100.
15   "Health of Americans", *The New York Times*, 16 July 1971, 30.
16   J E. Brody, "Cancer found in asbestos workers' kin", *New York Times*, 19 September 1974, 1.
17   P Brodeur, "The magic mineral", *New Yorker*, 12 October 1968, 117–165.

thousands of workers, and that the captains of industry who presided over it were the wholesale purveyors of a hideous legacy of disease, disability, and death."[18]

Central to Brodeur's 10,000–word *New Yorker* article, which appeared on October 12, is the clinical work and research of Irving Selikoff. Instead of relying solely on the doctor's famous one-liners, Brodeur also cites epidemiological statistics from the studies and he makes his own observations of the activities in the Mount Sinai School of Medicine research centre rooms and corridors.

Brodeur starts the piece at the beginning, as it were, with the history of asbestos from ancient times, when the mineral was first recognised for its fire-resistant properties, through to its modern day industrial applications. Assuming a level of sophistication in the reader, he ventures into the scientific phenomena and various medical conditions in the necessary, but esoteric, language of science and medicine. Still, he uses a journalist's eye to give dimension to the microscopic asbestos fibres: "... approximately a million individual fibrils lying side by side in a linear inch... [whereas]... six hundred and thirty human hairs can be aligned along the same distance."[19]

The article provides the most comprehensive history of the development of medical knowledge about asbestos disease that can be found in the press to that date. It is notably international in reach, picking out the major breakthroughs and writings from medical research in Britain, France, the US, and South Africa. Having cited Selikoff's expansive record of research, his latest findings, and his concerns about a "ripple" effect of indirect exposure in the community, Brodeur takes the liberty of musing about the everyday risks:

> There's no question in my mind that unsuspecting people are being exposed to small quantities of fibres from such sources as torn ironing-board covers and pot holders, and who knows how much asbestos is inhaled by hobbyists engaged in do-it-yourself projects around the house ...[20]

But the most poignant and powerful passage of his article is its final scene, which roots the piece in the city of its readers. Brodeur returns from the interview at the hospital by bus and on foot through the streets of

---

18 P Brodeur, *Secrets: a writer in the Cold War* (Boston: Faber and Faber, 1997), 143.
19 Brodeur, "The magic mineral", 117.
20 Brodeur, "The magic mineral", 161.

Manhattan noticing "for the first time" the builders and demolition workers in the streets spreading puffs of asbestos-laden plaster board dust and insulation spray across the sidewalks. He picks up some asbestos insulation that has fallen at his feet and crumbles the fibres in his fingers. Then, evoking the faintly falling snow all over Ireland in the final lines of James Joyce's "The Dead", Brodeur observes the asbestos insulation "blowing over the pavement like thistle down across a field" and away in the wind toward Central Park. "I was thinking about the children who play in Central Park, and about all the other children who live in this city and breathe its air."[21]

The article created interest and, later, action. In response to demand, the magazine reprinted the article in a booklet. It also published comments and letters about the piece. In 1972 asbestos fire-proofing spray on girders of high-rise buildings was banned. In announcing the law, the New York mayor at the time, John Lindsay, credited Brodeur's 1968 *New Yorker* article for raising the issue.[22]

The article also disturbed the forces of the asbestos industry. In his memoir, Paul Brodeur recalled personal pressure applied by PR operatives following the publication of "The Magic Mineral". On one occasion a staffer from the firm Hill and Knowlton, which had asbestos product manufacturer Johns Manville as a client, was snooping around colleagues of the *New Yorker* hoping to extract private dirt on the reporter. On another occasion in 1970 Brodeur was made an offer by an executive of Johns Manville to join their PR team for a salary of $45,000. "I looked straight ahead and pretended I hadn't heard him. The sum he mentioned was more than three times what I was making at the *New Yorker*."[23]

Books based on asbestos stories for the *New Yorker* over subsequent years garnered Brodeur a handful of national writing awards and international standing as a crusading environmental writer.[24]

1974: Australia discovers a killer in the home

The Australian post-war community had been a hive of residential construction, with the wonder building material asbestos being used in wall sheets, roofing, eaves, insulation, and fences across the country. While the

---

21   Brodeur, "The magic mineral", 165.
22   Brodeur, *Secrets: A writer in the Cold War*, 150.
23   Brodeur, *Secrets: A writer in the Cold War*, 149.
24   Paul Brodeur, Official website, http://www.paulbrodeur.net/. Accessed 13 October 2018.

mining industry and its workers were aware by then of some of the health hazards of asbestos exposure, others, like builders, were not; less so the general population.

In 1974 a cover story of the national public affairs weekly *The Bulletin* brought the matter home to Australian readers. Tim Hall, a British freelancer working in Sydney and a regular contributor to *The Bulletin*, wrote a feature under the heading "Is there a killer in your house?" The four-page feature gave national prominence to the wholesale threat:

> The children at Wittenoom, the souvenir shop keeper with her "shaggy" asbestos, the demolition contractor who ignores the dust and the handy man who saws up a sheet of asbestos are all taking an unnecessary risk.[25]

Hall tackles the issues broadly, from the recollections of state health and mines inspectors to workplace warnings from the International Labour Organizaton (ILO) in Geneva, to the latest medical research from as far away as Sweden, and the fears of chest specialists in major hospitals in different states. It marks a significant moment in the popular awareness of the asbestos hazard in Australia. And, as we shall see, it also has more personal significance for a couple of the key actors in the asbestos story.

Hall had been spurred to write a story after seeing an article on mesothelioma in *The Lancet*.[26] His editor Trevor Kennedy supported the assignment, which included paying expenses for travel to Western Australia. Kennedy hailed from WA and was familiar with the mining industry, having toured Wittenoom and the mineral-rich Pilbara region with the mining magnate (and first asbestos mine owner at Wittenoom) Lang Hancock. Kennedy saw in Hall "a crusader, who liked to get on a story that would get some results". He also felt the story fitted the new editorial temperament he was fostering for the magazine: "To break new ground. Get in front of the news, rather than simply follow". And in those hands-on days of editorial production, he lent his own practical support. In the absence of a suitable picture for the magazine's front page, Kennedy had a photograph taken of some busted up asbestos from his own home's verandah which was being demolished at the time.[27]

---

25   T Hall, "Is there a killer in your house?", *The Bulletin*, 6 Jul 1972, 33.
26   B Hills, *Blue murder: two thousand doomed to die—the shocking truth about Wittenoom's deadly dust* (Crow's Nest: Sun Books, 1989), 57.
27   Trevor Kennedy, interview with the author, 11 September 2015.

Hall's piece is critical of the Wittenoom mine operators, supported by evidence of advice from medical and mines department personnel that had been given to the company over the years. By 1974 these sources were prepared to go on the record. Director of Public Health Dr Jim McNulty called the Wittenoom mine the dirtiest mine he ever saw. He is described as a tireless critic of the mine, after diagnosing the first mesothelioma case as a chest physician at the Health Commission in 1960. He saw dozens more with various lung diseases. His frustration is conveyed in the article: "'Looking back now' he says 'I think I tried every legitimate means open to me. Perhaps I should have gone further and tried a few illegitimate ones.'"[28]

The article exhibits a number of elements present in the earlier Byrne (London) and Brodeur (New York) stories, and in stories by ABC radio reporter Matt Peacock that come later. These attributes include thorough research into the industrial situation that gave rise to asbestos diseases; an appraisal of up-to-date and international medical research; robust and erudite medical contacts who are prepared to speak up; and the editorial space and support to write a strong, exposé-style feature. Interestingly, the impact of the story went as far as Hancock himself. Kennedy recalls Hancock telling him that the mining mogul threw the copy of *The Bulletin* on his doctor's desk and demanded a chest examination.[29]

However, the revelations in Hall's story did not prompt follow-ups in the news media. Not even in those states with significant industrial activity, where asbestos was being mined or asbestos products manufactured. In his 1989 book *Blue murder*, newspaper journalist Ben Hills took aim at the institutions responsible for worker protection in the 1970s and also criticises the media of the day. "The Mines Department was useless, the Health Department powerless, and the union more concerned with money than the safety of its workers". He then asks: "So, as a last resort, where were the watchdogs of the media?" He notes in answer: "In the nine years to 1977... Western Australia's timid press carried just six stories about Wittenoom."[30]

This view of the Perth media of that time was echoed by Perth *Daily News* reporter George Williams, characterising the newspapers of the day as "generally well mannered, conservative and respectful of authority and government."[31] Originally from Perth, Williams had returned in the late

---

28 Hall, "Is there a killer in your house?", 32. For more on Jim McNulty see below, chapter 13.
29 Kennedy, interview with the author.
30 Hills, *Blue murder*, 56.
31 George Williams, email to the author, 30 October 2014.

1970s from seven years in Sydney where he had been assistant editor of *The Australian*, to report for the *Daily*. His new editor David Hummerston had greeted his return with the words "I want you to stick a finger up a lot of important noses in Perth," recalled Williams. The reporter began covering stories about former Wittenoom workers and their families seeking compensation for debilitating diseases, and investigating tip-offs about city offices whose ceilings of sprayed asbestos had started to deteriorate.

In an unusual move, the afternoon tabloid made space for a two-part feature for Williams. He leads his report with the effect on families and the way disease ravages its sufferers:

> A Perth woman and her two teenage children are waiting for her husband to die.
>
> The man, a non-smoker, has cancer.
>
> He worked for two years at the Wittenoom asbestos mine; 27 other former miners have died.
>
> The analysis of the cause of death is expected to become more detailed in future if more former Wittenoom workers are discovered with the disease.
>
> Doctors fear that a peak is coming with the disease showing itself in most workers up to 30 years after their exposure to asbestos.
>
> This latest man is dying quickly. He has pleural mesothelioma—cancer in the outer covering of his lungs.[32]

Exploiting good contacts with the unions and from inside government departments, Williams sought insights into the workplace and the family lives of workers.

> Asbestos was a very serious but potentially dull subject for a paper like the *Daily News*—a tabloid aiming at commuter readers in the afternoons and relying heavily on crime, courts and entertainment stories with a very quick buzz. Readers were not used to longer reports which required concentration on heavy, serious subjects. I decided early that it would be told best through people. I chased personal stories of people being affected by the sinister material.[33]

Following his editor's exhortation, Williams soon had noses out of joint. In the wake of revelations that the then Sir Charles Court government had had the state-owned R&I Bank building stripped of asbestos at night,

---

32   George Williams, "The deadly dust-cloud", *Daily News*, 14 September 1977, 8.
33   Williams, email to the author.

Williams' editor Hummerston told him that the senior management of the newspaper had been approached by an angry Sir Charles. The premier complained that Williams was "a muckraker from the eastern states, scaring people unnecessarily about asbestos".[34]

One of Williams' contemporaries, Catherine Martin, was medical reporter for the *Daily's* sister morning newspaper the *West Australian*. She soon made inquiries on her round. Martin was a fastidious reporter who cultivated her medical contacts in an era when doctors were suspicious of journalists. She took an interest in medical topics and devoted the time to get explanations from the medical practitioners who saw their work as important and wanted the public to understand it.[35]

She was told an epidemiological study had begun of Wittenoom mining families that showed an appalling rise in the incidence of asbestosis and cancers among people exposed to asbestos in the town some 30 years earlier. She followed up with a series of eight articles in 1978. This work won her the coveted national Walkley Award for best news story.[36]

Matt Peacock and the ABC

While Williams and Martin were reporting unfolding events in Perth, ABC radio reporter Matt Peacock was preparing programs about industrial safety. Peacock would go on to become the most acclaimed journalist in Australia at bringing the dangers of asbestos and corporate misdeeds to popular consciousness. He has maintained a vigilant interest in keeping asbestos in the public mind for 40 years. His exploits were dramatised in ABC's TV miniseries *Devil's Dust* (2012), in which a sneering James Hardie executive sledges the reporter for having built his journalistic career on asbestos. This is not fair. Peacock went on to report politics in Canberra and then Washington, New York, and London before returning to Sydney and a television career. Even then, he continued to bring stories about asbestos to light. Peacock's travails over those years, including his dealings with the asbestos industry's operatives, parallel in some ways those of Brodeur.

Peacock's first story mentioning asbestos was on the broader issue of occupational health, broadcast by ABC's Radio National science unit. After its airing, Peacock got a call from a PR firm working for the main

---

34 Williams, email to the author.
35 Margot Lang, former law reporter for the *West Australian* and colleague of Martin's, interview with the author, 26 November 2014.
36 J Hurst, *The Walkley Awards: Australia's best journalists in action* (Richmond, Vic: J. Kerr, 1988). 57.

manufacturer James Hardie seeking to use a section of the program. This rather unusual approach—PR firms were rarely this assiduous in their media monitoring, in Peacock's experience—served only to pique the reporter's interest. It set him on a path of investigations that included interviews with medical scientists, health officials, unions, lawyers, workers, company officials, disease sufferers, and their families.

Redolent of the private-investigator work of the PR agents in the US who stalked Brodeur, their counterparts in Australia were casing Peacock. Even before the next story had been written, James Hardie insiders were aware of his interviews with other sources, according to a company memo: "Mr Peacock of the ABC seems to have been most active in developing his proposed program on asbestos."[37]

The investigations did indeed lead to "his program"—the landmark four-part story in July 1977 "Work as a health hazard: asbestos" for ABC Radio National's *Broadband* program. The broadcasts elicited responses from sufferers, widows, workers, and others. These new leads opened more and more stories around the country for Peacock—in Melbourne, Baryulgil in country NSW, and Western Australia.

Given the relatively small audience enjoyed by Radio National, it was a bonus that the ABC's Double J youth channel played excerpts of the program to a bigger, younger community. Furthermore, an officer of a manufacturing union decided to copy the program onto cassettes and distribute them to workplaces—a 1970s version of today's online *liking*, though it involved hours of work with a tape recorder and then the good offices of Australia's postal system!

Peacock said he became obsessed by the subject and started to notice asbestos in buildings wherever he went. He was moved by the catastrophe facing an ignorant population and the efforts of the industry to maintain that state of ignorance. He embarked on what he called an "anti-PR campaign"—others might call it campaigning journalism. He said he never crossed the line to advocacy as a reporter. However, he was a co-founder of the Asbestos Diseases Society in Sydney, and attended meetings of fledgling ADS groups in Perth and Adelaide, though, it should be noted, at a time when he was "away from journalism".[38]

Despite his obsession and his relentless inquiries into every corner of the asbestos industry, Peacock did not himself see this as investigative reporting.

---

37   M Peacock, *Killer company: James Hardie exposed* (Sydney: ABC Books, 2009), 29.
38   Matt Peacock, interview with Gail Phillips for Australian Asbestos Network, 9 December 2009.

> It didn't take me long to find out the stuff, really, because it wasn't so much investigative journalism, it was a matter of finding out what people like Paul Brodeur... had been doing, getting his information and then trying to apply it to Australia. So it was very much a question of (overcoming) the concealment of the information from overseas.[39]

Peacock's journalistic contribution to public awareness in Australia of the dreadful plight of asbestos workers, the callousness of the industry, and the threat to public health is unparalleled. He chronicled his experience covering such stories, including his dealings with the firm James Hardie, in the 2009 book *Killer company* and he continued to report on asbestos issues until his retirement from the ABC in 2018.

Asbestos in Australia: A deadly secret for too long

By the late 1970s the story of asbestos risk was abroad in the Australian community. But the sorts of media stories Australians were seeing for the first time had been uncovered by the press in the UK and US in the previous decade; not to mention that the asbestos industry across the globe had known of the dangers for far longer. Peacock says the industry had simply been waiting and watching for the Australian media to finally cotton on.[40]

Why did the Australian media miss the story?

It can be explained in part by remoteness and provincial thinking. In this global age, it is hard to believe that an important story would not find its way either through the news media or just as likely through social media to other parts of the world. But that was the case. Daily newspapers in Australia's capital cities had provincial attitudes.[41] The asbestos industry and its conspiring spin machine were global, but Australian editors thought local. The national broadcaster, the ABC, was one of the few media organisations with genuine international reach and resources. Indeed it recorded and broadcast an interview with Irving Selikoff in 1977. But even the ABC had its blinkers. Peacock says:

> I'd do the story about the Baryulgil mine (in NSW), for example, and Victorians never heard about it. I'd do a story about the blue trains in Melbourne being lined with asbestos and the NSW people hadn't heard about it. Stories tended only to go in one state. Most people

---

39   Peacock, interview with Gail Phillips.
40   Peacock, *Killer company*, 26–32.
41   Williams, email to the author.

over on the east coast knew very little about Wittenoom. And the fact that we were doing a national program did make a difference and it did get the story around, and by then also I had a whole string of friendly journalists who'd also been following my work and were quite prepared to run with it themselves, so it just built up. But you've got to bear in mind, this was the avalanche that Hardie had been expecting for more than a decade. It was nothing particularly new, it was just that the information hadn't percolated through from overseas.[42]

The importance of mining in the Australian economy and its reach into the broader community cannot be under-estimated. Governments, like the one in Western Australia, were underwriting and promoting the development of their state's resources. While mining and manufacturing were known to be dangerous, the risks were thought to be limited to those working in the industry. Contacts within those industries were reluctant to blow the whistle. The unions were compromised or complicit.[43] Publishers and broadcasters were loath to risk their standing in the establishment by rocking the boat.[44] Asbestos executives had curried favour with media management and pursued advertising campaigns projecting James Hardie as patriotic and responsible.[45]

The vested interests in the asbestos industry—the keepers of the secret—acted to thwart public disclosure in manifold ways. To stack the odds against the possibility of damaging revelations, the asbestos industry managed its intelligence and its image very carefully. To ensure this, it engaged the services of public relations firms, and established medico-scientific industry bodies to do its bidding. The asbestos industry's strategy to keep its bad news away from its own workers and the public was developed very early on and adhered to scrupulously.

In 1935 US manufacturers Manville and Raybestos-Manhattan agreed to keep stories of disease out of the industry trade publications. And in the 1950s they "worked to suppress information that could have alerted the public to the crisis".[46] Those workers who had suffered the ill-effects of

---

42 Peacock, interview with Gail Phillips.
43 Hills, *Blue murder*, 55–6. Former ACTU president Greg Combet has a slightly different view: see below, chapter 18.
44 Williams, email to the author.
45 Peacock, *Killer company*, 148.
46 R L Heath, "Effects of internal rhetoric on management response to external issues: how corporate culture failed the asbestos industry", *Journal of Applied Communication Research*, 18, 2, 1990, 160.

asbestos and come to compensation settlements with their employers were invariably sworn to confidentiality. Such legal practices kept all sorts of maladies and dangers out of the public eye:

> If we were to rerun the film of the past fifty years, keeping everything constant but eliminating secrecy agreements respecting asbestos, Dalkon shield, Bridgestone/Firestone tire, and the like, earlier and more complete information about the dangers of these products would almost certainly have produced earlier recalls and withdrawals, thus reducing injuries and deaths.[47]

Once the media were eventually aware of the dangers of asbestos, the industry's PR strategy needed to change from secrecy to managing the message. One method was to seed scientific research or industry views that countered the medical reports and advocates' comments that linked asbestos to disease or hazard. In the 1980s, global firm Hill and Knowlton advised manufacturer and asbestos user US Gypsum to tackle the spread of damaging asbestos stories by making approaches at the local newspaper level and to offer Op-Ed pieces written by company-friendly experts. A Gypsum internal memo from 1985, revealed in court documents, is edifying:

> Attached is an excellent series run over four days, beginning March 3 in the *Detroit News*. Our consultant Jack Kinney, very actively fed much of this information to the special writer, Michael Bennett. SBA is exploring ways of more widely circulating these articles.[48]

Another element of the strategy was to put the language of industrial hygiene to the services of the manufacturers by using terms such as "acceptable" or "safe" levels of asbestos dust, or the "controlled use" of asbestos materials. Even as asbestos use declined in Western countries in the 1980s, Canada was marketing asbestos exports to developing countries under the marketing spiel that building products made from asbestos would be safe, provided they were subject to controlled use. This assumed the material would never be sanded, sawn, or drilled.[49]

---

47 D J Givelber and A Robbins, "Public health versus court-sponsored secrecy", *Law and Contemporary Problems*, 69, 3, 2006, 130–139, 135–6.

48 A Mundy, "Is the press any match for Powerhouse PR?", *Columbia Journalism Review*, 31, 3, 1992, 29.

49 M Huncharek, "Exporting asbestos: disease and policy in the developing world", *Journal of Public Health Policy*, 14, 1, 1993, 51–65.

Journalists have the duty to make sense of events and issues for their audience. In the field of scientific and medical reporting this means grappling with complex ideas and terminology, and interviewing experts who are in the business of qualifying their findings. Scientific and medical professionals are notoriously wary of the popular media for what they see not as distilling but as "dumbing down" issues and findings they report upon. The field of asbestos disease is a case in point. It is full of daunting terminology, from the names of minerals to the diseases:

> I spoke to a few medicos initially, and I got irritated at that point because not only did I have to learn how to pronounce "mesothelioma", which anybody coming to the subject has to, but these people would start talking about pneumoconiosis and they'd start using all these multi-syllabic words and it was clear they didn't want me to understand, they were just trying to intimidate me. And I started thinking, well, what would the workers who are being treated by these people be thinking? They're really just not being informed at all about what's going on.[50]

Just as journalists, editors, and their readers tend to seek clarity and certainty about the issues of public importance, so too do legislators and policy-makers. However, it runs counter to the cautiousness, qualification, and measured uncertainty that characterise scientific inquiry and debate. The "uncertainty" hand was played strongly by the asbestos companies and their hired professionals—scientific, legal, and promotional. For example, at the 1972 hearings of the Department of Labor in the US into the setting of appropriate dust levels in workplaces, asbestos industry representatives said there was too little scientific certainty about the causes of disease to warrant the kind of alarm being raised by other scientists. Such a requirement for scientific certainty was a ploy to impose an unnecessary standard from a different discipline (and purpose—namely, science) in an attempt to derail responsible policy-making based on "what reasonable people would believe on the basis of all available evidence."[51]

Another fairly effective strategy employed by the asbestos corporations, particularly in Canada, was the differentiation of the types of asbestos—crocidolite (blue), chrysotile (white), and amosite (brown). When it became accepted that the cancer mesothelioma had a direct link to exposure to the

---

50   Peacock, interview with Gail Phillips.
51   T H Murray, "Regulating asbestos: ethics, politics, and scientific values", *Science, Technology & Human Value*, 11, 3, 1986, 11.

asbestos mines of South Africa and Australia, the industry highlighted the point that those exposures were to blue asbestos, the type which constituted only a very small percentage of the international trade and use of asbestos. The industry adopted the "Chrysotile Defence", which portrayed soft and curly white asbestos as relatively safe compared with the needle-like crocidolite. This was not just a rhetorical ploy but was used in legal defences. The industry was successful also in fomenting scientific disagreement about the true danger of chrysotile.[52]

The PR assault was doomed to fail eventually, but the industry clung to it beyond what one might think was reasonable in the face of scientific evidence and general public awareness. In one analysis, Robert L Heath says the industry fell victim to its own rhetoric, which became embedded in the corporate culture and thereby coloured its ethical judgement and its relations with the workforce and others.[53] The industry held to the mantra that the product was so indispensable and beneficial to society that the hazards of production and other exposure were justified. So convinced were they of their beliefs and statements, the American corporations were stultified by them and unable to respond reasonably to mounting litigation, changes in liability law, and the ever-confirming scientific evidence of the hazard.

The reliance on spin, even after the hazard was known and production long ceased, was a critical element in the corporate manoeuvrings of James Hardie in the 2000s when it sought to separate its asbestos legacy from its ongoing operations. In 2001 PR firm Hawker Britton advised the company to avoid the (by then) hostile media by cultivating relations only with business journalists, keeping the message focused on financial implications, and communicating statements directly to government and other stakeholders, not through the media.[54]

The asbestos corporations and the strategies formulated by formidable legal, technical, and public relations advisers prevailed against poorly resourced and badly informed workers, their families, and those unions, journalists, and advocates who could see injustice, as well as misery, at the heart of the industry. The journalists who broke the story in various parts of the world, and those who followed in their footsteps, recognised their

---

52   J McCulloch and G Tweedale, *Defending the indefensible: the global asbestos industry and its fight for survival* (New York: Oxford University Press, 2008), 127.

53   R L Heath, "Effects of internal rhetoric on management response to external issues: how corporate culture failed the asbestos industry", *Journal of Applied Communication Research*, 18, 2, 1990, 153–67.

54   G Howell and R Miller, "Spinning out the asbestos agenda: how big business uses public relations in Australia", *Public Relations Review*, 32, 3, 2006, 261–66.

reliance on individuals who were brave enough to speak out; people like Dr Irving Selikoff, who warned passionately about the grave consequences of the continued use of asbestos. He was not only at the forefront of research in this field, but he was an effective orator, with a gregarious personality and a natural talent for publicity. He could speak in sound bites and was always available for the media. He wanted the dangers of asbestos made known to the world, beyond the secret confines of the industry and the esoteric medical forums. He was such a problem for the asbestos producers that he became a target of a campaign by them to silence him or, failing that, at least to smear him.[55]

No such Irving Selikoff-figure emerged from the medical profession in Australia, though a number of concerned practitioners and researchers were prepared to stand up and be quoted in their field of expertise. The sufferers needed a voice—a champion—to lift the lid on the industrial cruelty and warn Australians of the hazard residing in their homes and workplaces. That champion was Robert Vojakovic. A Croatian post-war immigrant, Vojakovic had worked for a short time at the Wittenoom mine in 1961. He became aware of the danger of asbestos in 1974 by reading the story by Timothy Hall in *The Bulletin*. Not normally a *Bulletin* reader, Vojakovic had bought the magazine because it had another story in that edition—about ASIO and Croatian terrorism. Vojakovic had recently been refused a government job in Canberra as a consequence (he was told confidentially) of his Croatian heritage and name. It was a few years after the article that Vojakovic got involved in advocating for the Wittenoom workers, some of whom he met in 1979 on a visit to the North Perth Migrant Centre, where they were meeting to discuss legal action for workers compensation. Vojakovic was dismayed at the poor legal advice and support the former workers were getting and decided to help out. He soon became the president of the fledgling Asbestos Diseases Society, which continues to support asbestos disease sufferers today with Vojakovic at the helm (see below, chapter 14). He had the courage and the self-proclaimed Croatian temperament to take on the insurance companies, the government, some quarters of the medical profession, and the industrial establishment. He was a fearsome negotiator and wily tactician and used the media as a tool in his fight for his members. He became familiar with the kinds of issues that piqued the interest of reporters and editors and was deft at contriving pictorial

---

55   McCulloch and Tweedale, *Defending the indefensible*, 84–96. See also Barry Castleman, interview with the author, 20 January 2015.

opportunities. He was as good as any newsroom chief-of-staff when it came to a story angle.[56] He always kept the media onside and provided reporters with people to interview and documents to support his claims. He understood the overbearing limitations that Australian libel laws placed on journalists, many of whom were threatened with or received defamation writs over such stories (none were successfully prosecuted).[57]

Conclusion

For too long the menace of asbestos had been carefully hidden from the public. The corporate resources and tactics of the holders of the secret—the asbestos industry—were substantial and global in nature. By using "hush" clauses in legal settlements with workers, by obfuscating and manipulating in scientific circles, and by applying spin in public discussion, the industry was able to keep its deadly secret for as long as it did. This endeavour was made easier because of the nature of the subject and the editorial diffidence and provincialism of the 20th century media in Australia. From our viewpoint in today's society, with its global, immediate news and social media networks, the idea of concealing an international scandal of this magnitude is hard to conceive. In this light, and given the internal and external forces arrayed against the truth, it is all the more important that the efforts of those pioneering reporters and their editors should be recognised.

---

56   N Aisbett, veteran journalist with the *West Australian*, interview with the author, 4 February 2016.

57   R Vojakovic, interview with the author, 3 February 2016.

Part 2
Asbestos Related Disease:
The Medical Journey

Chapter 5

MILESTONES IN THE KNOWLEDGE AND TREATMENT OF ASBESTOS RELATED DISEASES

A W (Bill) Musk

In his positions as a respiratory physician at Sir Charles Gairdner Hospital (1978-2017) and as Clinical Professor of Medicine and Population Health at the University of Western Australia (from 1992) Dr Musk has been a leader in Australian medical research on the asbestos related diseases. With training in clinical and occupational respiratory medicine, epidemiology and public health, and as an early anti-smoking activist, his research interests have been in clinical, epidemiological and preventive aspects of lung disease, particularly occupational and environmental lung diseases related to Wittenoom's blue asbestos workers and residents; Kalgoorlie goldminers; smoking; and in the Busselton population studies. In 1992 he was awarded Membership of the Order of Australia for services to medicine in the areas of asbestos related diseases and smoking control.

Introduction

The earliest mention of lung problems in people working with asbestos (weavers) in the medical literature seems to be in a *Handbuch der Hygiene* published by a Viennese physician Netolitsky in 1897.[1] The first patient with asbestosis for whom a record has been identified was a 33-year-old man who had worked in the carding room of an asbestos factory who was seen in 1899 by Dr Montague Murray at the Charing Cross Hospital in London.[2] The first pathological account of asbestosis was published in the

---

1   B I Castleman, *Asbestos: medical and legal aspects*, 4[th]ed. (New York: Aspen, 1996).
2   H M Murray, "Minutes of evidence, 21 December 1906", (*Report of the Departmental Committee on Compensation for Industrial Diseases*, London: HM Stationary Office, 1907), 127–28.

British Medical Journal in 1924.³ From that point knowledge of the health effects of exposure to asbestos has evolved with accelerating speed over the past century.

Research on asbestos related diseases in Australia more recently has tended to be led from Western Australia, followed by New South Wales because Australia's main asbestos mining ventures have been located there and these states have in addition seen significant residential usage of asbestos products. Western Australia's Wittenoom workers and township residents have sadly provided the basis for epidemiological and clinical studies of international scholarly significance because they have the dubious honour of being the only workers and residents in the world whose asbestos exposure has been exclusively to the blue variety of asbestos (crocidolite), and who can be effectively followed up for disease outcome with the establishment of well-identified cohorts which can be followed through mortality and morbidity records.

However, although medical knowledge of asbestos related diseases has evolved significantly, the problem has always been the slowness and ineffectiveness of dust controls in industry. In the 21st century, as the developed world has increasingly implemented restrictions to eliminate asbestos usage, the problem has moved to the developing world.

Asbestosis

Cases of severe pulmonary (lung) fibrosis in association with asbestos exposure and the pathological features of diffuse pulmonary fibrosis were first described in the early 1900s.⁴ An early scientific publication of an asbestos related disease was of asbestosis in a factory worker in England who made asbestos fabric, although Cooke stated that it had "long been suspected" that asbestos caused fibrosis. Over subsequent years an understanding of the subtleties of asbestosis as a disease entity and occupational health issue has emerged, but the initial clinical observations have been found to be correct and the general principles of prevention of asbestos related diseases have been confirmed repeatedly, although frequently ignored for commercial reasons at the expense of health.

---

3   W E Cooke, "Fibrosis of the lungs due to the inhalation of asbestos dust", *British Medical Journal*, 2, 3317, 1924, 147. D W Henderson, K B Shilkin, S le P Langlois, D Whitaker, eds, *Malignant mesothelioma*, (New York: Hemisphere Publishing Corp., 1992).

4   Cooke, "Fibrosis of the lungs due to the inhalation of asbestos dust", 140–2, 147. W E Cooke, "Pulmonary asbestosis", *British Medical Journal*, 2, December 1927, 1024–5.

The X-ray appearances and post-mortem changes of asbestosis were described accurately in the *British Medical Journal* by Cooke in 1924. In a subsequent publication in 1927 he described the clinical features, and differentiated asbestosis from other lung diseases resulting from a dusty environment at work and associated the disease with "badly ventilated" factories.[5] The characteristic pathological changes of asbestosis differentiating it from silicosis and the presence of "asbestos bodies" (and absence of silicotic nodules) in the lung tissues were described by McDonald in the same year as Cooke's article.[6] The relationship of asbestosis to tuberculosis (a disease that was common at the time) was also described (that tuberculosis was a "super-added infection"). The clinical aspects of asbestosis were described in the same year by Sir Thomas Oliver noting the frequency of breathlessness, lack of cough and sputum production, and the presence of "crepitations" on auscultation of the chest with a stethoscope (also the absence of tuberculosis bacteria in the patient's sputum).[7]

By 1930 it was recognised that lung impairment from the presence of asbestosis was related to the amount of asbestos to which a worker had been exposed, thus broadly describing the idea of a dose–response relationship that has subsequently been found to be a feature of the other asbestos related diseases as well.[8] Merewether also recognised the relatively different effects of chrysotile (a mineral of the serpentine variety) and of the amphibole varieties of asbestos (crocidolite or blue asbestos, amosite or brown asbestos, and anthophyllite). This issue has persisted to this day as most asbestos product manufacturers (as opposed to miners) have used whichever type of asbestos that has been cheapest at the time, so that identifying the relative pathogenicity of the different types and attributing disease to an exposure to one or other has often been difficult. Crude dust measurements were also made in the 1930s which showed that sack-filling by hand was the dustiest job in the textile factory and lower dust exposures could be achieved by wearing dust protection, wetting down, and exhaust ventilation or enclosing the working parts of the carding machines

---

5 Cooke, "Pulmonary asbestosis", 1024–5.

6 S McDonald, "Histology of pulmonary asbestosis", *British Medical Journal*, 2, 3491, 1927, 1025.

7 T Oliver, "Clinical aspects of pulmonary asbestosis", *British Medical Journal*, 2, 3491, 1927, 1026–7.

8 E R A Merewether, "The occurrence of pulmonary fibrosis and other pulmonary affections in asbestos workers", *Journal of Industrial Hygiene*, 12, 1930, 198–232, 239–257. E R A Merewether, C W Price, *Report on the effects of asbestos on the lungs and dust suppression in the asbestos industry* (London: HM Stationary Office, 1930), 1–34.

In 1930 it was already recognised that asbestosis progresses "inexorably" once it has started, underlining the need for prevention rather than simply removing a person from further exposure (a principle that was widely ignored by employers and regulatory authorities for very many years).

Although the condition of asbestosis was well recognised in 1942 when the Colonial Sugar Refining Company (CSR) took an option on the L G Hancock Asbestos Company's crocidolite plant and holdings in Wittenoom Gorge there was no acknowledgement in the Annual Report of the Western Australian Department of Mines for that year of the health risks that might result from expanding the operation.[9] The first asbestos related disease emerging from Wittenoom was indeed asbestosis.[10]

Dreesen first suggested in 1938 that an airborne asbestos dust concentration of less than 5 million particles per cubic foot (5mppcf) would protect against asbestosis but no legislation to regulate dustiness was introduced anywhere until 1945 when the "Dreesen Standard" was promulgated as an exposure standard in Victoria, Australia.[11]

Lung cancer

In 1933 Gloyne published a case of squamous cell lung cancer in a patient with asbestosis.[12] Between 1935 and 1955 further case reports and case series were published.[13] In 1938 there were also a number of papers from Germany and Austria reporting a link between asbestosis and lung cancer.[14] These were the first reports to suggest that asbestos may cause lung

---

9   Mines Dept of Western Australia, *Report of the Department of Mines for the year 1942* (Perth WA: Government Printer, 1944).

10 J Elder, "Asbestosis in Western Australia", *Medical Journal of Australia*, 2 (13) 1967, 579–83.

11 W C Dreesen, J M Dallavalle, T I Edwards, J W Miller, R R Sayers, "A study of asbestosis in the asbestos textile industry", *US Public Health Bulletin*, 241, 1938.

12 S R Gloyne, "The morbid anatomy and histology of asbestosis", *Tubercle*, 14, 11, 1933, 445, 493, 550.

13 D W Henderson and J Leigh, "The history of asbestos utilization and recognition of asbestos-induced diseases", in *Asbestos: risk assessment, epidemiology, and health effects*, R F Dodson, S P Hammar, eds, (CRC Press: Boca Raton, 2nd edn, 2011), 1–8.

14 K M Lynch and W A Smith, "Pulmonary asbestosis: III. Carcinoma of the lung in asbestos-silicosis", *American Journal of Cancer*, 24, 1935, 56–64. S R Gloyne, "Two cases of squamous carcinoma of the lung occurring in asbestosis", *Tubercle*, 17, 1935–6, 5–10. S R Gloyne, "A case of oat cell carcinoma of the lung occurring in asbestosis", *Tubercle*, 18, 1936–7, 100–1. D S Egbert and A J Geiger, "Pulmonary asbestosis and carcinoma: Report of a case with necropsy findings", *American Review of Tuberculosis*, 34, 1936, 143–50. M Nordmann, A Sorge, "Lungenkrebs durch Asbestsataub im Tierversuch", *Krebsforsch*, 51, 1941, 170.

cancer, and occurred well before the association of asbestos with lung cancer was more firmly established in a classic epidemiological study by Sir Richard Doll in 1955.[15] The association was seen to be between the presence of asbestosis (the disease) and lung cancer rather than between asbestos exposure (without the necessary presence of asbestosis) and lung cancer, a link that is important in endeavours to understand the mechanisms of cancer development that has been the focus of later studies in the Wittenoom cohorts, where measures of exposure have been available and it has been shown that the risk of lung cancer from asbestos exposure is related to the amount of asbestos inhaled and independent of the presence of asbestosis.[16] This is interpreted as indicating that one disease does not cause another but that asbestos causes both. This observation has also had important ramifications in medico-legal/compensation cases as defendants have been less able to claim that a cancer is not a result of asbestos exposure if no asbestosis has been identified. These epidemiological studies have also shown the inter-relationship of smoking and asbestos exposure in causing lung cancer; that is, that the two exposures multiply the risk of each other.[17] Later work has also shown that the amphiboles are more potent causes of lung cancer than chrysotile although the differential is less than for mesothelioma.[18] It has also been shown that the latent period between exposure and development of lung cancer in Wittenoom workers is several years, but is shorter than it is for mesothelioma.[19]

The causation of lung cancer by asbestos exposure has continued to be controversial for the same reasons that the causation of lung cancer by

---

15   R Doll, "Mortality from lung cancer in asbestos workers", *British Journal of Industrial Medicine*, 12, 2, 1955, 81–6.

16   N H de Klerk, A W Musk, B K Armstrong, M S Hobbs, "Smoking, exposure to crocidolite, and the incidence of lung cancer and asbestosis", *British Journal of Industrial Medicine*, 48, 1991, 412–7. N H de Klerk, A W Musk, J H Glancy, S C Pang, M S Hobbs, "Crocidolite, radiographic asbestosis and subsequent lung cancer", *Annals of Occupational Hygiene*, 41(supp) 1997, 134–6.

17   I J Selikoff, E C Hammond, J Churg, "Asbestos exposure, smoking and neoplasia", *Journal of the American Medical Assn*, 204, 1968, 106–12. G Berry, M L Newhouse, P Antonis, "Combined effect of asbestos and smoking on mortality from lung cancer and mesothelioma in factory workers", *British Journal of Industrial Medicine*, 42, 1985, 12–18.

18   J T Hodgson, A Darnton, "The quantitative risks of mesothelioma and lung cancer in relation to asbestos exposure", *Annals of Occupational Hygiene*, 44, 2000, 565–601. J T Hodgson, A Darnton, "Mesothelioma risk from chrysotile", *Occupational and Environmental Medicine*, 67, 2010, 432.

19   N H de Klerk, B K Armstrong, A W Musk, M S Hobbs, "Cancer mortality in relation to measures of occupational exposure to crocidolite at Wittenoom Gorge in Western Australia", *British Journal of Industrial Medicine*, 46, 8, 1989, 529–36

smoking has been: the defendants in compensation/litigation cases have a very real (financial) motive for denying that any link exists, or at least claiming that asbestos itself is not causative except when there is also asbestosis present in the lung tissue (as it was in the original reports when exposure could not be accurately measured). Because the fundamental mechanisms of carcinogenesis and fibrosis are not fully understood at a molecular level, it has not been possible to definitely attribute a given case of lung cancer to asbestos rather than tobacco smoke. The evidence to this time has been dependent on clinical and epidemiological observations (which the majority of scientists are willing to accept). This difficulty may have operated in favour of plaintiffs seeking compensation from the tobacco industry for lung cancer as the tobacco industry has managed to defend its behaviour more successfully than the asbestos industry. For individual cases of lung cancer it is agreed, based on epidemiological observations, that the risk from asbestos is doubled when there has been a cumulative exposure of 25 fibres per cubic centimetre per year (f/cc.yr), and a sufficient lag time.

Malignant mesothelioma

Malignant mesothelioma is a universally fatal disease that is almost exclusively related to asbestos exposure.[20] The occurrence of mesothelioma of the pleura in people exposed to blue asbestos (crocidolite) in the North-West Cape region of South Africa was first described by pathologist Dr Chris Wagner at a pneumoconiosis conference in Cape Town in 1959 and published in 1960.[21] There had previously been case reports in the medical literature dating back to 1943 but there was a great deal of scepticism about even the actual existence of the entity of mesothelioma because of the opinion and influence of an authoritative (Australian) pathologist of the time.[22] In the seminal article on lung cancer and asbestos exposure by Sir

---

20 A W Musk, N Olsen, H Alfonso, A Reid, R Mina, P Franklin, J Sleith, N Hammond, T Threlfall, K B Shilkin, N H de Klerk, "Predicting survival for malignant mesothelioma", *European Respiratory Journal*, 38, 2011, 1420–24. A W Musk, N Olsen, H Alfonso, S Peters, P Franklin, "Pattern of malignant mesothelioma incidence and occupational exposure to asbestos in Western Australia", *Medical Journal of Australia*, 203, 6, 2015, 251–2.

21 J C Wagner, C A Sleggs, P Marchand, "Diffuse pleural mesothelioma and asbestos exposure in the North Western Cape Province", *British Journal of Industrial Medicine*, 17, 1960, 260–71.

22 H W Wedler, *Deutsches Archiv für klinische Medizin*, 191, 1943, 189. H W Wedler, Deutsche Medizinische Wochenschrift, 69, 1943, 575. R A Willis, *The spread of tumours in the human body*, 1st edn 1934; 3rd edn (London: Churchill, 1984).

Richard Doll in 1955 one of the cases was "endothelioma of the pleura" which would now be called "malignant mesothelioma".[23] Since then Dr Wagner's observations have been born out repeatedly, especially in studies from Western Australia where crocidolite (blue asbestos) deposits also exist (at Wittenoom Gorge), and where it has been possible to identify and follow people who have been exposed because the employment records of the Australian Blue Asbestos Company have been preserved and subsequently made available for follow-up by researchers at the University of Western Australia.[24] The Wittenoom experience has been recognised and classified as a "Modern Industrial Disaster" internationally.[25] Dr Wagner's observations included mesothelioma in people whose asbestos exposure had been from contamination of the general environment as well as people who had been exposed occupationally. Thus the early observations were accurate and the absence of a safe level of asbestos has been confirmed repeatedly.

The first case of mesothelioma in Australia was in a Wittenoom worker and was published in the *Medical Journal of Australia* in 1962.[26] By this time Wagner had successfully induced mesothelioma experimentally in animals.[27] Irving Selikoff, an influential American from the Mount Sinai Hospital in New York, described mesothelioma in insulation workers exposed to another form of amphibole variety of asbestos—amosite (brown asbestos)—and pointed out that co-workers/bystanders could also contract the disease.[28] Thus most of the pertinent observations regarding asbestos and mesothelioma were available by the early 1960s: that mesothelioma exists, is a universally fatal cancer that results exclusively from asbestos exposure, that all types of asbestos can cause it, that it can occur from small doses of

---

23 R Doll, J Peto, *Effects on health of exposure to asbestos* (London: Health and Safety Commission, 1995).

24 B K Armstrong, N H de Klerk, A W Musk, M S Hobbs, "Mortality in miners and millers of crocidolite in Western Australia", *British Journal of Industrial Medicine*, 45, 1988, 5–13.

25 A W Musk, N H de Klerk, J L Eccles, M S Hobbs, B K Armstrong, L Layman, J C McNulty, "Wittenoom, Western Australia: a modern industrial disaster", *American Journal of Industrial Medicine*, 21, 5, 1992, 735–47.

26 J C McNulty, "Malignant pleural mesothelioma in an asbestos worker", *Medical Journal of Australia*, 49, 2, 1962, 953–4.

27 J C Wagner, "Experimental production of mesothelial tumours of the pleura by implantation of dusts in laboratory animals", *Nature*, 196, 1962, 180–1.

28 I J Selikoff, D H K Lee, *Asbestos and Disease* (New York: Academic Press; 1978). I J Selikoff, J Churg, E C Hammond, "The occurrence of asbestosis among insulation workers in the United States", *Annals of the New York Academy of Sciences*, 132, 1, 1965, 139–55. I J Selikoff, E C Hammond, "Asbestos-associated disease in United States shipyards", *CA: A Cancer Journal for Clinicians*, 28, 2, 1978, 87–99.

asbestos and takes many years to appear after exposure to asbestos has taken place, and that this "latent period" is not affected by the degree of exposure.[29] Subsequent research has repeatedly confirmed and refined these original observations.[30] Industry and governments throughout the world have been very slow to respond and have done so reluctantly. Occupational exposure standards have been slow to be introduced and even slower to be practised—and never enforced at Wittenoom as elsewhere—while dust measurements (particle counts) were poorly conducted in the industry and their results largely ignored, especially at Wittenoom. Only one adequate (by today's standards) survey of dustiness in the mine and mill at Wittenoom was ever carried out (methods for counting fibres were only just being invented by Gersh Major, an industrial hygienist at Sydney University) and took place only a few weeks before the mine closed down (for financial reasons) when it was too late to act on any findings. Whether particle counts or fibre counts were considered, the results showed gross levels of airborne dust in the mine, and this at a time when all dust suppression activities that had been considered possible/reasonable by the Australian Blue Asbestos company had been instituted.[31]

Epidemiological studies by Hansen *et al.* have shown that low levels of blue asbestos exposure such as were found in the general environment of Wittenoom are capable of causing mesothelioma.[32] Even when people with mesothelioma who do not appear after careful questioning to have been exposed to asbestos have their work histories scrutinised by expert industrial hygienists, they are almost invariably found to have evidence of likely exposure.[33]

---

29 de Klerk *et al.*, "Cancer mortality in relation to measures of occupational exposure to crocidolite at Wittenoom Gorge in Western Australia", 529–36. A Reid, G Berry, N K de Klerk, J Hansen, J Heyworth, G Ambrosini, L Fritschi, N Olsen, E Merler, A W Musk, "Age and sex differences in malignant mesothelioma mortality after residential exposure to blue asbestos (crocidolite)", *Chest*, 131, 2007, 376–82. A Reid, J Heyworth, N H de Klerk, A W Musk, "Cancer incidence among women and girls environmentally and occupationally exposed to blue asbestos at Wittenoom, Western Australia", *International Journal of Cancer*, 122, 2008, 2337–44.

30 G Berry, A Reid, P Aboagye-Sarfo, N H de Klerk, N Olsen, E Merler, P Franklin, A W Musk, "Malignant mesotheliomas in former miners and millers of crocidolite at Wittenoom (Western Australia) after more than 50 years follow-up", *British Journal of Cancer*, 106, 2012, 1016–20.

31 G Major, "Asbestos dust exposure", *Proceedings of the First Australian Pneumoconiosis Conference*, University of Sydney, 12–14 February 1968 (Sydney: Joint Coal Board, 1968), 467–74.

32 J Hansen, N H de Klerk, J L Eccles, A W Musk, M S Hobbs, "Malignant mesothelioma after environmental exposure to blue asbestos", *International Journal of Cancer Journal International du Cancer*, 54, 4, 1993, 578–81.

33 A W Musk, L Gordon, H Alfonso, A Reid, N Olsen, R Mina, P Franklin, S Peters, F Brims, J Hui, N H de Klerk, "Risk factors for malignant mesothelioma in people with no

Later work has refined knowledge on asbestos exposure and mesothelioma incidence: it has been shown that blue asbestos (crocidolite) is a much more potent cause than brown asbestos (amosite) which in turn is much more toxic than white asbestos (500;100;1).[34] Mesothelioma has become recognised as the symbol of past asbestos exposure (along with pleural plaques) and is particularly notable for its almost exclusive relationship to asbestos, although it has also been described in Turkey where it has been attributed to exposure to a similar highly durable non-asbestiform fibre that occurs in the Karain area, and also to another non-commercial amphibole in Montana (US), "Libby amphibole" which is found alongside deposits of vermiculite.[35] Its increasing occurrence rate many years after exposure has ceased and its uniformly fatal outcome is still observed despite advances in treatment modalities in the modern era.

The incidence of mesothelioma in Western Australia has been recorded carefully by the State's Health Department since the first case was identified by Dr James McNulty in 1962 by the setting up of a register of cases by Dr Janet Elder, a chest physician at the Sir Charles Gairdner Hospital where most cases were referred in the earlier days. Subsequently a dedicated expert committee comprising an occupational physician, a pathologist, and an epidemiologist was formed, and the state cancer registrar was set up when the Cancer Registry was established in 1981. In an attempt to identify all cases of mesothelioma that may have resulted from crocidolite exposure at Wittenoom, epidemiology researchers at UWA conducted an Australia-wide survey for cases prior to 1980.[36] Cancer became a mandatorily notifiable disease in 1980 so that the earlier statistics are as accurate and complete as they can possibly be and demonstrate the epidemic of mesothelioma that has been occurring in WA. While the number of cases has now ceased to increase, the sources of exposure have changed over the years: whereas in the first two decades of cases (1960–79) most resulted

---

known exposure to asbestos", *American Journal of Industrial Medicine*, 60, 5, 2017, 432–36.

34 Hodgson, Darnton, "The quantitative risks of mesothelioma and lung cancer in relation to asbestos exposure", 555–601. Hodgson, Darnton, "Mesothelioma risk from chrysotile", 432.

35 B Black, J Szeinuk, A C Whitehouse, S M Levin, C T Henschke, D F Yankelevitz, R M Flores, "Rapid progression of pleural disease due to exposure to Libby amphibole: 'not your grandfather's asbestos related disease'", *American Journal of Industrial Medicine*, 57, 2014, 1197–206.

36 A W Musk, P Dolan, B K Armstrong, J M Ford, N H de Klerk, M S Hobbs, "The incidence of malignant mesothelioma in Australia", *Medical Journal of Australia*, 150, 5, 1989, 242–6.

from work in the mining, milling, and transport of asbestos, during the 2000s the greatest proportion of cases resulted from exposure of builders and electricians doing maintenance work on old houses containing asbestos, boilermaker-welders, or do-it-yourself home handymen and women.[37] Epidemiological studies, especially those based on the Wittenoom people, have also shown that the incidence rate of mesothelioma does not continue to increase exponentially after about 40–50 years from first exposure.[38] This is thought to be a result of the death of more susceptible people and/or the clearance of fibres from the lungs, a process that takes place very slowly due to the indestructible properties of asbestos (from which it derived its name) and the fibrous shape of the particles.

Mesothelioma is universally fatal: half of patients die within 9–12 months.[39] The only treatment that has been shown to prolong survival at all is chemotherapy and then only by a few months. A massively large clinical trial was needed to show statistically that a combination of two modern chemotherapy drugs (cis-platinum and Pemetrexed) increased average survival by about three months.[40] Efforts at major surgery in relatively fit patients who have no evidence on detailed "staging" of extension beyond the pleura became increasingly invasive, with removal not only of the lung on the affected side but also the lining of the chest wall (the pleura), the

---

37 Berry et al., "Malignant mesotheliomas in former miners and millers of crocidolite at Wittenoom (WA) after more than 50 years follow-up", 1016–20. N J Olsen, P J Franklin, A Reid, N H de Klerk, T J Threlfall, K Shilkin, A W Musk, "Increasing incidence of malignant mesothelioma after exposure to asbestos during home maintenance and renovation", *Medical Journal of Australia*, 195, 2011, 271–4.

38 Z Xu, B K Armstrong, B Blundson, J M Rogers, A W Musk, K B Shilkin, "Trends in mortality from malignant mesothelioma of the pleura and production and use of asbestos in Australia", *Medical Journal of Australia*, 143(5) 1985, 185–87. A Reid, N H de Klerk, C Magnani, D Ferrante, G Berry, A W Musk, et al. "Mesothelioma risk after 40 years since first exposure to asbestos: a pooled analysis", *Thorax*, 69, 9, 2014, 843–50. A Reid, G Berry, N H de Klerk, J Hansen, J Heyworth, G Ambrosini, L Fritschi, N Olsen, E Merler, A W Musk, "Age and sex differences in malignant mesothelioma mortality after residential exposure to blue asbestos (crocidolite)", *Chest*, 131, 2007, 376–82. A Reid, J Heyworth, N H de Klerk, A W Musk, "Cancer incidence among women and girls environmentally and occupationally exposed to blue asbestos at Wittenoom, Western Australia", *International Journal of Cancer*, 122, 2008, 2337–44.

39 A W Musk, N H de Klerk, A Reid, G L Ambrosini, L Fritschi, N H Olsen, E Merler, M S Hobbs, G Berry, "Mortality in former miners and millers at Wittenoom", *British Journal of Industrial Medicine*, 65, 2008, 541–3.

40 N J Vogelzang, J J Rusthoven, J Symanowski, C Denham, E Kaukel, P Ruffie, et al. "Phase III study of pemetrexed in combination with cisplatin versus cisplatin alone in patients with malignant pleural mesothelioma", *Journal of Clinical Oncology: official journal of the American Society of Clinical Oncology*, 21, 14, 2003, 2636–44.

diaphragm and the pericardium (the wall of the sac that surrounds the heart), and the lymph nodes in the centre of the chest, followed (and sometimes also preceded) by chemotherapy and radiotherapy, with serious ill-effects from the treatments and no demonstrable survival improvement (and certainly no improvement in "quality of life").[41] Novel approaches to cancer treatment that focus on the genetic changes in cancer cells that have been successful in some cancers are being tried, as yet without success.

Pleural plaques

Hyaline and calcified pleural plaques were described as being a common finding at necropsy in cases of asbestosis in 1933.[42] They have been observed to occur on chest X-rays in people with exposure to asbestos and have been seen as an indicator of asbestos exposure for epidemiological studies for over 50 years.[43] They usually consist of smooth raised areas on the pleura of the chest wall rather than of the surface of the lung, although they are occasionally seen on the pleura between the different lobes of the lungs. They may appear within five to ten years of commencement of asbestos exposure, but are frequently overlooked on plain chest X-rays until they have calcium deposited in them to make them radio-opaque. Pleural plaques have also been associated with chest pain, especially in the people from Libby, Montana.[44]

As it has long been accepted that plaques are an index of exposure to asbestos it has raised concerns that they may become malignant; that is, develop into mesothelioma. While it is true that people with plaques are more likely to develop pleural mesothelioma than people without plaques, it has been shown in the Wittenoom studies that this association results from

---

41 J M Alvarez, T Ha, A W Musk, P Robins, M J Byrne, "Importance of mediastinoscopy, bilateral thoracoscopy and laparoscopy in correct staging of malignant mesothelioma before extrapleural pneumonectomy", *Journal of Thoracic and Cardiovascular Surgery*, 130, 2005, 905–16.

42 G Hillerdal, A Lindgren, "Pleural plaques: correlation of autopsy findings to radiographic findings and occupational history", *European Journal of Respiratory Diseases*, 61, 6, 1980, 315–319. S R Gloyne, in *Silicosis and asbestosis*, ed. A J Lanza (London: Oxford University Press, 1938).

43 D O'B Hourihane, L Lessof, P C Richardson, "Hyaline and calcified pleural plaques as an index of exposure to asbestos. A study of radiological and pathological features of 100 cases with a consideration of epidemiology", *British Medical Journal*, 1, 1069, 1966, 1069–74.

44 S Mukherjee, N H de Klerk, LJ Palmer, N J Olsen, S C Pang, A W Musk, "Chest pain in asbestos-exposed individuals with benign pleural and parenchymal disease", *American Journal of Respiratory and Critical Care Medicine*, 162, 5, 2000, 1807–11.

the dose of asbestos to which a person has been exposed and once this has been factored into the calculation there is no additional increase in the rate of pleural mesothelioma.[45] (Wittenoom's people have been ideal for this type of study because estimates of degree of exposure to asbestos have been made and validated by lung fibre content measurements.) Similarly lung cancer and asbestosis are more common in people with pleural plaques,[46] but this is also likely to be a result of greater exposure. It is difficult to envisage that a benign process that is taking place on the surface lining (pleural) cells of the chest wall could transform into a malignant process within the lung tissues or conducting airways.

Pleural plaques have been shown to have minimal effect on the function of the lungs and are not usually considered of themselves to be responsible for patients being disabled. They are frequently observed incidentally in people who have no relevant symptoms but undergo a plain X-ray or CT examination of the chest for unrelated reasons. When so found they can give rise to great anxiety in people who have been made aware of the long-term life-threatening effects of past asbestos exposure, especially asbestosis, lung cancer, and mesothelioma.

Diffuse pleural fibrosis

Diffuse pleural fibrosis/thickening has been a recognised effect of asbestos exposure for many years. "Old tough adhesions" were described at autopsy by Gloyne in 1933, but their significance was not appreciated and there was confusion with tuberculosis, a disease that was much more commonly seen at that time.[47] Diffuse pleural fibrosis is also especially common in people exposed to Libby amphibole.[48] It is a much less common effect of asbestos exposure than pleural plaques.[49] Pleural fibrosis may be on one

---

45 A Reid A, N de Klerk, G Ambrosini, N Olsen, S C Pang, "The additional risk of malignant mesothelioma in former workers and residents of Wittenoom with benign pleural disease or asbestosis", *Occupational and Environmental Health*, 62, 2005, 665–669.

46 F Brims, C Murray, N de Klerk, H Alfonso, D Manners, P Wong, N Olsen, A W Musk, "Ultra-low dose chest tomography screening of an asbestos-exposed population in Western Australia", *American Journal of Respiratory and Critical Care Medicine*, 191, 2015, 113–6.

47 Gloyne, "The morbid anatomy and histology of asbestosis".

48 Black *et al.*, "Rapid progression of pleural disease due to exposure to Libby amphibole", 1197–206

49 C P Murray, P M Wong, J Teh, N H de Klerk, T Rosenow, H Alfonso, A Reid, P Franklin, A W Musk, F J H Brims, "Ultra low dose CT screen-detected non-malignant incidental findings in the Western Australian Asbestos Review Program",

side of the chest (uni-lateral) or both sides (bi-lateral) and sequential. It is often preceded by benign asbestos pleural effusion although such effusion may not be observed before it spontaneously resolves. Its main effect is on causing "extra-pulmonary restriction"; that is, prevention of full expansion of the lungs. The restriction of expansion results in a decrease in the "vital capacity" with less effect on gas exchange in the lungs. This may result in breathlessness which may entitle the sufferer to compensation even if he/she doesn't have asbestosis in the underlying lung(s). Chest wall pain may be the predominating symptom (as seen in Libby, Montana).[50] On X-rays diffuse pleural fibrosis often mimics mesothelioma and care is needed to ensure which process is present: this may require repeated biopsies. CT and PET scans and MRIs are more definitive than plain chest X-rays as they can show malignant invasion of the chest wall (or diaphragm or other surrounding structures) which is a feature of mesothelioma as it advances.

Benign asbestos pleural effusion

"Asbestos pleurisy" was first described in 1964.[51] In 1971 American respiratory physicians Gaensler and Kaplan reviewed four thousand cases from their chest clinics and identified 57 cases with asbestos exposure, 14 of whom had pleural effusions with 12 of these determined to have benign asbestos pleural effusion.[52] This entity is now well accepted as an effect of asbestos exposure. It may occur on either side of the chest, but rarely on both sides at the same time.

Benign asbestos pleural effusion has no specific diagnostic features and is a diagnosis of exclusion of other causes of pleural effusion (for which specific diagnostic tests do exist) in people with a history of asbestos exposure. It must be distinguished from malignant effusions (mesothelioma or secondary malignancy), from effusions that occur as part of a "multisystem disease" such as rheumatoid arthritis, and from effusions associated with infections such as pneumonia or tuberculosis, by examination of the cells in the fluid and/or biopsy of the pleural tissue, and by culturing the fluid

---

Respirology, 21, 2016, 1419–24.
50   Black *et al.*, "Rapid progression of pleural disease due to exposure to Libby amphibole", 1197–206.
51   H B Eisenstadt, "Asbestos pleurisy", *Diseases of the Chest*, 46, 1964, 78–81.
52   E A Gaensler, A L Kaplan, "Asbestos pleural effusion", *Annals of Internal Medicine*, 74, 1971, 178–91.

for evidence of infection and testing its protein content and other special tests, as well as by observation of its natural history. The volume of fluid may be sufficiently large to displace enough lung to result in a reduced vital capacity and breathlessness requiring aspiration for relief.[53]

The onset of benign asbestos pleural effusion is usually earlier after first exposure to asbestos than mesothelioma.[54] Benign asbestos pleural effusion tends to resolve spontaneously although may need repeated aspirations or treatment with "pleurodesis" (with talc or other agent, or by operation) for control. It may be followed by the development of diffuse pleural fibrosis.

Rounded atelectasis

This almost unique asbestos-associated entity was first reported in the French literature in 1956 and in the German medical literature in 1971.[55] It has been called "infolding lung syndrome of Blesovsky" and consists of thickening (fibrosis) of the pleura of the lung surface with indrawing of the underlying lung tissue.[56] It is seen in people who have been exposed to asbestos, and has appearances that can be very similar to lung tumours or abscesses such that it may need to be biopsied in order to exclude the need for specific treatment.

Measurement of asbestos dust exposure

Gersh Major, a physicist/industrial hygienist who worked in the Occupational Health Unit of the School of Public Health and Tropical Medicine at the University of Sydney, described the intractable analytical difficulties of collecting and measuring airborne asbestos dust, particularly in relation to the Wittenoom crocidolite industry, at the First Australian Pneumoconiosis Conference in 1968.[57] At the time he was hopeful that

---

53   Mukherjee *et al.*, "Chest pain in asbestos-exposed individuals with benign pleural and parenchymal disease", 1807–11.

54   W O Cookson, N H de Klerk, A W Musk, J J Glancy, B K Armstrong, M S Hobbs, "Benign and malignant pleural effusions in former Wittenoom crocidolite millers and miners", *Australian and New Zealand Journal of Medicine*, 15, 1985, 731–37.

55   G Roche, J Parent, P Daumet, "Atelectasis parcellaires du lobe interieur et du lobe moyen au cours du pneumothorax therapeutique", *Revue De Tuberculose Et De Pneumologie* (Paris) 29, 1956, 87–93. R Hanke, ["Round atelectasis (spherical and cylindrical atelectasis). Contribution to the differential diagnosis of intrapulmonal round foci"], *Fortschritte auf dem Gebiete der Röntgenstrahlen und der Nuklearmedizin*, 114, 2, 1971, 164–83.

56   A Blesovsky, "The folded lung", *British Journal of Diseases of the Chest*, 60, 1966, 19–22.

57   Major, "Asbestos Dust Exposure".

these problems could be resolved "in the near future". The measurements that he had made in Wittenoom in 1966 almost immediately prior to the closure of the industry were the only "fibre" (as opposed to "particle") measurements ever conducted there and his methods have survived the test of time and have been used elsewhere ever since. Nevertheless his reservations have been highlighted (unsuccessfully) by litigation defendants in damages claims against the Australian Blue Asbestos Company and its parent company CSR who have described them as being inaccurate by "orders of magnitude". These same measurements however have been validated repeatedly by demonstrating that they are associated with risk of various asbestos related diseases and have proven vital for understanding dose-response relationships for crocidolite in numerous epidemiological studies ever since.[58]

Exposure standards and disease

In the United Kingdom official action to control exposure to asbestos was initiated in 1930, based on a 1928–29 study of Mereweather and Price (1930) which showed that asbestosis was indeed an industrial disease and concluded that there was no substitute for dust control at source. The UK Asbestos Regulations (1931) were introduced along with a scheme of compensation of workers developing asbestosis.

The first recommendations for control of asbestos exposure in the United States were made in 1938 following a study of 541 employees in four asbestos textile plants.[59] It was recommended that an air concentration of 5 million particles (not fibres) per cubic foot (mppcf), as measured by the midget impinger technique and counted by light microscopy, be established. In 1946 the American Conference of Government Industrial Hygienists adopted 5mppcf as a threshold limit value (TLV). This level was adopted by the Health Department in New South Wales in 1938, and in Victoria in 1945.

In 1956 the asbestos industry in Western Australia was declared to be a "dangerous trade" (under the Health Act). Thus in Western Australia knowledge of the harmful effects of asbestos existed in the responsible instrumentalities during the time that the Wittenoom industry was operating. However the National Health and Medical Research Council in Australia

---

58 N H de Klerk, A W Musk, V Williams, P R Filion, D Whitaker, K B Shilkin, "Comparison of measures of exposure to asbestos in former crocidolite workers from Wittenoom Gorge, W. Australia", *American Journal of Industrial Medicine*, 30, 5, 1996, 579–87.

59 Dreesen *et al.*, "A study of asbestosis in the asbestos textile industry".

did not make a recommendation on asbestos exposure limits until 1964. It suggested a limit of 5mppcf, which approximately equates to 30 fibres per millilitre (f/ml) and applied it to all types of asbestos. It was reduced to 4mppcf (12 f/ml) in 1969 (after Wittenoom had closed down) and then 4 f/ml in 1973. In 1974 it was further reduced to 2 f/ml for chrysotile and 0.1 f/ml for crocidolite. Western Australia was even slower to act and did so in the Factories and Shops Act of 1978. Responsibility for health and safety in the WA mining industry was the statutory responsibility of the Mines Department which resisted interference from the Health Department. Thus no legislative restrictions were ever imposed on the industry at Wittenoom. Dust measurements using a konimeter (which counts any particles, be they fibres or not) were conducted but there was no dust control that could be enforced. The literature at the time discussed only asbestosis as a disease which occurred only after lengthy exposure, and lung cancer as occurring only in people with asbestosis. Although high particle counts were recorded no action was taken.

The *Western Australia Mines Regulation Act, 1946–1974 and Regulations* stipulated that

> where rock containing asbestos or fibrous talc is mined the long term average fibre concentration shall not exceed four fibres per cubic centimetre of air as measured by the membrane filter method of the British Occupational Hygiene Society or by any other method acceptable to the Ventilation Board.

This was amended in the *Mines Regulations Amendment 1984 Regulations* to indicate that

> where rock containing asbestos or fibrous talc is mined the air in the working place shall not contain more than - (i) 0.1 fibre of crocidolite; or (ii) 1.0 fibre of chrysotile, amosite or fibrous talc, per millilitre of air as calculated from measurements made by the National Health and Medical Research Council Membrane Filter Method for estimating air-borne asbestos dust over a sampling period of not less than 4 hours, or by some other method approved by the Ventilation Board.

By this time Wittenoom crocidolite production had well and truly ceased and no other crocidolite mine was operating in the State.[60]

60　*Western Australia Mines Regulation Act 1946–1974* and *Regulations*, amended 1984, 42.

Treatment

With the exception of lung cancer for which the treatment principles are the same as for lung cancers of any cause (usually smoking but also other exposures such as silica or radiation), the treatments of asbestos related diseases are mainly palliation (that is, relief of symptoms and complications). Pain relief for patients with mesothelioma is paramount and opiates are almost universally used, the problem of addiction being unimportant as life expectancy is so limited. Chronic pain presents a problem when it is due to benign processes such as diffuse pleural thickening (especially a problem with Libby amphibole exposure) and other measures for control are required; for instance, nerve blocks and non-steroidal anti-inflammatory analgesics. Thus palliative care is important and has been improved over the years to the extent that this discipline is now a specialty in its own right.

Surgery for some lung cancers has improved, especially in the area of selection of suitable candidates who may tolerate/survive resection of lung tissue by the use of more accurate staging of the extent of disease and the use of video-assisted procedures which allow removal of lobes or whole lungs with small incisions.

Chemotherapy has advanced and expanded for the treatment of all cancers in recent decades, especially for small cell lung cancer. Chemotherapy has never been useful for mesothelioma until relatively recently when new chemotherapy drugs have been introduced and shown on average to improve survival by an average of three months.[61] There is now a great deal of interest in "biologicals" for the treatment of mesothelioma. These agents utilise the rapidly expanding knowledge of the cancer process which involves DNA mutations/alterations at a molecular level.

Advanced asbestosis results in the need for oxygen replacement, and ambulatory devices are now available to help patients remain active/mobile and maintain an optimal quality of life. This is often associated with the need to treat "heart failure" which results from the added strain on the (right) heart ("cor pulmonale") resulting from the presence of severe lung disease. Medications for this disease process have improved markedly over the period that asbestos related diseases have been extant and survival has been improved, although never usually measured in such a way as to know what any particular medication the improvement is attributable to.

---

61   Vogelzang *et al*. "Phase III study of pemetrexed in combination with cisplatin versus cisplatin alone in patients with malignant pleural mesothelioma".

Conclusion

Medical knowledge of asbestos related diseases has been accumulating since the late 19th century. The risks of exposure to asbestos have been slow to be acknowledged by the medical profession, as evidenced by the absence of any consideration of asbestos related diseases by Associate Professor Bryan Gandevia in the Annual Postgraduate Oration delivered on 26 May 1971 in the Great Hall of the University of Sydney to commemorate those who have advanced the art and science of medicine in New South Wales where asbestos exposure was known to be an occupational health issue.[62] However the emergence and recognition of these risks has ultimately resulted in a complete ban on the importation and use of asbestos of any variety in Australia, but not in many other countries where economic factors are seen as being more important than health considerations.

To a large extent the asbestos industry in Western Australia has resulted in there being a better understanding of asbestos dose-response relationships for the different mineral types.

The final milestone will be the extinction of asbestos related diseases in the community which will occur at a point when all asbestos has been removed from the environment so that it can no longer be inhaled and the latent period between exposure and disease has passed for those who have already been exposed.

---

62   B Gandevia, "Occupation and disease in Australia since 1788", Annual postgraduate oration. *Bulletin of the Postgraduate Committee in Medicine*, University of Sydney, 27, 1971, 157–97, 199–228.

Chapter 6

ASBESTOS AND MESOTHELIOMA —FIFTY YEARS ON

Geoffrey Berry

Geoffrey Berry has worked as a biostatistician in medical research for almost a half century; first from 1966 to 1982 at the British Medical Research Council's Pneumoconiosis Unit in Penarth, Wales; then from 1982 to 2001 at the University of Sydney; and since his retirement he has remained active in research on the health effects of asbestos exposure, including working with the University of Western Australia's research group on the Wittenoom workers and residents. A major part of his work has been in the area of health hazards associated with asbestos, including collaborative research on the epidemiological studies of the Cape and Ferodo factories in the UK set up by Dr Molly Newhouse; the Nottingham women gas mask workers initiated by Dr Stephen Jones; the Wittenoom cohorts of former workers at the mine and mill and residents of the town; and projections of future mesothelioma numbers in Australia. In this chapter Emeritus Professor Berry tells of the researchers with whom he has worked as well as others, and their contributions to a growing understanding of the lethal asbestos disease, mesothelioma.

In February 1959 a Pneumoconiosis Conference was held in Johannesburg. The major theme was on silicosis, but two presentations that formed a minor part of the conference have proved to be the first presentation of a ground-breaking discovery that led to much research work worldwide, and to changes on the use of asbestos in many countries.[1] From their titles the papers' main emphasis appears to be asbestosis, but it was the observations

---

1   J C Wagner, "Some pathological aspects of asbestosis in the Union of South Africa", in *Proceedings Pneumoconiosis Conference, Johannesburg, 1959*, ed. A J Orenstein (London: J & A Churchill Ltd, 1959), 373–82. C A Sleggs, "Clinical aspects of asbestosis in the Northern Cape", in *Proceedings Pneumoconiosis Conference, Johannesburg, 1959*, ed. AJ Orenstein (London, J & A Churchill Ltd, 1959), 383–90.

on mesothelioma that were to have such far-reaching and long-lasting effects. In these papers Wagner and Sleggs described for the first time the occurrence of pleural mesotheliomas in the Northwest Cape crocidolite mining area in South Africa, and that some of these cases arose from environmental exposure to crocidolite asbestos.

Dr Sleggs described the Northern Cape asbestos hills situated 100 miles west of Kimberley where Cape Blue asbestos had been mined for several decades. At Prieska there was a crushing plant and dump since 1930, and at Kuruman there were cobbing activities during the 1920s and a mill from 1926 to 1930. There were 20 confirmed cases of pleural mesothelioma and fourteen of these were associated with the Kuruman district. They suggested that exposure to asbestos was the cause of the mesotheliomas, although they were cautious in this claim, both Wagner and Sleggs saying the association "has not been proved".

> We believe, though we readily admit that the contention has not been proved, that in some way inhaled asbestos is the cause of the mesotheliomas which we see in the Northern Cape.

A year later Wagner, Sleggs, and Marchand extended the results in a classic paper, generally regarded as the key paper on the discovery of the link between exposure to crocidolite asbestos and mesothelioma.[2] There had been earlier papers but they had little impact at the time they were published. This paper became a Citation Classic in 1979 and is probably the most cited paper in occupational medicine with well over a 1000 citations.[3]

The researchers summarised the history of mining in the Asbestos Hills to the west of Kimberley. The mining of crocidolite, known as Cape Blue Asbestos, started at Prieska in 1893 and moved northwards reaching Kuruman by 1908, and continuing further northward to near the border with Bechuanaland by 1950. Initially quarrying was in open cast workings, followed by shallow mining and shafting after 1930. Men quarried the rock in the open cast workings, and women and children were then involved in sorting the rock and cobbing it by hand, which involved striking the rock with a hammer to separate out the asbestos fibre. After the 1939–45 war with an increasing demand for crocidolite

---

2   J C Wagner, C A Sleggs, P Marchand, "Diffuse pleural mesothelioma and asbestos exposure in the North Western Cape Province", *British Journal of Industrial Medicine*, 17, 1960, 260–71.

3   This Week's Citation Classic CC/Number 32, 6 August 1979.

the mining and milling operations became more mechanised with deeper mining and the establishment of more mills reducing the need for hand cobbing.

There were 33 confirmed cases of diffuse pleural mesothelioma. Thirty-two of these—that is, all except one—had probably been exposed to Cape Blue crocidolite asbestos. For 28 cases the exposure was in the Asbestos Hills west of Kimberley, and for four cases exposure was in industry. For those whose exposure was in the Asbestos Hills about half had occupational exposure either as a miner or in transporting asbestos, but for the other half the exposure was environmental through living in a mining area, and in four cases playing on the dumps as a child. In an Addendum to the paper it was reported that, by June 1960, 47 cases of mesothelioma had been identified, including one of the peritoneum, and a possible association with crocidolite asbestos established for 45 of the 47 cases.

The whole process had been started by what Dr Chris Wagner almost three decades years later described as a "lucky break", when in February 1956 he carried out a necroscopy examination of a 'Bantu" man who had worked as a shower attendant at a Witwatersrand gold mine.[4] He was thought to have died of tuberculosis pleurisy but at post-mortem Dr Wagner was amazed to find a huge gelatinous tumour.[5] This case was described by Martiny in 1956.[6] Perhaps it was a lucky break, but the conversion of this piece of luck into a major discovery involved much detailed work by himself and Drs Sleggs and Marchand.

It may now seem surprising but at the time a diagnosis of mesothelioma was not recognised by some of the leading pathologists of the day. Indeed, because of this, Dr Wagner had difficulty in finding a journal willing to publish the paper. So an important contribution was to obtain recognition of "mesothelioma" as a distinct pathological entity, as well as, of course, the discovery of the link with blue or crocidolite asbestos.

As noted by Wagner in 1991 and McDonald and McDonald in 1996 there had been earlier reports on mesothelioma associated with asbestos exposure, but they had little impact at the time, possibly because of the

---

4   J C Wagner, "Mesothelioma and mineral fibers (Charles S. Mott Prize)', *Cancer*, 57, 1986, 1905–11.

5   J C Wagner, "The discovery of the association between blue asbestos and mesothelioma and the aftermath", *British Journal of Industrial Medicine*, 48, 1991, 399–403.

6   O Martiny, "Report on a case of mesothelioma", *Proceedings of the Transvaal Mines Medical Officers Assn*, 35, 1956, 355–63.

small number of cases.[7] The first such report was by Gloyne on two cases in Britain in 1935.[8] This was followed by two cases in Germany reported by Wedler in 1943,[9] two cases in Canada reported by Cartier in 1952,[10] a case in a naval dockyard worker by Weiss in 1953,[11] a peritoneal mesothelioma reported by Leicher in 1954,[12] and three cases in Holland reported by Van der Schoot in 1958.[13]

A few years before the link between crocidolite asbestos and mesothelioma was established the link between asbestos exposure and bronchial cancer was confirmed. As for mesothelioma there were early reports that did not attract much attention at the time.[14] Nordmann knew of about eight cases with an average latency of 18 years and suggested that asbestos related lung cancer should be recognised as an occupational disease.[15] E R A Merewether in his position as the Chief Inspector of Factories in Britain reported in 1947 that on death certificates for men on which asbestosis was mentioned the cause of death was recorded as bronchial cancer in 13 per cent of cases compared with 1 per cent in cases of silicosis.[16] Then in 1955

---

7   J C Wagner, "How the relationship between mesothelioma and asbestosis was first discovered", in *Asbestos-related cancer*, ed. M Sluyser (New York, Ellis Horwood, 1991), 9–12. J C McDonald, A D McDonald, "The epidemiology of mesothelioma in historical context", *European Respiratory Journal*, 9, 1996, 1932–42.

8   S R Gloyne, "Two cases of squamous carcinoma of the lung occurring in asbestosis", *Tubercle*, 17, 1935, 5–10.

9   H W Wedler, "Über den Lungenkrebs bei Asbestose", *Deutsches Archiv für klinische Medizin*, 191, 1943, 189–209. H W Wedler, *Deutsche Medizinische Wochenschrift*, 69, 1943, 573.

10   P Cartier, "Abstract of discussion", *Archives of Industrial Hygiene and Occupational Medicine*, 5, 1952, 262.

11   A Weiss, "Pleurakrebs bei Lungenasbestose in vivo morphologisch gesichert", *Medizinische*, 1, 1953, 93–94.

12   F Leicher, "Primärer Deckzelltumor des Bauchfells bei Asbestose", *Arch Gewerbepath Gewerbehyg*, 13, 1954, 382–93.

13   H C M Van der Schoot, "Asbestosis and pleural tumours", *Ned T Geneesk*, 102, 1958, 1125–26.

14   Aa Wolff, "Asbestos pulmonum", *Nord Hyg Tidsskr*, 21, 1940, 1–48. S R Gloyne, "The asbestosis body", *Lancet*, 219, 1932, 1351–6. K M Lynch, W A Smith, "Pulmonary asbestosis III: carcinoma of lung in asbesto-silicosis", *American Journal of Cancer*, 24, 1935, 56–64. W B Wood, S R Gloyne, "Pulmonary asbestosis, a review of one hundred cases", *Lancet*, 224, 1934, 1383–85. D S Egbert, A J Geiger, "Pulmonary asbestosis and carcinoma", *American Review of Tuberculosis*, 34, 1936, 143–50.

15   M Nordmann, "The occupational cancer of asbestos workers", *Zeitschr Krebsforsch*, 47, 1938, 288–302.

16   Ministry of Labour and National Service, *Annual Report of the Chief Inspector of Factories for the year 1947* (Cmd. 7621) HMSO, London, 1949.

Doll published results from a study of workers at an asbestos textile factory at Rochdale in the north of England.[17] He reported on the mortality experience of a group of 113 men who had worked for at least 20 years in areas scheduled by the Asbestos Industry Regulations of 1931 as being dusty. Out of 39 deaths there were 11 due to lung cancer compared with an expected number of 0.8. The asbestos used at this factory was mainly chrysotile but a smaller amount of crocidolite was used. This finding confirmed the link between asbestos exposure and lung cancer.

Mesotheliomas had only been found associated with Cape blue crocidolite asbestos. Two other commercial asbestos types, amosite and chrysotile, were also mined in South Africa. A natural question was—does exposure to these two types also cause mesothelioma? Dr Wagner was always interested in the differences between fibres types. His father, Dr Percy Albert Wagner, was a distinguished geologist and so he was well aware of the geological differences between asbestos types. His knowledge that the serpentine asbestos, chrysotile, was quite distinct geologically from the amphibole types (crocidolite, amosite, tremolite) led him to compare the health effects. He was critical of the tendency of some to ignore the structural differences and assume all types of asbestos as equal in effect. Although the name "asbestos" is in common usage there are differences between the types—differences of chemistry, of aerodynamics in industrial use, and in solubility or biopersistence. Dr Chris Wagner therefore saw no *a priori* reason that their health effects would necessarily be similar.

Mesotheliomas had been observed mainly in the mining areas. So another natural question arose—what is the situation in industries using asbestos? Much of the asbestos mined in South Africa was at that time exported to the United Kingdom for industrial use. Wagner later wrote that "by 1962 it became obvious that these investigations should be continued in the United Kingdom".[18] And so in 1962 Wagner moved to the Medical Research Council's Pneumoconiosis Research Unit in Penarth in South Wales, at the invitation of Dr J C Gilson, the Director of the Unit, and a new area of research began.

I have been privileged to work with these researchers at the Pneumoconiosis Research Unit and others and will concentrate mainly on the contributions

---

17   R Doll, "Mortality from lung cancer in asbestos workers", *British Journal of Industrial Medicine*, 12, 1955, 81–86.

18   Wagner, "The discovery of the association between blue asbestos and mesothelioma and the aftermath", 399–403.

of those I knew, given that a full review would be well beyond the space available, but fuller details are available elsewhere.[19] My introduction to research on the health effects of asbestos was about 50 years ago when I took up an appointment in 1966 at the Pneumoconiosis Research Unit in Penarth, South Wales.

The Director Dr John Gilson and Dr Chris Wagner were giants in the asbestos area. Dr John Gilson had recognised the importance of the health effects due to asbestos exposure and steered the Unit into research to investigate this problem, and an important step in this was his active recruitment of Dr Chris Wagner. Dr Gilson did a lot of work developing objective ways of reading chest radiographs and developing the international UICC classification system. He also had astute insights into epidemiology and the "big picture".

John Gilson and Chris Wagner were very active in encouraging and facilitating research by other groups, and mesotheliomas associated with asbestos exposure were soon identified. It became apparent however that the type of asbestos responsible was difficult to assess because many of those working with asbestos had exposure to more than one of the three main commercial types (amosite, chrysotile, and crocidolite).[20] Dr Gilson was one of the first to suggest, as early as 1965 in the Wyers Memorial Lecture, that, of the three major commercial types of asbestos, crocidolite resulted in the highest rate of mesothelioma, with amosite next, and chrysotile resulting in a much lower risk.[21] Through their efforts and encouragement many well-known studies that made important contributions were initiated, including Molly Newhouse's studies of hospital records and the Barking (Cape) and Ferodo factories; Stephen Jones's study of the Nottingham gas mask workers; Corbett McDonald and colleagues' study of the Canadian chrysotile mines; and Peter Harries' study of Naval Dockyard workers.

Another giant in asbestos research at that time was Dr Irving Selikoff. He had set up a research group at the Mt Sinai Hospital in New York and worked closely with the late Dr Cuyler Hammond, a statistician. The group was highly prolific over many years and reported studies of

---

19 G W Gibbs, G Berry, "Mesothelioma and asbestos", *Regulatory Toxicology and Pharmacology*, 52, 2008, S223–31.

20 Wagner, "Mesothelioma and mineral fibers", 1905–11.

21 J C Gilson, "Health hazards of asbestos: recent studies on its biological effects", (Wyers Memorial Lecture 1965)", *Transactions of the Society of Occupational Medicine*, 16, 1966, 62–74.

US insulation workers in the New York area, [22] shipyard workers,[23] and workers at a factory using amosite asbestos.[24] Selikoff, Hammond, and Churg also presented the first evidence of the important synergistic effect between asbestos exposure and smoking in the causation of lung cancer.[25]

The mortality of a group of insulation workers in Belfast was investigated by Elmes and Simpson,[26] and of workers at the Devonport Naval Dockyard in England by Harries and colleagues.[27]

The 1964 Conference in New York on the Biological Effects of Asbestos was a major event in putting the health related consequences of asbestos exposure on the map – not just mesothelioma but also the increased incidence of lung cancer.[28]

Dr Newhouse, invariably known as Molly, has been described as a "Doyenne of Occupational Medicine" in a biographical article by Salerno

---

22   I J Selikoff, J Churg, E C Hammond, "Asbestos exposure and neoplasia", *Journal of the American Medical Assn*, 188, 1964, 22–26. E C Hammond, I J Selikoff, J Churg, "Neoplasia among insulation workers in the United States with special reference to intra-abdominal neoplasia", *Annals of the New York Academy of Sciences*, 132, 1965, 519–25. I J Selikoff, E C Hammond, H Seidman, "Mortality experience of Insulation workers in the United States and Canada", *Annals of the New York Academy of Sciences*, 330, 1979, 91–116. I J Selikoff, H Seidman, "Asbestos-associated deaths among insulation workers in the United States and Canada, 1967–1987", *Annals of the New York Academy of Sciences*, 643, 1991, 1–14. S B Markowitz, S M Levin, A Miller, A Morabia, "Asbestos, asbestosis, smoking and lung cancer; new findings from the North American insulator cohort", *American Journal of Respiratory and Critical Care Medicine*, 188, 2013, 90–96.

23   I J Selikoff, R Lilis, W J Nicholson, "Asbestos disease in United States shipyards", *Annals of the New York Academy of Sciences*, 330, 1979, 295–311.

24   I J Selikoff, E C Hammond, J Churg, "Carcinogenicity of amosite asbestos", *Archives of Environmental Health*, 25, 1972, 183–86. H Seidman, I J Selikoff, E C Hammond, "Short-term asbestos work exposure and long-term observation", *Annals of the New York Academy of Sciences*, 330, 1979, 61–89.

25   I J Selikoff, E C Hammond, J Churg, "Asbestos exposure, smoking and neoplasia", *Journal of the American Medical Assn*, 204, 1968, 106–12.

26   P C Elmes, M J C Simpson, "Insulation workers in Belfast. 3. Mortality 1940–66", *British Journal of Industrial Medicine*, 28, 1971, 226–36. P C Elmes, M J C Simpson, "Insulation workers in Belfast. A further study of mortality due to asbestos exposure (1940–75)", *British Journal of Industrial Medicine*, 34, 1977, 174–80.

27   P G Harries, "Asbestosis hazards in naval dockyards", *Annals of Occupational Hygiene*, 11, 1968, 135–45. P G Harries, "Experience with asbestos disease and its control in Great Britain's naval dockyards", *Environmental Research*, 11, 1976, 261–67. C E Rossiter, R M Coles, "HM Dockyard, Devonport: 1947 mortality study", in *Biological effects of mineral fibres*, ed. J C Wagner (IARC Scientific Publications No. 30, Lyon, 1980), 713–21.

28   "Biological Effects of Asbestos", *Annals of the New York Academy of Sciences*, 132, 1965, 5–705.

and Feitshans.[29] She did not start her research career until she was in her early fifties. She had served in the Royal Army Medical Corps during the war, going into Europe soon after D-Day, and later served in India and Singapore where she treated rescued prisoners of war. She reached the rank of full Colonel, the highest rank then available to a female medical officer. So she came into research quite late in her career but produced some very important work.

The case control study of Newhouse and Thompson, first presented at the New York Conference, showed mesotheliomas in women who had laundered their husband's work clothes and those living close to a factory.[30] Out of 83 mesothelioma patients at the London Hospital, there were 7 women whose relatives worked with asbestos.

> The most usual history was that of the wife who washed her husband's dungarees or work clothes. In one instance a relative said that the husband, a docker, came home "white with asbestos" every evening for three or four years and his wife brushed him down.[31]

There were also cases with no direct exposure who lived within half a mile of an asbestos factory, thus providing evidence of mesotheliomas due to environmental exposure. This was an extremely important paper, as was recognised by its reprinting in 1993.

Molly Newhouse also conducted historical cohort studies at the Cape factory in Barking in east London and the Ferodo friction products factory in the north of England. In the study at the Cape factory over 5000 workers were followed up for more than 30 years. It was shown that the mesothelioma rate increased with both the intensity and the duration of exposure. This was a very important finding when it was published in 1976 as at that time there was a widely held view that mesothelioma was not dose related.[32] Up to 1980 by which time a quarter of the cohort had died (1249) there had

---

29 D F Salerno, I L Feitshans, "Influential women in occupational health – Muriel (Molly) Lina Newhouse, MD: British doyenne of occupational medicine", *Journal of epidemiology and community health*, 58, 2004, 17.

30 M L Newhouse, H Thompson, "Epidemiology of mesothelial tumors in the London area", *Annals of the New York Academy of Sciences*, 132, 1965, 579–88.

31 M L Newhouse, H Thompson, "Mesothelioma of pleura and peritoneum following exposure to asbestos in the London area", *British Journal of Industrial Medicine*, 22, 1965, 261–69 (reprinted 50, 1993, 769–78).

32 M L Newhouse, G Berry, "Predictions of mortality from mesothelial tumours in asbestos factory workers", *British Journal of Industrial Medicine*, 33, 1976, 147–51.

been 98 deaths due to mesothelioma out of 537 deaths due to cancer; that is, 8 per cent of deaths were due to mesothelioma.[33]

At the Ferodo factory friction products were produced. A total of 13,460 workers were followed up. There were 1,633 deaths including 149 due to lung cancer and 10 from pleural mesothelioma.[34] There was no increased risk of lung cancer since the observed number of 149 was similar to the 151 that would have been expected in a population of that size over the time period of the follow-up. The asbestos used in the manufacture of the friction products was almost entirely chrysotile, except that between 1929-33 and 1939-44 there was one contract that specified the use of crocidolite. The majority of those with mesothelioma (8/10) had worked on the crocidolite contract compared with few of the controls (3/40), providing evidence that crocidolite is more potent than chrysotile in producing mesothelioma.

Asbestos type and mesothelioma

Various studies have been carried out over the years providing evidence of mesotheliomas after exposure to each of the three commercial asbestos types. These are just some of the critical studies.

Crocidolite

In addition to the original findings in South Africa, confirmation that crocidolite can produce mesotheliomas in substantial numbers came from a study of former miners and millers at the Wittenoom crocidolite mine where 26 mesotheliomas were reported on in 1980.[35] These results have been updated over the years and the most recent update gave 316

---

33   M L Newhouse, G Berry, J C Wagner, "Mortality of factory workers in east London 1933–80", *British Journal of Industrial Medicine*, 42, 1985, 4–11. G Berry, M L Newhouse, J C Wagner, "Mortality from all cancers of asbestos factory workers in east London 1933–80", *Occupational and Environmental Medicine*, 57, 2000, 782–85.

34   M L Newhouse, G Berry, A W Skidmore, "A mortality study of workers manufacturing friction materials with chrysotile asbestos", *Annals of Occupational Hygiene*, 26 1982, 899–909. G Berry, M L Newhouse, "Mortality of workers manufacturing friction materials using asbestos", *British Journal of Industrial Medicine*, 40, 1983, 1–7.

35   M S T Hobbs, S D Woodward, B Murphy, A W Musk, J E Elder, "The incidence of pneumoconiosis, mesothelioma and other respiratory cancer in men engaged in mining and milling crocidolite in Western Australia", in *Biological Effects of Mineral Fibres*, ed. J C Wagner (IARC Scientific Publications No. 30, Lyon, 1980), 615–25.

mesotheliomas in a group of 6,489 former male workers.[36] Mesotheliomas have also occurred in residents of the township of Wittenoom who were not exposed in the mine or mill. The town was about 12 km from the mine. Tailings that contained residual crocidolite fibre were used throughout the town for paving roads, parking areas, the school playground, and the racecourse, and spread on the yards of houses to suppress the red dust. Asbestos was trucked through the town past the primary school and houses, and the workers took their dusty work clothes home for washing. Hansen and colleagues reported 27 cases in 4,659 former residents to the end of 1993.[37] A more recent follow-up showed 67 cases of mesothelioma in 4,768 former residents of the town to the end of 2002.[38] Musk and colleagues described the health consequences of exposure to crocidolite asbestos at Wittenoom as a "modern industrial disaster".[39]

Another important study was in Nottingham where Dr Stephen Jones collected cases of mesothelioma over thirty years and identified many in women who during the Second World War, between 1940 and 1944, had worked in a factory that had been requisitioned for the assembly of military gas masks, using filter pads prepared from 80 per cent merino wool and 20 per cent crocidolite asbestos. Jones in 1980 reported 16 mesotheliomas in 727 women who had been exposed only to crocidolite.[40] Shortly before his death Jones handed over the records to Dr Corbett McDonald and this facilitated some further epidemiological study of this rich data source of 1,154 employees (mainly women) and it is now known that 65 mesotheliomas have occurred in the total group employed on gas mask production

---

36 G Berry, A Reid, P Aboagye-Sarfo, N H De Klerk, N J Olsen, E Merler, P Franklin, A W Musk, "Malignant mesotheliomas in former miners and millers of crocidolite at Wittenoom (Western Australia) after more than 50 years follow-up", *British Journal of Cancer*, 106, 2012, 1016–20.

37 J Hansen, N H de Klerk, A W Musk, M S T Hobbs, "Environmental exposure to crocidolite and mesothelioma – exposure-response relationships", *American Journal of Respiratory and Critical Care Medicine*, 157, 1988, 69–75.

38 A Reid, G Berry, N H de Klerk, J Hansen, J Heyworth, G L Ambrosini, L Fritschi, N Olsen, E Merler, A W Musk, "Age and sex differences in malignant mesothelioma after residential exposure to blue asbestos (crocidolite)", *Chest*, 131, 2007, 376–82.

39 A W Musk, N H de Klerk, J L Eccles, M S Hobbs, B K Armstrong, L Layman, J C McNulty, "Wittenoom, Western Australia: a modern industrial disaster", *American Journal of Industrial Medicine*, 21, 5, 1992, 735–47.

40 J S P Jones, P G Smith, F D Pooley, G Berry, G W Sawle, B K Wignall, R J Madeley, A Aggarwal, "The consequences of exposure to asbestos dust in a wartime gas mask factory", in *Biological effects of mineral fibres*, ed. JC Wagner (IARC Scientific Publications No. 30, Lyon, 1980), 637–53.

at that factory.[41] The first occurred in 1963 and the most recent in 1994. It was found that the mesothelioma rate was fairly stable between 30 and 50 years after exposure. After about the first 20 years, during which there were no cases, the rate increased rapidly up to 30 years from exposure but then remained fairly steady for the next 20 years. No mesothelioma was identified between 1996 and 2003. This is evidence that the mesothelioma rate does not increase indefinitely with time since exposure.

Another group of workers assembled military gas masks to the same specification in Canada and by the end of 1975, 9 mesotheliomas had occurred in a group of 199 persons.[42] Acheson and colleagues found 5 mesotheliomas out of 219 deaths in women working with crocidolite in the assembly of gas masks in Lancashire, England, compared with one in 177 deaths in women working with chrysotile.[43]

Amosite

Seidman and colleagues followed a group of 933 men employed during the Second World War at a factory in Paterson, New Jersey, producing insulation for ships with amosite asbestos. Fourteen mesotheliomas were found in 528 deaths[44], later updated to 17 in 593 deaths.[45] There were 5 mesotheliomas in 333 deaths among a group of 4,820 men producing insulation board from amosite at a factory in Uxbridge, England.[46] Sluis-Cremer and colleagues linked an increased risk of mesothelioma in mining[47] and increased risks have been reported in manufacturing industries processing amosite.[48]

---

41   J C McDonald, J M Harris, G Berry, "Sixty years on: the price of assembling military gas masks in 1940", *Occupational and Environmental Medicine*, 63, 2006, 852–855.

42   A D McDonald, J C McDonald, "Mesothelioma after crocidolite exposure during gas mask manufacture", *Environmental Research*, 17, 1978, 340–46.

43   E D Acheson, M J Gardner, E C Pippard, L P Grime, "Mortality of two groups of women who manufactured gas masks from chrysotile and crocidolite asbestos: a 40 year follow-up", *British Journal of Industrial Medicine*, 39, 1982, 344–48.

44   Seidman, Selikoff, Hammond, "Short-term asbestos work exposure and long-term observation", 61–89.

45   H Seidman, I J Selikoff, S K Gelb, "Mortality experience of amosite asbestos factory workers: dose-response relationships 5 to 40 years after onset of short-term work exposure", *American Journal of Industrial Medicine*, 10, 1986, 479–514.

46   E D Acheson, M J Gardner, P D Winter, C Bennett, "Cancer in a factory using amosite asbestos", *International Journal of Epidemiology*, 13, 1984, 3–10.

47   G K Sluis-Cremer, F D K Liddell, W P D Logan, B N Bezuidenhout, "The mortality of amphibole miners in South Africa 1946–1980", *British Journal of Industrial Medicine*, 49, 1992, 566–75.

48   J L Levin, J W McLarty, G A Hurst, A N Smith, A L Frank, "Tyler asbestos workers: mortality experience in a cohort exposed to amosite", *Occupational and Environmental Medicine*, 55, 1998, 155–60.

Chrysotile

A large follow-up study of miners and millers from the Quebec mines has been conducted over several decades by McDonald and colleagues.[49] In a follow-up of 11,000 workers they found 10 mesotheliomas out of 4,463 deaths.[50] To the end of 1988 there had been a total of 33 mesotheliomas in 6,091 deaths; 28 of these were in miners and millers and 5 in workers at a small factory where commercial amphiboles had been used.[51] A later follow-up gave 38 mesotheliomas in 8,009 deaths up to the end of 1992.[52] In the Balangero chrysotile mine in Italy there were 2 mesotheliomas reported in 427 deaths,[53] recently updated to 7 in 722 deaths.[54]

Commercial chrysotile may contain a small proportion of tremolite, a non-commercial amphibole, which may have contributed to the mesothelioma risk observed in some of the workers exposed to chrysotile asbestos. Evidence that exposure to tremolite can cause mesothelioma comes from a study of workers in a vermiculite mine in Montana where asbestiform "tremolite" (soda tremolite) is associated with the vermiculite. There was a high risk of mesothelioma and it was concluded that the potency for mesothelioma of this asbestiform mineral from the Montana vermiculite mine was similar to that of crocidolite.[55]

---

49 J C McDonald, A D McDonald, G W Gibbs, J Siemiatycki, C E Rossiter, "Mortality in the chrysotile asbestos mines and mills of Quebec", *Archives of Environmental Health*, 22, 1971, 677–86.

50 J C McDonald, F D K Liddell, G W Gibbs, G E Eyssen, A D McDonald, "Dust exposure and mortality in chrysotile mining, 1910–75", *British Journal of Industrial Medicine*, 37, 1980, 11–24.

51 J C McDonald, F D K Liddell, A Dufresne, A D McDonald, "The 1891–1920 birth cohort of Quebec chrysotile miners and millers: mortality 1976–88", *British Journal of Industrial Medicine*, 50, 1993, 1073–81.

52 F D K Liddell, A D McDonald, J C McDonald, "The 1891–1920 birth cohort of Quebec chrysotile miners and millers: development from 1904 and mortality to 1992", *Annals of Occupational Hygiene*, 41, 1997, 13–36. A D McDonald, B W Case, A Churg, A Dufresne, GW Gibbs, P Sébastien, J C McDonald, "Mesothelioma in Quebec chrysotile miners and millers: epidemiology and aetiology", *Annals of Occupational Hygiene*, 41, 1997, 707–19.

53 G F Rubino, G Piolatto, M L Newhouse, G Scancetti, G A Aresini, R Murray, "Mortality of chrysotile asbestos workers at the Balangero mine, northern Italy", *British Journal of Industrial Medicine*, 36, 1979, 187–94. G Piolatto, E Negri, C La Vecchia, E Pira, A Decarli, J Peto, "An update of cancer mortality among chrysotile asbestos miners in Balangero, northern Italy", *British Journal of Industrial Medicine*, 47, 1990, 810–14.

54 E Pira, C Romano, F Donato, C Pelucchi, C La Vecchia, P Boffetta, "Mortality from cancer and other causes among Italian chrysotile asbestos miners", *Occupational and Environmental Medicine*, 74, 2017, 558–63.

55 J C McDonald, J Harris, B Armstrong, "Cohort mortality study of Vermiculite miners exposed to fibrous talc: an update", *Annals of Occupational Hygiene*, 46 (Suppl. 1), 2002,

J C McDonald and A D McDonald in 1995 reported that the risk of mesothelioma in the Canadian chrysotile mines at Thetford was four times higher in a localised area of five mines compared with the other ten mines, and this difference corresponded to a similar four-fold difference in the concentration of tremolite found in the lungs of miners in the two areas who had died of causes other than mesothelioma.[56] In view of the fact that fibrous tremolite can cause mesothelioma and is a more durable amphibole fibre than chrysotile fibre it is not surprising that there is a risk of mesothelioma with chrysotile containing fibrous tremolite, but the level of risk of chrysotile in the absence of any tremolite is a matter of debate.[57]

The asbestos textile factory in Rochdale, England is important because exposure was mainly to chrysotile and for a time it was considered valid to attribute any asbestos related health effects entirely to chrysotile.[58] In 1985 it was reported that there were 17 mesotheliomas in 850 men who had died more than 20 years after first exposure,[59] but by this time it had been reported in 1979 that an average of 60 tonnes a year of crocidolite had been processed over a 40-year period,[60] and a study of the asbestos in the lungs at post-mortem in former workers showed an average crocidolite content of 300 times that of the general population.[61]

93–94. J C McDonald, J Harris, B Armstrong, "Mortality in a cohort of vermiculite miners exposed to fibrous amphibole in Libby, Montana", *Occupational and Environmental Medicine*, 61, 2004, 363–66.

56   J C McDonald, A D McDonald, "Chrysotile, tremolite, and mesothelioma (letter)", *Science*, 267, 1995: 775–76.

57   C M Yarborough, "Chrysotile as a cause of mesothelioma: an assessment based on epidemiology", *Critical Reviews in Toxicology*, 36, 2006, 165–87.

58   Doll, "Mortality from lung cancer in asbestos workers", 81–85. J F Knox, S Holmes, R Doll, I D Hill, "Mortality from lung cancer and other causes among workers in an asbestos textile factory", *British Journal of Industrial Medicine*, 25, 1968, 293–303. J. Peto, R. Doll, S V Howard, L J Kinlen, H C Lewinsohn, "A mortality study among workers in an English asbestos factory", *British Journal of Industrial Medicine*, 34, 1977, 169–73. J Peto, "The hygiene standard for chrysotile asbestos", *Lancet*, 1 March 1978, 484–89.

59   J Peto, R Doll, C Hermon, W Binns, R Clayton, T Goffe, "Relationship of mortality to measures of environmental asbestos pollution in an asbestos textile factory", *Annals of Occupational Hygiene*, 29, 1985, 305–55.

60   Health and Safety Executive (HSE). *Asbestos—final report of the advisory committee*, vols 1 and 2 (London: HMSO, 1979). G Berry, J C Gilson, S Holmes, H C Lewinsohn, S A Roach, "Asbestosis: a study of dose-response relationships in an asbestos textile factory", *British Journal of Industrial Medicine*, 36, 1979, 98–112.

61   J C Wagner, G Berry, F D Pooley, "Mesotheliomas and asbestos type in asbestos textile workers: a study of lung contents", *British Medical Journal*, 285, 1982, 603–06.

Exposure to mixed types of asbestos

These studies are often less useful for distinguishing between the mesothelioma rates of different types of asbestos because in most cases it is impossible to disentangle the contributions of the different types to the risk of mesothelioma. This was the situation at the Barking factory mentioned earlier. But there are exceptions where some discrimination is possible because of a separation of fibre types either in time or space and one of these is the Ferodo friction materials factory in England referred to earlier. Here it was possible to identify a subgroup of workers who had been exposed to crocidolite whilst working on a special project. The majority (8/10) of those with mesothelioma had worked on this contract compared with 3/40 of controls, contributing evidence of the higher mesothelioma risk of crocidolite compared with chrysotile. Alies-Patin and Valleron reported four mesotheliomas in a French asbestos cement factory in which mainly chrysotile was used, but three of these cases had come from the minority who had worked with crocidolite throughout their employment.[62]

A D McDonald, Fry and colleagues compared asbestos workers in three factories in the US.[63] In an asbestos textile factory where only chrysotile was processed there was one mesothelioma in 570 deaths. In a friction products factory using only chrysotile there were no mesotheliomas in 803 deaths. In the third factory where crocidolite and amosite were used as well as chrysotile there were 14 mesotheliomas out of 895 deaths.

The relative risk of mesothelioma with respect to exposure to the different types of asbestos was controversial over many years. The controversy is less now, with general agreement that crocidolite and amosite are much more potent than chrysotile, and that crocidolite has a higher risk than amosite, a position first suggested by Gilson as early as 1966.[64] Almost 20

---

62 A M Alies-Patin, A J Valleron, "Mortality of workers in a French asbestos cement factory 1940–82", *British Journal of Industrial Medicine*, 42, 1985, 219–25.

63 A D McDonald, J S Fry, "Mesothelioma and fiber type in three American asbestos factories – preliminary report", *Scandinavian Journal of Work, Environment and Health*, 8 (Suppl. 1), 1982, 53–58. A D McDonald, J S Fry, A J Woolley, M C McDonald, "Dust exposure and mortality in an American chrysotile textile plant", *British Journal of Industrial Medicine*, 40, 1983, 361–67. A D McDonald, J S Fry, A J Woolley, J C McDonald, "Dust exposure and mortality in an American factory using chrysotile, amosite, and crocidolite in mainly textile manufacture", *British Journal of Industrial Medicine*, 40, 1983, 368–74. A D McDonald, J S Fry, A J Wooley, J C McDonald, "Dust exposure and mortality in an American Chrysotile Asbestos Friction Products Plant", *British Journal of Industrial Medicine*, 41, 1984, 151–57.

64 Gilson, "Health hazards of asbestos: recent studies on its biological effects", 62–74.

years later Doll and Peto gave a table summarising the mortality experience of cohorts of asbestos workers pooled over a range of exposure conditions according to asbestos type.[65] They found that the ratios of the proportions of mesothelioma deaths are 1:6:17 for chrysotile, amosite, and crocidolite respectively.

In 2000 Hodgson and Darnton reported a quantitative meta-analysis in which, after taking account of the amount of exposure and the age at first exposure, the relative mesothelioma-causing potencies of the commercial asbestos types, crocidolite, amosite and chrysotile were in the ratio of 500:100:1 respectively.[66] In a draft report prepared for the US EPA, it was suggested that the best estimate of the potency for amphibole was 750 times that of chrysotile,[67] whilst Leigh and Driscoll concluded that the relative mesothelioma carcinogenicity for crocidolite: amosite: chrysotile were 26:14:1 respectively.[68]

That is history—what about the future? Over the last 30–50 years new use of crocidolite asbestos has been discontinued in many industrial countries, also amosite, and more recently chrysotile. So there will be a consequent marked reduction in mesotheliomas, but this effect will be delayed because of the long latent period between exposure and the occurrence of mesothelioma.

In Australia, there was no new use of crocidolite after about 1970, amosite was phased out in early 1980s, and a very limited use of chrysotile was discontinued in 2003. However, asbestos remains present particularly in buildings erected in earlier years and this involves some risk to those involved in maintenance work, a risk that can be minimised through recognition of the presence of asbestos and compliance with recommended and regulated working practices.

Whilst the ban on the new use of asbestos means that there will be a marked reduction in mesotheliomas arising from exposure to asbestos, unfortunately this effect will take another 20 years or longer because of the long latent period between exposure and the occurrence of mesothelioma.

---

65   R Doll, J Peto, *Asbestos: effects on health of exposure to asbestos* (London: Health and Safety Commission, HMSO, 1985).

66   J T Hodgson, A Darnton, "The quantitative risks of mesothelioma and lung cancer in relation to asbestos exposure", *Annals of Occupational Hygiene*, 44, 2000, 565–601.

67   D W Berman, K S Crump, *Final Draft: Technical Support Document for a protocol to assess asbestos related risk. Prepared for the Office of Solid Waste and Emergency Response* (US Environmental Protection Agency, Washington, 2003).

68   J Leigh, T Driscoll, "Malignant mesothelioma in Australia, 1945–2002", *International Journal of Occupational Medicine and Environmental Health*, 9, 2003, 206–17.

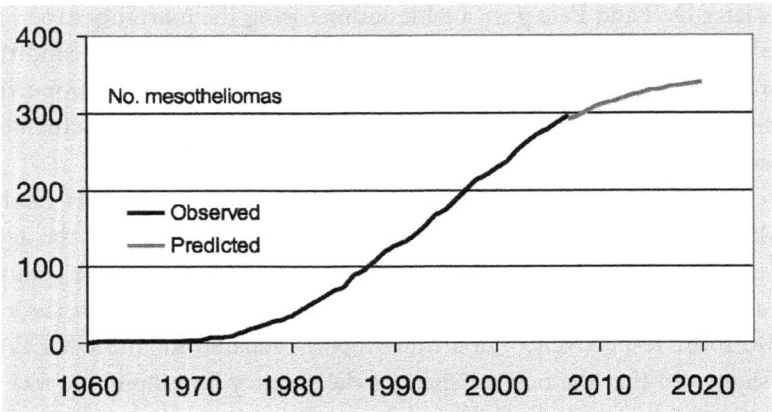

Figure 6.1: Wittenoom workers (men): increases in cases of mesothelioma in male workers up to 2007, and predicted to 2020

An example showing this is the miners and millers at Wittenoom. The mine and mill were closed in 1966. The first known mesothelioma occurred in 1960 and from the 1970s the numbers in men and women climbed steadily, to 46 by 1980, 139 by 1990, 247 by 2000, and 329 by 2008. The majority occurred long after the mine and mill had closed. Figure 6.1 shows the increasing number of mesotheliomas in the male workers over time to 2007, and the projected number up to 2020.

For Australia as a whole Figure 6.2 shows the predicted annual number of mesotheliomas in men due to asbestos exposure based on an analysis of mesothelioma incidence for 1983-2003.[69] The peak was estimated by about 2017 but the numbers were expected to remain appreciable for a further 30 years after the peak. Projections showing fairly similar patterns have been published for the US, UK and several other European countries.

---

69 M Clements, G Berry, J Shi, "Actuarial projections for mesothelioma: an epidemiological perspective", *Institute of Actuaries of Australia XIth Accident Compensation Seminar 1–4 April 2007, Melbourne*, 1–17. Institute of Actuaries of Australia, Sydney, 2007, 1–17. M Clements, G Berry, J Shi, S Ware, D Yates, A Johnson, "Projected mesothelioma incidence in men in New South Wales", *Occupational and Environmental Medicine*, 64, 2007, 747–52. G Berry, M Clements, "Mesotheliomas and asbestos exposure – historical aspects and future projections", *Proceedings of 25th Annual Conference of the Australian Institute of Occupational Hygienists 2007*, ed G Benke, D Collins, 130–137. Australian Institute of Occupational Hygienists Inc, Tullamarine, Victoria (ISBN-10 0-9803010-9-2).

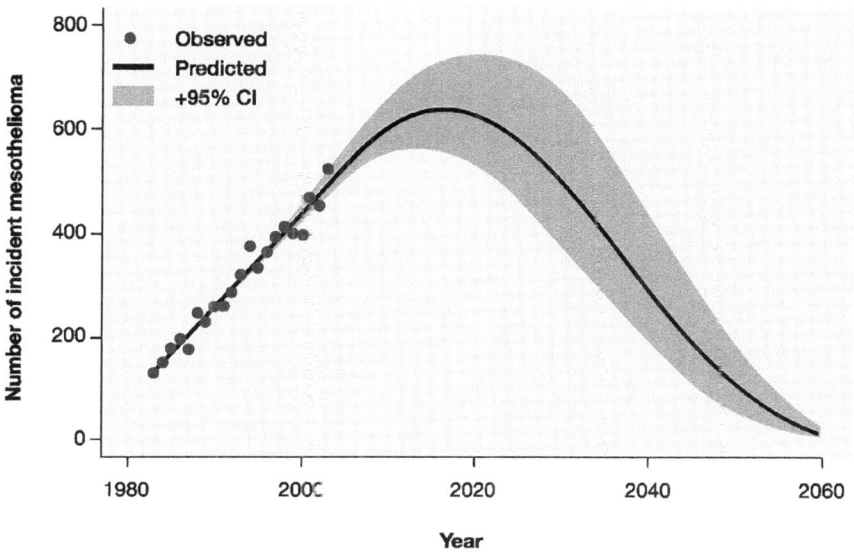

Figure 6.2: Australian workers (men): predicted annual number of incident mesotheliomas to 2060
SOURCE: Berry, Clements, 2007, based on model in Clements, Berry, Shi, Ware, Yates, Johnson, 2007.

Conclusion

The discovery of the link between crocidolite exposure and mesothelioma made almost 60 years ago has led to an enormous amount of research worldwide over five decades, and a phasing out and banning of asbestos use in many countries, but despite this the mesothelioma "epidemic" has many years to run because of the delay between exposure and mesothelioma occurrence.

Chapter 7

HEALTH OUTCOMES OF THE WOMEN AND CHILDREN WHO LIVED AT WITTENOOM

Alison Reid

As well as workers who were employed in the mining and milling operations at Wittenoom, there were an estimated further 5000 people who also lived at Wittenoom. Half of these were women and children. This chapter outlines their living conditions at Wittenoom and how they were exposed to asbestos. It explains how the cohort studies were established and used to track the Wittenoom women and children, and then describes their health outcomes.

Most of what we know about the impact of asbestos exposure on human health has come from cohort studies of men exposed to asbestos in their workplace. However, most women and children have been exposed to asbestos in their general environment, rather than in their job. We do not know if these studies of men, with different exposure profiles, sufficiently describe the risks of asbestos exposure for women and children. Studies of men cannot tell us about possible associations with reproductive cancers, in particular if asbestos exposure causes ovarian cancer. Susceptibility and carcinogenicity may differ in men, women, and children. The Wittenoom cohort studies (sadly) have been integral to answering these important questions.

Women and children at Wittenoom

Apart from a small number of State Government employees, for example teachers and nurses, most women who came to Wittenoom were wives and partners of Australian Blue Asbestos Company (ABA) workers. The sex ratio in the township was 2:1 in favour of men, as the majority of workers were young and transient and, if they had families, they came to Wittenoom without them. The families that were at Wittenoom were mostly young couples with small children. In 1953 there were 130 women and 200 children in the town, the majority of children being less than school age.[1]

Living and housing conditions in the town were basic. By 1958 the township had a general store, State and Catholic schools and kindergarten, a hospital, police station, post office, and hotel. Other amenities included a café, library and cinema, billiard room, tennis courts, a racecourse, and cricket and football ovals.[2] The government provided houses that consisted of one sheet of asbestos cement on the inside and the wooden framework on the outside, so houses quickly heated during the day, but had the benefit of cooling quickly at night. Each house was equipped only with a wood stove for cooking, in a climate where the daytime temperature rose to more than 38°C (100° Fahrenheit) for eight months of the year. The house water supply pipes were located just below the ground's surface and baths had to be run in the morning so that they would be cool enough to use at night. Showers could not be taken as the water was scalding hot.[3] There was no swimming pool located in the township, rock pools were present in the gorges but most residents did not have access to a car to get to them. There was no air conditioning, no radio and no television and the closest town (Port Hedland) was 300 kilometres away, accessible only by unsealed road/track that often became impassable in the rainy season.

Women often were initially dismayed on their arrival at Wittenoom. Many are recorded as having wept when they saw the bush, their houses and the township itself. They were not acclimatised to the heat, the physical environment or the local fauna: snakes, centipedes, and racehorse goannas, and were socially isolated. For many women, Wittenoom was a place to be "endured". Some took in laundry and boarders so they could "get out of there quicker". Wittenoom was perceived as being too isolated, male dominated, and primitive, and the way of life too centrally focused on alcohol and the hotel. Heavy drinking and broken relationships were not infrequent occurrences.[4]

---

1 L Layman, "Work and workers' responses at Wittenoom 1943–1966", *Community Health Studies*, 7, 1, 1983, 1–18.

2 A W Musk, N H de Klerk, J L Eccles, M S Hobbs, B K Armstrong, L Layman, *et al.*, "Wittenoom, Western Australia: a modern industrial disaster", *American Journal of Industrial Medicine*, 21, 5, 1992, 735–47.

3 S Lovenfosse, interview with L Layman, 28 October 2003. S Lovenfosse, "The children of Wittenoom. A social and environmental history", History Honours thesis, Macquarie University, 2000.

4 Layman, "Work and workers' responses at Wittenoom", 1–18.

The Australian Blue Asbestos Company was the largest employer in town and most of its jobs were for male workers. Those women who worked for ABA were mostly the wives of ABA employees. A few women were employed sewing the hessian bags in which the asbestos was transported between 1960-1966, and small numbers of other women worked in the company office, town store, and hotel. No more than 20 women at one time worked for ABA.[5] While chest X-rays were mandatory, women who worked for ABA were rarely offered annual chest X-rays.[6]

Exposure to asbestos was a feature of all aspects of life at Wittenoom. Tailings from the mine, rich in crocidolite fibres, were used throughout the town to pave roads and footpaths, parking areas, school playgrounds, and for reducing the red dust in backyards in the dry and the mud in the wet, as substitute for gravel and sand. The local shire (Ashburton) used the tailings on town roads, at the golf course, racecourse, airport, drive-in cinema, and caravan park. The use of tailings in the town did not stop until the mid-1960s. Vehicle movement over the roads raised a great deal of dust. Airline pilots claimed they honed in on Wittenoom from considerable distances by identifying the blue haze emanating from the mill on the horizon.[7] Similarly crocidolite contamination existed in areas outside the town; at the mine and mill sites, the tailings dumps in the Eastern and Western Gorges and their surrounds. The tailings have also washed into local creek beds.[8] Recreational pastimes included asbestos: the racecourse was covered with tailings from the mine and clouds of blue dust were raised when the horses raced past, and a competition filling 44-gallon (200 litre) drums with tailings was popular. Former Wittenoom residents vividly recall the asbestos dust that permeated the town.[9] In summary, asbestos was prevalent at work, in the home, and in the general environment and was an accepted part of everyday life.

Research study of Wittenoom Women and Children

In order to examine the health of former Wittenoom workers and residents, two cohort studies were established. ABA employment records were used

---

5   Layman "Work and workers' responses at Wittenoom", 4.
6   J McCulloch, "The mine at Wittenoom: blue asbestos, labour and occupational disease", *Labor History*, 47, 1, 2006, 1–19.
7   Musk *et al.*, "Wittenoom, Western Australia: a modern industrial disaster".
8   B Snell, J Langley, *Reading - the Wittenoom disaster*, Perth: Worksafe, Department of Consumer and Employment Protection, Govt of Western Australia, January 2007.
9   L Layman, "The blue asbestos industry at Wittenoom in Western Australia: a short history", in D W Henderson, D Whitaker, S L P Langlois (eds), *Social-Historical, medicolegal, and ethical aspects of mesothelioma* (New York: Hemisphere, 1989), 305–27.

to establish the Wittenoom workers cohort study in 1974. Information provided on the employment record included start and end date of employment and all the jobs each worker undertook whilst working for ABA.[10]

Then, in the early 1990s, a range of public and private records was searched to identify the former residents of Wittenoom, those who did not work for ABA. These sources included: state primary school records, admission and outpatient records from the Wittenoom hospital and General Practitioner, the State electoral roll for the Pilbara district, and a questionnaire to participants in a cancer prevention program established for former Wittenoom workers and residents in 1990. From 18,553 records collected, 5,097 individuals were identified. Between 1991 and 1993 a questionnaire was sent to all former Wittenoom residents traced to an address in Australia asking about their date, length, and place of residence at Wittenoom, their occupation at Wittenoom, and whether they lived with an asbestos worker and washed the clothes of an asbestos worker. Smoking and medical history information was also sought.[11]

Estimates of asbestos exposure

An important strength of the cohort studies, and what makes them unique globally, is the estimates of the levels of asbestos exposure that were derived for each worker and resident individually. These estimates have permitted the examination of the exposure-response relationship between asbestos exposure and disease outcome, but have also allowed the examination of disease patterns and susceptibility that may vary across sex and age groups. How these exposures were derived for workers and residents is briefly outlined below.

Several surveys of dust exposure were conducted by the Mines Department of Western Australia in the mine and mill between 1945 and 1958, and in 1966 airborne fibres were measured in various workplaces in the mine and mill and in the township. Using the information from those surveys, and the dates of employment and jobs indicated on the ABA employment record, each worker was assigned an exposure measured in fibres per ml years (f/ml years).[12]

---

10   B K Armstrong, N H de Klerk, A W Musk, M S Hobbs, "Mortality in miners and millers of crocidolite in Western Australia", *British Journal of Industrial Medicine*, 45, 1, 1988, 5–13.

11   J Hansen, N H de Klerk, J L Eccles, A W Musk, M S Hobbs, "Malignant mesothelioma after environmental exposure to blue asbestos", *International Journal of Cancer*, 54, 4, 1993, 578–81.

12   Armstrong *et al*, "Mortality in miners and millers of crocidolite in WA".

To estimate the exposure for former residents, information was derived from the surveys that used personal and fixed positional monitors to measure environmental levels in the township in 1973, 1977, 1980, 1984, 1986, and 1992, and the earlier surveys conducted by the WA Mines Department. From this information, residents were assigned an intensity of exposure of 1.0 fibre per ml of air (f/ml) when resident between 1947 and 1958, 0.5 f/ml between 1958 and 1966 when the mine and mill closed, and decreasing to 0.10 f/ml in 1992. For each individual resident, duration of residence was combined with the intensity of exposure to provide a measure of cumulative exposure (f/ml years) similar to that derived for the workers.[13]

Levels of asbestos exposure in the Wittenoom women and children.

Since their inception both cohort studies have been linked to national and state death and cancer registries to identify the cases of asbestos related diseases. To examine the health outcome of the women and children (those aged less than 15 years at the time of arrival at Wittenoom), women and children were identified from both cohort studies. According to the data 416 women had worked for ABA over the lifetime of the mine. A further 1746 women, 1222 girls, and 1279 boys had lived at Wittenoom and not been employed by ABA.

The majority of women arrived at Wittenoom in the 1950s and 1960s, of whom 45 per cent lived there for less than one year, 41 per cent between one and five years and 12 per cent for five or more years. Most women at Wittenoom were exposed to asbestos from their general environment. Thirty-five per cent of women were estimated to have exposure levels of < 2 f/ml and 62 per cent were estimated to have exposure levels between 2 f/ml and less than 5 f/ml. Cumulative exposure levels (duration of residence x intensity) estimated 85 per cent of women had exposure levels of <10 f/ml years.[14]

---

13   J Hansen, N K de Klerk, A W Musk, M S Hobbs, "Environmental exposure to crocidolite and mesothelioma: exposure-response relationships", *American Journal of Respiratory and Critical Care Medicine*, 157, 1, 1998, 69–75. J Hansen, N K de Klerk , A W Musk, M S Hobbs, "Individual exposure levels in people environmentally exposed to crocidolite", *Applied Occupational and Environal Hygiene*, 12, 7, 1997, 485–90.

14   A Reid, J Heyworth, N K de Klerk, A W Musk, "Cancer incidence among women and girls environmentally and occupationally exposed to blue asbestos at Wittenoom, Western Australia", *International Journal of Cancer*, 122, 10, 2008, 2337–44.

All the Wittenoom children incurred their asbestos exposure from their general environment at Wittenoom. In this cohort 63 per cent arrived before the age of five years (including 463 (30 per cent) who were born there). As for period of residence, 55 per cent stayed at Wittenoom for less than two years, 28 per cent between two and five years, and 16 per cent greater than five years. In relation to exposure, 62 per cent of children had an estimated cumulative asbestos exposure of < 5 f/ml years, 19 per cent between 5 and 10 f/ml years, and 17 per cent > 10 f/ml years.[15]

Health outcomes of women

Mesothelioma

Between 1960 and 2005 there were 47 cases of malignant mesothelioma diagnosed among the Wittenoom women, 11 in the former workers. The time from first exposure to onset of mesothelioma was shorter in the workers (median 34.1 years) compared with the residents (39.3 years). The first case occurred in a worker 24.6 years after first exposure compared with 23.5 years in a resident. The incidence rate among workers appears to have peaked at 30-39 years since first exposure (304 per 100,000), while for residents peak exposure occurred 40-49 years since first exposure (275 per 100,000). At every 5 year period since 1975, the mesothelioma incidence rate was higher in workers than residents, and appears to be still increasing among workers (542 per 100,000 compared with 150 per 100,000 respectively, in the period 2000-2005).

Based on 40 deaths from mesothelioma that occurred among the Wittenoom women to the end of 2004, we estimated the future number of mesotheliomas that might occur in this group, using models that take into account time since first exposure, level of asbestos exposure, and competing risks from other diseases. We estimate that between 66 and 87 more mesotheliomas will develop among the Wittenoom women, to the end of 2030.[16]

Susceptibility to mesothelioma

Several studies[17] have suggested that women are more susceptible to mesothelioma than men, but none of these studies has been able to account for

---

15   A Reid, P Franklin, N Olsen, J Sleith, L Samuel, Aboagye-Sarfo P, *et al*. "All-cause mortality and cancer incidence among adults exposed to blue asbestos during childhood", *American Journal of Industrial Medicine*, 56, 2, 2013, 133–45.

16   A Reid, G Berry, J Heyworth, N K de Klerk, A W Musk, "Predicted mortality from malignant mesothelioma among women exposed to blue asbestos at Wittenoom, Western Australia", *Occupational and Environmental Medicine*, 66, 3, 2009, 169–74.

17   M L Newhouse, G Berry, J C Wagner, M E Turok, "A study of the mortality of female asbestos workers", *British Journal of Industrial Medicine*, 29, 2, 1972, 134–41.

the degree of asbestos exposure. Examining 67 cases of mesothelioma that occurred among the Wittenoom residents to 2000 showed that women residents are not more susceptible to mesothelioma than their male counterparts. Women residents had a steeper exposure–response curve but consistently lower rates of mesothelioma mortality compared with male residents. Although the exposure-response curve was steeper among the women the overall risk of mesothelioma was greater among men with exposures of 50 f/ml-years and less, a dose which covered 99 per cent of the residents.[18]

How patterns of mesothelioma in women differ from those of Wittenoom men

We found that the pattern of mesothelioma incidence differed in the Wittenoom women from that of the male ABA workers. The first cases of mesothelioma in the Wittenoom women developed 20-29 years since first exposure which was longer than the male ABA workers at 10-19 years. Male ABA workers had considerably higher asbestos exposure with an average cumulative exposure of 6 f/ml years compared with 0.5 f/ml years for a female ABA worker. The rate of malignant mesothelioma continued to increase among male ABA workers with 40 or more years since first exposure (364 per 100,000), in contrast to the women's rate for the same period which declined (114 per 100,000).[19]

Lung cancer

There were 55 lung cancers diagnosed between 1960 and 2005 (37 in residents). Of residents, the risk of lung cancer was two-and-a-half times greater in women who reported living with an ABA worker, but not increased among those women who reported washing the clothes of an ABA worker. Former Wittenoom workers had a greater incidence of lung cancer than former residents. However, we did not find an association with asbestos exposure and lung cancer in the Wittenoom women.[20]

    E Pira, C Pelucchi, L Buffoni, A Palmas, M Turbiglio, E Negri, *et al.*, "Cancer mortality in a cohort of asbestos textile workers', *British Journal of Cancer*, 92, 3, 2005, 580–6. S Metintas, M Metintas, I Ucgun, U Oner, "Malignant mesothelioma due to environmental exposure to asbestos: follow-up of a Turkish cohort living in a rural area", *Chest*, 122, 6, 2002, 2224–9.

18   A Reid, G Berry, N K de Klerk, J Hansen, J Heyworth, G Ambrosini, *et al*, "Age and sex differences in malignant mesothelioma after residential exposure to blue asbestos (crocidolite)", *Chest*, 131, 2, 2007, 376–82.

19   Reid *et al*, "Cancer incidence among women and girls environmentally and occupationally exposed to blue asbestos at Wittenoom, WA".

20   Reid *et al*, "Cancer incidence among women and girls environmentally and occupationally exposed to blue asbestos at Wittenoom, WA".

Reproductive cancers

Between 1960 and 2006 145 cases of breast or gynaecologic cancers were diagnosed among the Wittenoom women; 16 ovarian, 19 cervical, 14 uterine, and 96 breast cancers. In order to examine the specific question of whether asbestos exposure was associated with ovarian cancer, we reviewed the pathology of all cases of ovarian, colon, and peritoneal cancers and found that no cases had been misclassified. There was no difference in the incidence of ovarian, uterine, cervical, or breast cancer in the Wittenoom women compared with the Western Australian female population. Among the Wittenoom workers, cervical cancer was twice that of the WA female population, whilst ovarian was 40 per cent less, but these differences were not statistically significant. Women who lived with or washed the clothes of an ABA asbestos worker did not have an increased risk for any of these cancers. Age at first exposure was associated with cervical cancer with women who arrived at Wittenoom aged 40 years or above having a two-fold increased risk compared with those who were first exposed aged less than 15 years. Excepting time since first exposure, ovarian, uterine, and breast cancer were not associated with any measure of asbestos exposure. Overall, we found no increased risk for gynaecologic or breast cancers among the Wittenoom women compared with the WA female population, and no suggestion that asbestos exposure was associated with these cancers.[21]

Gestational trophoblastic diseases

Among the Wittenoom women we identified several cases of a very rare cancer, and its precursor, not previously associated with asbestos exposure.

Gestational trophoblastic disease (GTD) names a spectrum of abnormally proliferating trophoblasts from malignant choriocarcinoma (cancer of the placenta) to hydatidiform moles, most commonly occurring after a pregnancy. They are very rare.[22] In Australia in 2003 there were six cases of malignant choriocarcinoma and 540 hospital separations where hydatidiform mole was listed as the principal diagnosis. Known risk factors include maternal age (aged between 20 and 40), having a history of a hydatidiform mole, and use of oral contraceptives, the risk increasing with a longer duration of use.[23]

---

21 A Reid, N K de Klerk, A W Musk, "Does exposure to asbestos cause ovarian cancer? A systematic literature review and meta-analysis", *Cancer Epidemiology, Biomarkers & Prevention*, 20, 7, 2011, 1287–95.

22 S K Khoo, "Clinical aspects of gestational trophoblastic disease: a review based partly on 25-year experience of a statewide registry", *Australian & New Zealand Journal of Obstetrics & Gynaecology*, 43, 4, 2003, 280–9.

23 A Reid, J Heyworth, N K de Klerk, A W Musk, "Asbestos exposure and gestational trophoblastic disease: a hypothesis", *Cancer Epidemiology, Biomarkers & Prevention*,

There were three cases of malignant choriocarcinoma among women residing in Wittenoom in 1963. According to our records, there were 302 women of reproductive age living in Wittenoom in 1963, giving a crude incidence rate for malignant choriocarcinoma of 3/302=9.9 per 1000 women of reproductive age. In addition, three cases of hydatidiform moles were also found in the Wittenoom women, giving a crude incidence rate of 1.7 per 1000 deliveries. These rates were considerably higher than that for Australian women as a whole, at 0.08 and 1.4 per 1000 confinements for choriocarcinoma and hydatidiform mole respectively.[24]

There is some biological plausibility for an association of these rare diseases and asbestos exposure. International work has reported the presence of asbestos fibres in the placental digests of live and stillborn infants, and further found that the transplacental transfer of fibre occurs via the maternal circulation.[25] The women who developed choriocarcinoma were residents of Wittenoom at the time the disease developed, whereas the cases of hydatidiform moles occurred many years later among women who had first been exposed to asbestos as young girls (all three were born at Wittenoom). Four of the six cases had lived with ABA workers, and the three choriocarcinoma cases worked for ABA. It may be that the placental burden of asbestos fibres is greater in women with known, heavy asbestos exposure such as occurred at Wittenoom, therefore increasing their risk for these diseases.[26]

Cancer incidence compared with Western Australian population

There were 437 incident cancers in the Wittenoom women diagnosed between 1960 and 2005, 84 (20 per cent) in the former ABA workers, and 303 in the former residents. Of the former residents, 72 per cent of cases had lived with an asbestos worker and 35 per cent reported washing the clothes of an asbestos worker. Compared with the WA female population, the Wittenoom women had excess risk of all cancers, lung cancer, and mesothelioma. Specifically, the excess risk of all cancers in the Wittenoom women was between 12 and 51 per cent greater, and the incidence of lung

---

  18, 11, 2009, 2895–8.
24 Reid *et al*, "Asbestos exposure and gestational trophoblastic disease: a hypothesis".
25 A K Haque, M G Mancuso, M G Williams, R F Dodson, "Asbestos in organs and placenta of five stillborn infants suggests transplacental transfer", *Environmental Research*, 58, 2),1992, 163–75. A K Haque, D M Vrazel, K D Burau, S P Cooper, T Downs, "Is there transplacental transfer of asbestos? A study of 40 stillborn infants", *Pediatric Pathology & Laboratory Medicine*, 16, 6, 1996, 877–92. A K Haque, D M Vrazel, T Uchida, "Assessment of asbestos burden in the placenta and tissue digests of stillborn infants in South Texas", *Archives of Environmental Contamination & Toxicology*, 35, 3, 1998, 532–8.
26 Reid *et al*, "Asbestos exposure and gestational trophoblastic disease: a hypothesis".

cancer was between 84 and 254 per cent greater than the Western Australian female population. The incidence of malignant mesothelioma was between 55 and 77 times greater in the Wittenoom women than the WA female population.[27]

Mortality compared with Western Australian population

Similar to cancer incidence, the excess risk of mortality was greater in the Wittenoom women than the WA female population. Among residents, there were 425 deaths between 1950 and 2004. Compared with the WA female population, Wittenoom residents had excess deaths from all causes, all cancers, mesothelioma, lung cancer, pneumoconiosis and symptoms signs and ill-defined conditions. Specifically, mortality was 13 per cent greater for all causes, 42 per cent greater for all cancers, 215 per cent greater for lung cancer, 635 per cent greater for symptoms signs and ill-defined conditions and 1180 per cent greater for pneumoconiosis than that for the WA female population.[28]

Among Wittenoom workers, excess deaths were found for all causes, all cancers, mesothelioma and lung cancer compared with the WA female population. Specifically mortality was 35 per cent greater for all causes, 207 per cent greater for all cancers and 423 per cent greater for lung cancer than that for the WA female population.[29]

Health outcomes of children

Almost 2500 children lived at Wittenoom over the period of the mining and milling operation. They have been followed up as part of the residents' cohort study, and their health tracked over time. We report on their health status as adults.

Mesothelioma

To the end of 2009, there had been 42 cases of mesothelioma among the Wittenoom children, 29 in males. For every level of cumulative asbestos exposure, males had higher incidence rates than females, although the difference was not statistically significant. There was no difference in the incidence rate in those who were first exposed at Wittenoom aged less than

---

27   Reid *et al*, "Cancer incidence among women and girls environmentally and occupationally exposed to blue asbestos at Wittenoom, WA".

28   A Reid, J Heyworth, N K de Klerk, A W Musk, "The mortality of women exposed environmentally and domestically to blue asbestos at Wittenoom, Western Australia", *Occupational & Environmental Medicine*, 65, 11, 2008, 743–9.

29   Reid *et al*, "The mortality of women exposed environmentally and domestically to blue asbestos at Wittenoom, WA".

5 years, between 5 and 9 years, and between 10 and less than 15 years, although again, males had double the rate than females. No cases of mesothelioma occurred in childhood, the youngest case was diagnosed at age 26 years. However, 17 per cent of all deaths to the end of 2009 in the former children were due to mesothelioma.[30]

Susceptibility to mesothelioma

Children in general appear to be more susceptible to exposure to environmental pollutants, than adults.[31] Work from the UK has suggested that children have a greater susceptibility to mesothelioma than adults.[32] We have examined this issue several times among those who were first exposed to blue asbestos as children. Follow up of the residents to the end of 1993 and an examination of 27 cases of mesothelioma found a 30 per cent reduced risk for mesothelioma in those first exposed aged 10 years or less compared with those first exposed at older ages.[33] Further follow up of the residents' cohort to 2000, and an examination of 64 deaths from mesothelioma, found that those first exposed as children had a lower rate of mesothelioma than those first exposed as adults. The mesothelioma mortality rate in children (47 per 100,000) was 40 per cent that of those first exposed as adults (112 per 100,000), and 25 per cent after adjusting for exposure and sex. No difference in the slope of the exposure-response relationship was found between the two groups.[34] Follow up of the Wittenoom children to the end of 2009 and an examination of 42 mesotheliomas found a similar rate of 44.6 per 100,000.[35] The most recent follow up to examine this question, with 119 mesotheliomas to the

---

30 Reid *et al*, "All-cause mortality and cancer incidence among adults exposed to blue asbestos during childhood".

31 W A Suk, H Ahanchian, K A Asante, D O Carpenter, F Diaz-Barriga, E-H Ha, *et al.*, "Environmental pollution: an under-recognized threat to children's health, especially in low- and middle-income countries", *Environmental Health Perspectives*, 124, 3, 2016, A41–A5.

32 *Committee on Carcinogenicity of Chemicals in Food Consumer Products and the Environment. Statement on the relative vulnerability of children to asbestos compared to adults. 2013.* Contract No.: CC/13/S1). United Kingdom Department for Education. The management of asbestos in schools. A review of Department for Education policy. London, 2015.

33 Hansen *et al*, "Malignant mesothelioma after environmental exposure to blue asbestos".

34 Reid *et al*, "Age and sex differences in malignant mesothelioma after residential exposure to blue asbestos".

35 Reid *et al*, "All-cause mortality and cancer incidence among adults exposed to blue asbestos during childhood".

end of 2014, found a rate of 76.8 and 121 per 100,000 among Wittenoom children and adults respectively.[36]

Overall, we do not find that those who were first exposed to asbestos as children at Wittenoom have a greater risk of mesothelioma than those first exposed as adults. However, given the long latency of mesothelioma, and the greater years of life yet to be lived by the Wittenoom children, it is likely that there will be more cases of mesothelioma in the future among those first exposed as children.

Lung cancer

Few lung cancer cases were found in the Wittenoom children to the end of 2009, three in males and five in females. Neither incidence nor mortality from lung cancer was in excess in the male and female Wittenoom children, compared with the WA population.[37]

Cancers compared with Western Australian population

The risk of developing cancers, other than lung cancer, was considerably greater in the former Wittenoom children than the WA population. To the end of 2009 there were 215 cases of cancer diagnosed in those first exposed to asbestos as children. Among females, there were 95 cancers, with the first case being diagnosed in 1970. The most frequent cancers were breast (28), mesothelioma (13), melanoma (11) and ovarian (6). Compared with the WA female population, former female children from Wittenoom had excess risks of mesothelioma (between 70 and 113 times greater risk), all cancers (between 12 and 72 per cent excess risk), brain cancer (four-fold excess risk), and ovarian cancer (four-fold excess risk).[38]

Among males, there were 114 cases of cancer and the most common were mesothelioma (29), melanoma (17), prostate (12), colorectal (10), and leukaemia (7). Compared with the WA male population, former male children from Wittenoom had excess risks of all cancers (between 70 and 292 per cent greater), mesothelioma (between 45 and 78 times greater) leukaemia (four- to five-fold increase), prostate (two-fold

---

36   A Reid, P Franklin, G Berry, S Peters, N Sodhi-Berry, F Brims, A W Musk, N de Klerk, "Are children more vulnerable to mesothelioma than adults? A comparison of mesothelioma risk among children and adults exposed non-occupationally to blue asbestos at Wittenoom", *Occupational and Environmental Medicine*, July 2018. http://dx.doi.org/10.1136/oemed-2018-105108.

37   Reid *et al*, "All-cause mortality and cancer incidence among adults exposed to blue asbestos during childhood".

38   Reid *et al*, "All-cause mortality and cancer incidence among adults exposed to blue asbestos during childhood".

increase), brain (four-fold increase) and colorectal (two-fold increase) cancers.[39]

Mortality compared with the Western Australian population

Mortality was also increased among the former Wittenoom children compared with the WA population.

To the end of 2007 there were 228 deaths among the former Wittenoom children. Seventy females had died. The main causes of death were cancer (20 deaths including 9 from mesothelioma), symptoms signs and ill-defined conditions (10 deaths), and accidents, injuries and poisonings (9 deaths including 5 transport accidents). Compared with the WA female population, former Wittenoom girls had an excess risk of dying from all causes (47 per cent excess), all cancers (between 66 and 224 per cent excess), mesothelioma (between 76 and 99 times greater), cancers other than mesothelioma and lung cancer (69 per cent excess) and symptoms signs and ill conditions (approximately five-fold excess).[40]

One hundred and forty eight males had died over the same time period. The main causes of death were cancers (49, including 23 mesotheliomas), circulatory system (17 deaths) and accidents, injuries and poisonings (55, including 25 transport accidents). Compared with the WA male population, former Wittenoom boys had an excess risk of dying from all causes (between 50 and 83 per cent excess), all cancers (three- to four-fold excess), mesothelioma (56 to 79 times greater), diseases of the nervous system (two- to three-fold excess), diseases of the circulatory system (two-fold increase) and accidents, including transport accidents (50 per cent excess).[41]

Mental health

Studies of people impacted by other technological disasters have reported short-term negative impacts on mental health and in particular on a person's sense or locus of control.[42]

Sense of control refers to the notion that individuals have control over their own lives and act with authority and influence over it. Sense of control varies among individuals, wherein some feel they can achieve anything

---

39   Reid *et al*, "All-cause mortality and cancer incidence among adults exposed to blue asbestos during childhood".

40   Reid *et al*, "All-cause mortality and cancer incidence among adults exposed to blue asbestos during childhood".

41   Reid *et al*, "All-cause mortality and cancer incidence among adults exposed to blue asbestos during childhood".

42   M S Gibbs, "Factors in the victim that mediate between disaster and psychopathology: A review", *Journal of Traumatic Stress*, 2, 1989, 489–514.

and their successes and failures lie with them (internal sense of control), while others feel that good or bad luck, or powerful others, are responsible for the things that happen to them, and that they themselves have little control (external sense of control).[43]

In 2007, we examined the sense of control and wellbeing of Wittenoom workers and residents, four decades after the closure of Wittenoom. We found that younger Wittenoom residents (aged 30–64 in 2007) had poorer wellbeing compared with the same age group in the Western Australian population, and a more external sense of control than younger Wittenoom workers. We also found that being an adult at the time of first arrival in Wittenoom was associated with better wellbeing than being a child at first arrival, although this difference was not statistically different after adjusting for other demographic variables. Overall, residence at Wittenoom may have had a detrimental impact on the mental health of those who first arrived at Wittenoom as children.[44]

Conclusion

The Wittenoom Cohort studies have provided the most comprehensive information on the health outcomes of women and children exposed to asbestos. Clearly, exposure to asbestos from the general environment, at levels lower than that incurred occupationally, has had a catastrophic effect. Compared with the Western Australian population, Wittenoom women have a greater risk of dying from malignant mesothelioma, lung cancer, all cancers, and all causes of death. Wittenoom children have a greater risk of dying from malignant mesothelioma, all cancers, and all causes. The brief period of crocidolite mining in Western Australia's history will continue to exert a detrimental impact upon the future of the women and children who lived there, with a further 66 to 87 mesotheliomas predicted to occur in the women alone to the end of 2030.

---

43   C R Anderson, "Locus of control, coping behaviors, and performance in a stress setting: a longitudinal study", *Journal of Applied Psychology*, 62, 4, 1977, 446–51. J Mirowsky, Age, subjective life expectancy, and the sense of control: the horizon hypothesis", *The Journals of Gerontology. Series B, Psychological Sciences and Social Sciences*, 52, 3, 1997, S125–34. J B Rotter, "Generalized expectancies for internal versus external control of reinforcement", *Psychological Monographs*, 80, 1, 1966, 1–28. K A Wallston, B S Wallston, S Smith, C J Dobbins, "Perceived control and health", *Current Psychological Research and Reviews*, 6, 1, 1987, 5–25.

44   A Reid, H Alfonso, T S Ti, E Wong, N Klerk, A W Musk, "Sense of control and wellbeing decades after exposure to blue asbestos at Wittenoom, Western Australia", *International Journal of Occupational & Environmental Health*, 18, 2, 2012, 116–23.

Part 3
Damaged Communities

Chapter 8

MEMORIES OF WITTENOOM

Compiled by Gail Phillips

Wittenoom in the remote north of Western Australia was the site of a small asbestos mine and mill run by the CSR company, operating through its wholly owned subsidiary Australian Blue Asbestos, from 1943 to 1966. As the mine and mill operations expanded the township of Wittenoom grew. Unemployed people and new migrants fleeing war-torn Europe took up the opportunity for employment. Set in a beautiful part of the country, Wittenoom appeared to offer welcome opportunities to communities desperate for work. However CSR, inexperienced in mining work and eager for quick profits, ignored the basic safety and dust control standards. Furthermore, it also ignored warnings about the particular and grave health hazards from asbestos, even though these were known by the 1930s. As a result, the residents of Wittenoom suffered an appalling legacy, with men, women, and children falling victim to asbestos related diseases, including mesothelioma, over the following decades. In this chapter some of the former workers and their families recall their experiences of life in Wittenoom.

For two decades Wittenoom was the site of a working asbestos mine and mill. The town was in many ways an archetypal Australian country town with a lively social life and a diverse but close community. However everyone, managers, workers, wives, and children, lived surrounded by a pall of asbestos dust. In the years that followed no one was immune to the range of diseases that were linked to this toxic exposure. As people became aware of the toll in illness and death there was growing anger as they realised the dangers of asbestos were known at the time the mine was given the go-ahead. Those who sought compensation often found themselves bound to silence through confidentiality clauses. So the voices of Wittenoom remained largely silent. This chapter is based on oral history interviews conducted with former residents in which they have the chance to tell the story of Wittenoom in their own words at last. The interviews were collected by the Australian Asbestos Network research group.[1] The contributors are:

> Jack Carroll [JC] millworker
> Celestina Delpero [CD] wife of Wittenoom mineworker Spero Delpero
> Ted Grant [TG] child of Wittenoom and Port Samson worker
> Silvia Lovenfosse [SL] nurse and widow of Phil Lovenfosse, surveyor
> Angela Napolitano [AN] widow of miner Liborio Napolitano
> Margaret Page [MP] child of Wittenoom
> Rod Powell [RP] bogger and mill worker
> Clive Rutty [CR] truck driver
> Joseph Schrott [JS] miner
> Clarence Taylor [CT] mine worker
> Robert Vojakovic [RV] mine and mill worker

Who went to Wittenoom

In the immediate postwar period times were hard in Australia. Unemployment was high and returning soldiers and newly arrived migrants searched for jobs. The remote and somewhat hostile location of Wittenoom was not immediately appealing, but many had little choice.

> If you went up there looking for work it wasn't an adventure, was it, it was a case of that was all you could find for work. The migrants, the vast majority of them, were assisted migrants, and one of the part of their contract for the government paying their fare out there, they had to work wherever the government sent them for two years. The attitude was: "Well, it was really hard to find work, and we knew the money was good, so we went there." [SL][2]

Clive Rutty emigrated as a teenager to Australia from England in 1951 and worked in Wittenoom from 1951 to 1952.[3] He recalls the lure of the promise of employment:

---

1 The Australian Asbestos Network was a project undertaken at Murdoch University under the leadership of Professor, now Emeritus Professor Bill Musk, with support from the National Health and Medical Research Council, with the aim of collecting asbestos stories from people whose lives had been touched by it. They can be accessed at www.australianasbestosnetwork.org.au.
2 Interviewed by Mia Lindgren, 1 February and 4 July 2008.
3 Interviewed by Raymond Grenfell, 4 June 2008.

> When you stop and think that we'll fly you up and it won't cost you anything and when you have been here for six months we'll fly you back and you'll be back where you started, so it meant that people who had no money would get on a plane and go and earn good money and put up with the conditions up there and then be flown back. So it was pretty clever. The other thing is that people came from all over the world, virtually every country was represented at Wittenoom Gorge. I used to help write letters, they had come out of the war, they were very poor, they had been able to migrate out here for nothing, and with them not being able to speak the language going to Wittenoom was perfect. [CR]

Later in the 1950s the overtime available at Wittenoom and the contract payments for underground mining made it appear an attractive proposition for young men trying to set themselves up in life. Liborio Napolitano was aged 21 and engaged to his future wife Angela when he decided to take up a contract there:[4]

> At that time he knew nothing whatsoever of the impact of asbestos. All they knew was that these mines were very low, they were only a metre high, they didn't have to go deep down like they do for gold mines, so they thought the mines were quite safe. There was nothing at all mentioned about the actual product. It was very dusty but all the men didn't worry about the dust because the money was good and they had no idea whatsoever that the dust was dangerous. Deadly. [AN]

Wittenoom, the place

The tragic legacy of Wittenoom has obscured the fact that for many of the new residents it was a beautiful place. Ted Grant experienced Wittenoom as a child:[5]

> It was fantastic, it was beautiful, the most beautiful scenery I've ever seen. I was fascinated with it. I used to climb Mt Hamersley every Friday if I could, go up into the gorge with the dog, swimming in the pools. I had a friend who lived up in the gorge itself, and it was a great place to be as a kid. [TG]

---

4   Interviewed by Mia Lindgren, 24 September 2008.
5   Interviewed by Mia Lindgren, 11 March 2008.

Celestina Delpero was a young wife when her family arrived from Italy in 1951:[6]

> The accommodation was very good, the houses very nice. We got tap water everywhere, we got bath, we got toilet, and then we started the normal routine of life. We settled down, the house was there, the children was there, they built a new hospital there, we were quite happy. [CD]

Celestina and the other migrants from Europe found Wittenoom a haven after the depredations of war:

> If you came from war-torn Europe and you came to this little place in the middle of nowhere that was so beautiful, and you'd get enough to eat, your kids were being educated…as one of them said, "We were happy, we were free". We'd sit outside at night and just have a couple of slices of ham and a beer and…you know, to them it was just the most peaceful, lovely place, and that's why they stayed. [SL]

Mine work

Both mine and mill quickly gained a bad reputation for dust. Workers were used to working in dusty mine sites where the risk of various forms of lung disease was an acknowledged part of the job; nevertheless they thought Wittenoom was much worse than the rest. Rod Powell describes the conditions he encountered as a working miner:[7]

> It would have been one of the worst things in my life. The area you worked in was about four foot high, and you had to climb up a 60 foot ladder through a round hole to get to where you worked in a stope. No lights. All you had was a light on your helmet and that's what you worked in all day long. [RP]

Sylvia Lovenfosse's husband Phil was a surveyor who moved from Broken Hill to Wittenoom in the late 1950s. The mining operations differed from what Phil had been used to:

> In Broken Hill everybody is out of the mine by three o'clock and they fire and you don't go back down until four o'clock. That gives the mine time to vent and the dust to settle, and the same in the afternoon,

---

6 Interviewed by Tristan Broomhall, 20 May 2008.
7 Interviewed by Caitlin Hawkins, 5 May 2008.

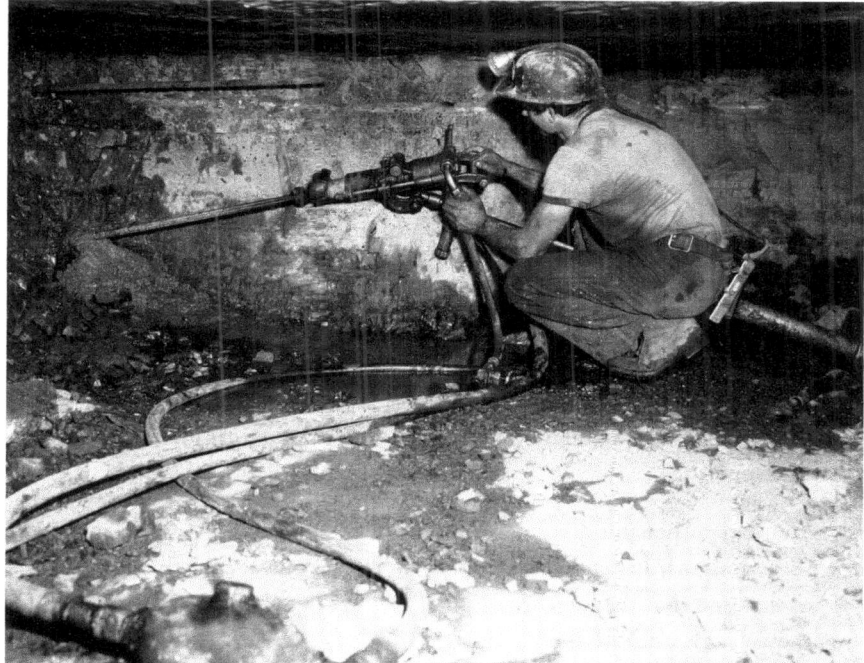

Figure 8.1: A miner drills in the narrow stope of the Australian Blue Asbestos mine, Wittenoom.
Courtesy: State Library of Western Australia.

> they come out at 11:00 and they fire as soon as everyone is out and then they don't go down until midnight. At Wittenoom he said they come out, they fire, and you go back in again. And he used to come home and the fracture fumes would make him nauseated and his back would be scratched through his clothes, he'd actually have skin off from where the backs had been...little bits that stick down had been scratching his back. [SL]

Rod Powell's work as a bogger was hard and dangerous:

> After they had exploded the face I had to shovel back 15 foot all the material that had been blown down, set up bollards like steel jacks, and feed cables through for the winches to be able to pull the metal through a big hole and drop it through into the main tunnel. After I set up the pillars they start the scraper going and it pulls a bucket over to a big hole and all the asbestos goes through this big hole and drops down onto a thing they called a grizzly [a sifting grid] underneath.

> When I first started there they put me on a grizzly and told me "all the big rocks that hadn't gone through, break them". And I thought the loco came and tipped the rocks out. They didn't tell me they were going to come down from up the top, and ten tonnes of rocks come crashing down onto this grizzly where you're standing. They only lost one person, he got pushed through and came out in pieces on the belt. That was about the spookiest part working on that.
>
> You worked on your backside. You had to shovel on your backside. A lot of the guys up there got gout because they were working in water too, and some of them had their feet wrapped up in big rags and towels and they looked like giant footballs because of the gout. [RP]

The pressure to produce was intense, and was reinforced by Rod's co-workers:

> You had to put out a certain amount of tonnes. I was working with some Italians, I was on wages, they were on contract for the amount of tonnage that they put through. If I didn't put the tonnage through they would probably shoot me! [RP]

Lack of communication with the rest of the team increased the risks of this working environment:

> It was a bit frightening because you never had any communication with them—the only communication you had was the light on your hat and you shook your hat to let them know that everything was ready to start pulling. But if you were pulling with steel cables wrapped around your shoulder and you might be 200 metres away from them and you slip and your helmet goes blink blink then they start the winch up and you've got a steel cable wrapped around your shoulder they are pulling you to a hole in the ground until you start screaming and they realise, gee whiz, stop! That happened to me a couple of times. You'd have whip marks across your shoulder. [RP]

Rod recalls one particularly dangerous episode:

> I was underground with two Italian blokes who didn't speak English and I didn't speak Italian, and we were in our stope and what we didn't know was the mine was empty and they had set off all the charges so we had to slide down this ladder to the bottom because everything started to shake and rocks started falling everywhere and we were

about one-and-a-half to two miles underground so we dropped down to the main tunnel and ran like the devil to the front entrance. And when we got up to the front main entrance they were just opening the gates to come back and look for what was left of us. [RP]

Mill work

Jack Carroll, who worked in the mill for two years from 1947, describes the job:[8]

> The asbestos came out of the mine mouth and the trucks would tip it in a great bin at the top of the crusher, then through the crusher, and sometimes they had to blast the rock in the crusher to break it, then into the next crusher, and then out onto these rotary screens, and all the mullock fell through and the asbestos stayed on top of the screen and was lifted off by suction, and that was where it started coming down these chutes. Any that fell off the conveyor belts it was one of my jobs to get under and bog it out. It just came down the chute, and you pulled it out of the chute and into the bag and round it off with a stick until what we reckoned there was enough in the bag and then sew the bag. [JC]

Rod Powell describes the bagging process:

> All the guys were standing there—there was a big long trough—I suppose it would be at least 20 foot long—and after the asbestos was teased up it came down conveyor belts into this hopper and the guys just stood there, the bag was on the floor before you, and you just pulled it with your hands and shoved it down the bag and that's what they did all day long. And you had to bag and bag otherwise it would just build up. So you had to work like a devil to get it out of the way. [RP]

Jack Carroll recalls the dust:

> They had 25 bags to the tonne and you had to ram it in pretty hard to get the bag full—it was pretty spongy stuff. There was a lot of dust. It was all dust, because it was dry mining, no sign of water anywhere. Once the bags were full they were carted away to the coast. It had to be dry because the whole mill worked on a suction process lifting the fibre out of the rock. [JC]

---

8   Interviewed by Denise Ross, 16 June 2009.

Robert Vojakovic, who emigrated to Australia from Croatia in the early 1960s, worked at Wittenoom for three months in 1961.[9] On his first day he experienced for himself the rigours of the bagging job:

> They had a cluster of people who were bagging the asbestos with their hands as it was coming down the chute. There were four of us and when one person would go to the loo or for a smoke or for a walk they wanted to make sure the asbestos was being bagged all the time so I was asked by the foreman to go and do the job, which was more or less to fill a bag with asbestos. That process seems to be pretty simple, but it is not. I think I filled half a dozen bags that first day because you would be at all times ramming with a stick because asbestos is kind of like wool and to get it to weigh 100 pounds you've got to ram it pretty hard to make it fit. I think I weighed my bag about 20 times hoping it would weigh 100 pounds! [RV]

There was little or no protective gear provided to minimise exposure to the dust:

> No protective gear I can remember except for boots which we had to buy ourselves, no gloves, no overalls. They'd never get away with it today. [JC]
>
> You never got issued with a new mask, it was just an old mask and you couldn't wear them, you'd sweat if you put that thing on. If they had been little air conditioned ones like they have now it might have been a different thing. It was a very choking sort of job. [RP]

The accommodation for the miners was primitive. Josef Schrott, an experienced miner who migrated from Austria in 1962 aged 29, was far from impressed with the living conditions for the single men:[10]

> My first impression was it looked a quite nice mining town, but the reality was it only looked good. Married people had a reasonable standard of accommodation, single men an iron hut, no inside lining, eight beds in a room of say six by four metres, the shared toilets 50 metres away in the open, semi-enclosed. My opinion then was that refugees after the war in Europe in the late 1940s, early 50s were better accommodated than the mining accommodation for single people. [JS]

---

9   Interviewed by Chris Smyth, 3 February 2016.
10   Interviewed by Linda Toovey, 14 May 2008.

From mill to port

The bags of asbestos were loaded onto trucks and transported to Port Samson where they were transferred onto ships. Clive Rutty's job was to collect bags of asbestos from the mill:

> One of the things that I remember so much was going up to the mine and getting the bags of asbestos. And the smoke in there and the asbestos dust flying around there was unbelievable. So what happened was when I went up to where the crushing mill was I had to back in so they could load all these bags of the asbestos and the dust was so bad that I couldn't see the back of my truck, so I had one bloke alongside of me while I sat in the driver's seat, one halfway down, and one at the back, and they would tell me to go righthand down or lefthand down or whatever to guide me up to where the bags were, and then they all were loaded on to the truck. I had a shirt that I used to put over my head and at the end of every day I used to wash the pillowcase and it used to be absolutely blue from the stuff out at the mill. [CR]

Ted Grant remembers the dusty conditions during the process of transferring the bags from the shed at Port Samson to the boats.[11]

> When the trucks came down from Wittenoom with the asbestos which was in wheat bags, we used to unload them onto railway trucks and into the storage sheds off conveyor belts. Dust everywhere. Working on the railways trucks there was not so much dust because the wind used to blow it away, but in the sheds it was just total dust. Dust, dust, dust.
>
> I was always in the hold. They empty the bags out of the nets into the hold and we have to pick the bag up and stow it in the hold. So every corner of the ship had a bag of asbestos in it, from the bottom of the deck right to the top. [TG]

Government monitoring of the mine site was far from rigorous:

> When the people working up there started to complain about the dust, when the inspector came up they made everything clean. The inspector is supposed to come up without giving them any warning. [CD]

---

11   Interviewed by Mia Lindgren, 11 March 2008.

Josef Schrott holds the government responsible:

> I would blame the government, not for not giving me the information, but for not enforcing the law. The company had warnings, they were told the inspectors will arrive within a day or two, so they made every effort to minimise the visual impact on the inspectors. When you spoke to the inspectors they said well it looks alright while they were there, but what happened the day or week afterwards is a different story. [JS]

The tailings

The mill generated a huge amount of waste in the form of tailings which were liberally distributed around the town, serving a variety of functions. Jack Carroll remembers the process for spreading the tailings:

> There was one old fellow there, he was a truck driver, and he had to park his truck just under the tailing chute, and all this dust pouring into the back of his truck. It was the tailings and he used to go along the road and put the tip up and pour it out on the road. So everywhere you went was covered in the stuff. [JC]

The tailings were used as a readily available building and surfacing material.

> They used it in the cement to build our houses, the floors in our houses, it was used in the septic tanks, it was used in our dry wells in the yard, and there was also quite a bit of it scattered around our yards. We had it wherever we looked. [MP][12]

According to Sylvia Lovenfosse,

> It was in the bitumen on the roads, the tennis courts, the airport, the picture theatre. The picture theatre was open-air and the little canvas chairs were sitting on the tailings, so the kids scooted down the aisles, the dust was flying up. And most of all, it was on both the schoolyards. [SL]

A feature of Wittenoom town life was the dust from the mine and mill.

---

12   Interviewed by Mia Lindgren, 4 April 2008.

> The asbestos used to hang in the trees like cobwebs. We'd go there and knock it down. The next morning, the next day, a couple of days later, it would all be back up there again. In the gorge itself, when the wind was in a certain direction blowing down from the mill towards the mine township, the atmosphere was blue, it was a blue, blue haze. You just had to be there to see it, everything was covered in this blue haze. You could be hanging the clothes on the line and it would have a blue dust on it, and that's why most of the mums succumbed to asbestos, shaking the dust off the clothes. [TG]

The weather conditions exacerbated the problem:

> The willy willies were unbelievable, wherever they went they just picked it all up and dumped it somewhere else. It was amazing. [CR]

Daily life

The houses in Wittenoom were very basic in design and construction.

> Our house consisted of a kitchen, dining room, two bedrooms, and a sleep-out. The houses weren't much chop, they didn't have any outside walls on them. You had your timber frame and you could see the actual wall of your rooms from the outside of your house. I think the only room in the house that I can recall having outside walls was the kitchen, but all along the veranda you could see all the woodwork in the inside walls. So it was really slapped together houses, throw them up there! I know we had the actual pieces of rock with the blue asbestos and the white asbestos, we had them as ornaments in our house, as doorstops, and people that came up there used to bring them home with them. [MP]

Cooking was a challenge.

> The worst thing for me was the wood stove. All those little houses had a wood stove in them, up there in those conditions. There was nothing, only a wood stove. We just turned around, went down to the store and bought ourselves a little Primus, and that's all I had. I learned to cook cakes in the little frypan. I had a frypan I'd brought with me and I had the little Primus that we brought and our jug and that's what we

used all the time. I used to cook the veggies on the Primus and put the meat in the frypan. [SL]

For the women dust was a feature of their lives no less than their husband's. As Celestina Delpero recalls,

> They used to wear this special flannelette t-shirt, very thick grey with three buttons, because they absorb. They used to take the clean shirt up, have a shower, and bring the dirty home. I tell you what, thank god I am here today because when I saw him take his clothing off and put it in the corner of the laundry, believe me or not the dust was like this on the floor. I used to put it on top of the big rubbish drum we had outside and shake it, but before I touched it I put a big scarf around myself because after a while I would start sneezing. So that was my protection. [CD]

According to Margaret Page,

> The men used to come home filthy, and of course naturally your kids go up and hug your dads. When they come home from work naturally we'd get all their filth on our clothes, not that we weren't already filthy anyway from playing in the tailings up there. Mum got a washing machine when we were up there, but up until then she used to do it all by hand, boil everything, scrub everything, and boil it up in the copper. And it didn't matter how careful you were up there, you tracked the dust and yuck through your houses all the time. Mum was forever dusting. You used to get the red dust and the asbestos dust, especially when the trucks were dumping it. [MP]

Residents also had to adapt to a rather quirky running water system which added to the challenge of keeping clean.

> The water was appalling. The pipes weren't actually on top of the ground but they must have only been about two inches under because the water was always really, really hot. Our kids had one of those little wading pools we bought for them, we got that sent up from Perth, and you would put the water in first thing in the morning and you would empty it out at night, or you refilled it again at night if you wanted to so it was nice and cool so they could play in it, because it was too hot for them to get in. And I used to fill the bath up and leave that all day because it was the only way that I could bath the kids

because the water was too hot. And if you ask any of the women from Wittenoom, they'll tell you the same thing, we had hot water but we didn't have cold. [SL]

There was little in the way of locally grown produce and food had to be brought in from elsewhere:

> I used to get our fruit and vegetables sent up every week, I had a continuous order from Boans in Perth, it would come up on the plane. When the plane came in you had to run down to the store and get in the queue, and we wouldn't get any fruit and vegetables because the store never bought enough, so they ran out the first day. It was a company store and there was nothing else there, so if you didn't get them sent up from Perth you probably didn't get any some days. We grew a few things. I remember we found beetroot grew very well in Wittenoom. And we had our own chickens. [SL]

Medical services were very basic at first:

> When we arrived at Wittenoom there was no hospital. We got a sister there—she was like a doctor—she got the company house, and on one side there was a big room like a first aid room, and up at the mine there was a first aid room in case there was an accident. The doctor came on Tuesday and Friday. [CD]

There was entertainment—dances, soccer competitions, race meetings—like so many country towns. Asbestos featured even during leisure time:

> We had shovelling competitions out in the open. It was pretty good prize money, 100 quid or something, to shovel a tonne of asbestos metal the fastest. They'd put a tonne in a heap, and the Italians used to cheat, they made themselves wider shovels so they could move more with a shovel-full! So we didn't have much chance of beating those guys. But they could throw it 15 foot, no worries—there were some pretty tough guys up there in those days [RP]

In 1948 when Margaret Page was in Wittenoom there was no dedicated school building:

> The school that we attended was one room in the staff accommodation out at the staff quarters at the mine. It was just one classroom and they were from first stage school until grade six. Most of the other

kids were the mine bosses' kids that lived out at the mine settlement and that's where the store used to be and staff accommodations and of course our school room. Of course you had all the tailings and everything from the mine all around the place. [MP]

They didn't escape the tailings on their way to school:

We went out to school on the back of the ute, sometimes the same bus the miners used which was full of asbestos dust. In the township itself where they were building there was heaps and heaps of tailings which naturally all us kids played in, and yes we used to get so dirty, and of course we didn't know no dangers. [MP]

By the time Ted Grant came Wittenoom in the 1960s a school had been built:

I think it was purposely built there, with shutters and everything and a veranda all the way around with oleander growing all the way around it and water cooler out the back made out of spinifex and the water used to run through the spinifex so you can get cold water, go out and have a cold drink. [TG]

Childhood in Wittenoom

As far as the children were concerned, Wittenoom was a paradise.

I loved the place. I'm a person that likes outdoors and scenery, and to me that was an ideal scenic spot for me. Even at ten I loved the hills and the scenery, I loved to go out to the swimming holes and go swimming. And when I left there I always swore and declared I was going back there. On the weekends I used to love hill climbing, so when all my chores were done Mum used to let me go for a walk up the hills, and I loved it up on the hill, but little did I know the higher up I was getting the more I was exposing myself to all the dust and that. When we got the dust storms you couldn't see a thing, it was so thick and bad. [MP]

I never wore shoes. The only reason I wore shoes was when I was climbing Mt Hamersley because of the spinifex. The view from the top of Hamersley was fantastic, I still remember looking out there, seeing the willy-willies, watching the planes come and land, and you could see forever, forever. The eagles flying. It was always blue sky, always. [TG]

The swimming hole was a favourite place for the children:

> They didn't have a swimming pool at Wittenoom but up the road to the mine there was different pools that you could go swimming in. And from the township to the mine was seven miles, so it wasn't hard to get on your bicycle and ride up there. So we'd ride up there a couple of times a week. I'd go up there and go swimming in the river just at the bottom of the mine. [TG]

The asbestos bags and tailings featured in many of the children's games.

> The bags that we used to play bag races in, they all came from the mine. Nobody knew any of the dangers that we're up there living… what the companies knew were going to kill us, and yet they didn't tell anybody or do anything. And they just let us play in the bags. Unreal. Because every time we had sports day we were in our bags, jumping around. [MP]

Ted Grant recalls playing with the tailings:

> It was soft, stopped you getting sore feet, that's about all it is. You threw it at one another, sucked it, played in it, rolled in it. We'd throw the stuff at one another, didn't hurt, it was just dusty. We'd break the limbs off the oleander to make them into golf clubs and knock a tennis ball around the yard. Wrestle in it. It was about four inches thick. And you didn't play anywhere else except on that because it was pea gravel and that's not nice to walk on, it's like being on roller skates without being on roller skates. It couldn't do you any harm. There was nothing ever said, nobody knew. [TG]

Wittenoom's deadly legacy

The time at Wittenoom was to cast a shadow over the lives of all its residents. As the years went by, people started to die of asbestos related diseases, including the deadly cancer mesothelioma. Twenty years after working as a miner at Wittenoom Josef Schrott was diagnosed with asbestosis. As he looked about him he saw he was not alone:

> In the time I was up there I made good friends with probably a dozen people and there is none of them alive at the present time. This is hard to express. I accept that I worked in an environment where I should

have had more warning. It was my decision to work at Wittenoom. Would it have been fully explained to me what the after effects were of working in that environment in hindsight I might have said I will go back to another mining environment where the risk is less. I knew there were certain risks involved, but being young, ten foot tall, I said "well, I take the risk and whatever happens, bad luck". [JS]

Ted Grant, both a child and then a worker at Port Samson, saw the writing on the wall in what had happened to his own father who died of mesothelioma:

I saw Dad and I knew that my turn will come because I was at Wittenoom and I worked at it, in Samson, in the sheds and on the ships. For Dad it was 20 years, for me it was 50 years. Asbestos is a time bomb, so it just takes time, it will catch up with all of us some time or other. [TG]

While Rod Powell escaped the disease many of his co-workers were not so lucky:

A few of the young blokes that I worked with lost their lives because when they finished work they would hop in the top of the big semi-trailers loaded with asbestos, lay on top of the bags, nice and comfortable, and sleep all the way to Port Hedland. So they were laying on it breathing it in because there were no warnings about it, they didn't know. I suppose you get a little bit angry when you think about it that you weren't told—I am just lucky I am still healthy. [RP]

Hardly a family escaped—and cases of asbestos related disease were not confined to the older generation. The former children of Wittenoom began to get sick.

There was a boy I interviewed who lost his sister with meso. She died about 36, leaving behind two small children. We knew that some of the wives were dying, and they were saying it was because they washed their husbands' clothes, but we didn't know the children were dying until then. [SL]

The survivors live with a permanent sense of dread that they would be next.

I have lost quite a few of my family with it, which is sad. From a family of 11 that went up that way, there's only six of us left, and there's

> only two of my sisters that have not been diagnosed with it as yet. And because I've flared up now, well, I should say they're living in fear waiting for the results of whether they're going to get it. But you just never know when it's going to come, it just hits you. [MP]
>
> It's really hard to come to grips with it, it's sort of like having a big horrible bird sitting on your shoulder all your life and you're looking over your shoulder wondering when it's going to pounce on you. [SL]

For former Wittenoom miner Liborio Napolitano a sense of impending doom ruined his life. When in the 1970s the media began to report cases of asbestosis and cancer in former Wittenoom workers he began to worry obsessively about the chances of his life being cut short, as his wife Angela recalls.

> At that time he was in his 20s and he thought by the time he was in his 40s he would be ill with asbestosis or get cancer. He became very fearful. It was very hard to live with because at the time we had a child that we knew we were going to lose and this also made things even worse because he thought "if something happens to me my wife's going to be left with this sick child on her own". [AN]

His fears were exacerbated by what he observed amongst his circle of ex-Wittenoom workers:

> As the years went by in the 70s we started to lose friends and by the 80s we had lost quite a few that had actually been working alongside him in the mines, and this was very, very frightening as it was like "my turn will be next". He tried not to think about it, but we found as our friends were getting sick and some were dying it became harder to disassociate yourself from these fears because you could see it happening in front of your very eyes. [AN]

It impacted on their social life as he began to dread being in their company:

> We went dancing a lot to the Italian clubs and that's where most of our friends went, and a lot of our friends were the people from Wittenoom and it became a place where we didn't want to go anymore because when he got there, there was always someone who knew of someone who had just got sick, and then he would come home and he found he couldn't sleep at night because he was worrying about

what had happened to his friend and that he may be next. It was just frightening. [AN]

In the end in 1994 Liborio's worst nightmare was realised and he contracted mesothelioma. Before succumbing to the disease he fought successfully in court for compensation for the blight the fear of sickness had cast over his life.

For Sylvia Lovenfosse the cause of the epidemic among former Wittenoom residents was evident:

> The reason that the incidence of mesothelioma is so high in the town is that the town was 13 kilometres from the mine and they effectively moved the mine to the town when they brought all those tailings in. They just brought it in by the truckload and put it everywhere. If that hadn't moved off the lease, it would have been like most things, it would have been the men that got affected, the workers, but they've had school teachers, they've had the postman, the children should never have been affected. They have had lots of people like that that lived and worked in the town and never went near the mine, die of meso. [SL]

This led to a terrible sense of regret amongst former residents:

> We do have our regrets that we were ever taken up to Wittenoom Gorge, and it's a terrible shame that this thing has come from Wittenoom Gorge with Wittenoom being such a beautiful place. It's an absolutely tremendous place, and it's just a shame that it was such a killer of a place. [MP]

Clarence Taylor, who worked in Wittenoom in the 1960s, lost both his wife and his son to mesothelioma, for which he carries a huge burden of guilt:[13]

> What I had was about three-and-a-half years of happiness [living in Wittenoom] and I am paying very dearly for it now. How can you lose one of your children and your wife and say I'm in front. You're not. Your life is destroyed. I wish to God I had never gone to that damned place. I feel as though I murdered my wife and I murdered my son. I was the one that took them. [CT]

Many felt a great sense of anger at being left in ignorance:

---

13   Interviewed by Lim Phaik Chien, 17 May 2008.

There was nothing ever said, nobody knew. And then I find out in later years that in 1898 they knew about it, in 1926 they had a symposium, in 1936 they also had another one. So they knew in 1956 the dangers of asbestos and they were still mining it. [TG]

The pain felt by these casualties of Wittenoom was exacerbated by the lack of government assistance:

I got sick and had to stop work, so because I was not gainfully employed I don't get the same sort of payout as if you're still working and get a payout. So you've got to try and survive on what's the minimum that they give, whereas I think everybody who was up there, we've all been given a life sentence, and we should be treated accordingly. [TG]

That the sufferers had to engage in long legal battles that were necessary to receive even meagre amounts of compensation added to their bitterness:

I never really had any knowledge of it being dangerous. It was only years and years later that people started protesting and people were dying with it. I even lost a brother who died from asbestos. That has gone over my mind so many times, laying in bed and going back, just laying there and thinking about the past.[CR]

Like so many others ex-Wittenoom worker Robert Vojakovic was ignorant of the risks attached to asbestos exposure:

I had no idea of asbestos dangers. I didn't know of asbestos dangers until around seven years later when I was reading about it in one of the magazines. [RV]

Robert gradually became aware of the toll asbestos was taking on the former Wittenoom community and with his wife Rose Marie founded the Asbestos Diseases Society of Australia to provide advocacy, advice and assistance (see chapter 14 in this book). For them the battle is ongoing:

Rosemary and I only got involved to save lives. People are dying around us, uncompensated, but I am more interested in saving lives. I got involved in this conundrum but the job is not finished. I am just locked into a system and every day I am hoping that something will change, but generally speaking I am just as much involved as any other person who is sick, the only thing is, he is worried about himself and the family, and I worry about him and many others. I am disappointed I didn't save more lives. [RV]

Chapter 9

WORKING AND LIVING IN BARYULGIL

Compiled by Lenore Layman

> It seems our Kooris were working in mines for over forty years and they've been dying from lung diseases. Down there in Sydney they're screamin' bloody blue murder about it. Asbestos is in ships and school classrooms and the workers won't touch it! What about our poor blackfellas, aye? Nobody cares about them! ... That's the story of our lives, us Kooris. Look at all that mob that can get sick from it. Not only that! How about the kids?
>
> Ruby Langford Ginibi[1]

Baryulgil on the Clarence River near Grafton in northeastern New South Wales is home to Bundjalong Aboriginal people. Baryulgil Square was created in 1918 as a settlement to accommodate Bundjalong people no longer needed to work on Yulgilbar Station as well as those camped along the Clarence River. It was a Koori community linked in kinship networks and was gazetted an Aboriginal Reserve in 1960.[2] As in the rest of Australia, the community faced racial segregation

---

1   Ruby Langford Ginibi, *My Bundjalung people* (St Lucia: Uni of Qld, 1994), 167.
2   House of Representatives Standing Committee on Aboriginal Affairs, "Effects of asbestos mining on the Baryulgil community", *Report* (Canberra: Australian Government Publishing Service, 1984), 11. Also transcript of evidence, 6 February – 23 August 1984, 2392.

until recently with Aboriginal children removed from the state school in 1935 and separately schooled, the latter mainly through the efforts of Jack Patten.[3] *Discrimination was common and living conditions poor.*[4] *However people were proud to have steady work—at the white asbestos (chrysotile) open cut mine and mill.*[5] *Mining began during the First World War but ceased in the mid-1920s. The mine was revived and expanded from 1942 when the Wunderlich company resumed mining. It became a joint venture with James Hardie from 1944 until 1953 when James Hardie purchased Wunderlich's interest. James Hardie ran the mine through a wholly-owned subsidiary until 1976 when Woodsreef acquired the venture.*[6] *The mine was shut down in 1979; the asbestos tailings that had been spread throughout the community were covered over, and the site was remediated, but concern for the health of residents resulted in the establishment of a new centre five kilometres away at Malabugilmah to which many remaining residents moved. Only a few families remained at the Square. In this chapter Baryulgil workers and residents tell of life and death amid a sea of white asbestos.*

Family lives damaged by asbestos

Generations of the large Mundine family lived at Baryulgil. For Michael (Mick) Mundine memories are mixed:

> There were nine of us: six brothers and three sisters. We lived in a house with a dirt floor, no electricity, no sewerage. We lived the hard life but there were good times as well. In summertime, at lunch break, we'd run to the creek and have a swim. I remember playing rounders with our granny, and dancing while she played the piano accordion. We might have been poor but there was a lot of love and caring and sharing in those days. My dad, uncles, cousins, my brother, Tony, they all worked at the mine. When we were kids, we'd take lunch out there for the men and we'd play in the asbestos tailings. Family and friends have died as a result of the asbestos. Their deaths were slow and painful, and a lot of them never got compensation for it.[7]

Brother Tony Mundine, who found success in boxing, remembered "hard times".

---

3   *Daily Examiner*, 13 August 1935, 3; 21 September 1935, 4; and 5 November 1938, 7. *Koori Mail*, 29 February and 8 March 2016.
4   *Truth* (Sydney), 20 June 1954, 47.
5   For a history of the mine, see J McCulloch, "The mine at Baryulgil: work, knowledge and asbestos disease", *Labour History*, 92, 2007, 113–29.
6   1984 Inquiry, *Report*, 41.
7   *The Saturday Paper*, 12 July 2014.

> My dad was 6ft 3in (190 cm) and solid. When he died at 51 he was like a bloody matchstick. The cancer killed a lot of his brothers too and some of my sisters. Where I grew up we had no electricity. After my youngest brother Leon was born my mother's spine was damaged and she lost the use of one of her legs. She had to raise nine kids in a shack dad built at Baryulgil. We had no running water either, and when she had to wash she used to drag herself on one leg to the creek and sit there from daylight to dusk.[8]

He also reflected on the toll asbestos had taken on his family.

> I've lost my father, the five uncles, all of my three sisters and two of my four brothers. It's something you never really get over, and to walk through the graveyard knowing so many of the people who are buried there is just too hard to see. Money doesn't mean much when you look what the mine has done to the community, the ones who will receive it won't have long to live anyway.[9]

Cousin Warren Mundine explained:

> All my uncles worked there. My aunts used it [asbestos tailings] to stuff into sewn sheets to make eiderdowns to keep them warm. Mothers and sisters would wash the asbestos dust out of the men's work clothes. They used the asbestos bags to line the inside walls of their homes. The kids walked across the asbestos-filled earth, kicking up the dust and fibres, and played in the asbestos dunes at the mine. It was soft and fluffy and fun and, although we didn't know it then, it was death. All Dad's brothers died in their forties and early fifties from mesothelioma, asbestosis and other dust diseases. As did most of his brothers-in-law and many other family members.[10]

Lillian Williams, a Yaegl elder, raised her family at Baryulgil. Her husband Norrie, who worked at the mine, died of suspected asbestos related disease in 2010 and her son Ffloyd Laurie, who played as a child in the tailings, was diagnosed with mesothelioma in 2016.[11] He did not work at the mine. She remembered an environment suffused with asbestos.

---

8   *Courier Mail*, 4 March 2017.
9   *Daily Examiner*, 20 March 2006.
10   Warren Mundine, *Warren Mundine in black + white: race, politics and changing Australia* (Sydney: Pantera Press, 2018).
11   ABC North Coast, 30 September 2016; www.abc.net.au/news/2016-09-30/baryulgil-facing-more-asbestos-illness/7892452. Accessed 11 October 2018.

> When you looked up in the skies some days all glitter. All us women there we would do washing for our kids, the men that worked there we had to wash their clothes. We went through a lot with asbestos too. I'm suffering with chest trouble, everything. I was a healthy girl, runner in my day, healthy; but today I can't even travel too far in the car. All in my reports I've got "asbestos related". I can't shake what I've got. There's no escape, because this was there. The kids used to play in it, they used to build sandcastles up near the mine. The trees, the lemon trees, they all had the dust on them too. And the fruit and the water what they got from up at the mine. It's always going to be in your mind that it's going to come at you; it's going to hit you. We all loved it, my kids call it home today, but the danger was there.[12]

Lillian's son Ffloyd grew up amid that danger.

> We used to have it all around our yard—we used to play marbles, we used to make pancakes and we didn't know what it was.[13]
>
> My father worked on the mine and we used to go up and see him where he was working. Dust would float around us and we'd ride on the equipment. We used to eat the fruit near the mine; we never used to wash it off.[14]

White dust everywhere

Pauline Gordon was married to Ken who worked at the mine for 20 years and they raised their family in Baryulgil. Here she describes the contamination that surrounded them in 1977 when the mine was still operating.

> When he comes home to me of an evening he's covered from head to foot with white dust. It is on his clothes; he's got it all through his hair! You can see the fine pieces of fibro all through his hair and in his nose and in his ears, in his clothes, and when I wash his clothes you've got to soak them and rinse them about ten times.
>
> Oh the wind just blows the dust and it comes in on your clothes, in through your window and in on your cups and plates and everything because the housing facilities are no good, you know. They're just rough; we just built them ourselves, and made do. And our

---

12   ABC North Coast, 30 September 2016.
13   ABC North Coast, 30 September 2016.
14   *The Guardian. The Worker's Weekly*, 12 October 2016.

children—well, ever since my kids were born, ever since they could walk, they've been playing in heaps of shivers and coming in snow white, covered in dust. They've been in with bronchitis all the time.[15]

The spread of asbestos tailings

Tailings or "shivers" were spread around the entire community from the commencement of mining until 1977 when the practice was ended. Roads were surfaced with tailings for 25 years to stop them becoming boggy. The foundations of buildings, children's play pits, footpaths, road verges, driveways and backyards were all covered.[16] "Makes me shudder", Pauline Gordon said of these past actions.[17]

> We told the children to play in the white dust as we thought it was cleaner than the red dust. People from the mine used to deliver piles of tailings to each house for the kids and the street used to be completely white from the dust.[18]

Scott Monaghan who went to school at Baryulgil remembers the tailings spread everywhere:

> At the school the foundations and inside the footings of the building, works were conducted and asbestos was used in and around the school quite widely—in the sandpit; on sports days it was used for the high jump pit and long jump pit. And basically there wasn't a road in Baryulgil that wasn't covered in asbestos tailings simply because it was free and the overburden pit at the mine was large. It's always in the back of your mind. You try and block it out but I think for most people up here it's simply a fact of life.[19]

Poor living conditions

In its submission to the federal government's 1984 inquiry into the effects of asbestos mining on the Baryulgil community, Sydney's Public Interest Advocacy Centre highlighted the poor living conditions at Baryulgil.

---

15   M Peacock, researcher and presenter, *Asbestos—work as a health hazard* (Sydney: Australian Broadcasting Commission, 1978), 105–06.
16   1984 Inquiry, *Report*, 13.
17   *Asbestos—work as a health hazard*, 106.
18   *Daily Examiner*, 20 March 2006
19   ABC North Coast, 30 September 2016.

Houses were modest to say the least, the roads were dirt tracks, overcrowding was common, running water was not available until 7 years ago [1977], and electricity was connected in May this year.

Baryulgil was an Aboriginal reserve and therefore severely disadvantaged but its access to employment gave it a marked sense of independence and pride that it had left "the welfare time" behind, as Rex Marshall explained to the 1984 inquiry.

It has only been 17 years since the referendum to give Aboriginals equal rights. A lot of us worked before that time at the mines. We were still working under the system of the old Aboriginal rights, the welfare time. One thing I could say about the reserve over here and the people is that they are very independent people.[20]

An Aboriginal workforce

Over the life of the mine Aboriginal workers made up 85-95 per cent of the labour force.[21], One of those long-time Aboriginal workers, Neil Walker, expressed both pride and disillusionment at the situation.

I suppose if we knew the dangers then and we knew what we know now then there would have been no mine operating because the mine was wholly and solely run by Aboriginal people. The only jobs that they did not handle were the engineer's job and the manager's job. That is because they would not give us a go at it.[22]

The workforce was never large, for instance numbering 35 in 1949, 46 in 1961, and 63 in 1972, before falling to 14 by 1975.[23]. There was a core of long-time workers. In 1972, of the mine's 63 employees, 29 per cent had worked there for more than 10 years and two of these for 28 years. Another group were very recent (and perhaps transient) employees—27 per cent had been employed for a year or less.[24] It was a more stable workforce than

---

20   1984 Inquiry, transcript of evidence, 170.
21   1984 Inquiry, *Report*, 12. In 1961 87 per cent of the labour force was Aboriginal; *The Dawn*, 10, 7, July 1961, 22.
22   1984 Inquiry, transcript of evidence, 169.
23   *Daily Examiner* (Grafton), 29 October 1949, 11. *The Dawn*, 10, 7, July 1961, 21–23. 1984 Inquiry, transcript of evidence, 677, and document submission, 2295 and 2933–35.
24   James Hardie Baryulgil Plant, April 1972. Aboriginal Legal Service of NSW, 1984 Inquiry, document submission, 2933-35.

Wittenoom's where the average length of employment was 4 months.²⁵ Total numbers of workers at Baryulgil over the mine's 37 years of operation are difficult to gauge, estimates varying between 200 and 300 men.²⁶

Poor working conditions

The plant buildings were primitive, showers cold and mine site regulations inadequately unobserved. With no dust extraction systems the old mill was so dusty "it was impossible to see anywhere".²⁷ Although the new mill (operational from 1959) was less dusty, both mills and quarry were very dusty workplaces with few amenities, as Neil Walker recalled:

> Terribly dusty it is. Down in the quarry it's dusty and up in the mill it's worse…you can see it in the air, travelling through the air all the time whether it's windy or it's a clear day. The dust is there. It's there all the time.²⁸

By the dust standards of the time—million particles per cubic foot in the 1960s and 4 fibres per cubic centimetre in the early 1970s—it was an excessively dusty workplace. Masks, sometimes called half-face respirators, were supposed to be worn by all those working at dusty stations. However, as at Wittenoom, these mill and mine workers could not do their manual work, indeed could not breathe, in masks that quickly clogged up, as Greville Torrens described:

> It was definitely no good having protection and that on you when you work and lose a bit of sweat. It needs a little bit of sweat to get wet and you start to suck it back. That's how bad they were. I chucked them away.²⁹

Almost all workers held this opinion of dust masks, even management conceding that they provided only 10–15 minutes protection before becoming clogged and choking the wearer. They also increased sweating and discomfort, especially during the summer heat.³⁰

---

25 L Layman, "Work and workers' responses at Wittenoom 1943–1966", *Community Health Studies*, 7, 1, 1983,1–18.
26 *Asbestos—work as a health hazard*, 110.
27 1984 Inquiry, G F Burke, transcript of evidence, 178.
28 *Asbestos—work as a health hazard*, 113.
29 1984 Inquiry, transcript of evidence, 154
30 1984 Inquiry, transcript of evidence, 706–11.

Bagging

Bagging was the dustiest job at the mine and its danger was increased because management sometimes re-used the hessian fibre bags, introducing both brown and blue asbestos into the workplace.[31] This raised the risk of mesothelioma. Greg Harrington who worked as a bagger in the mill from 1962 to 1968 remembered the practice.

> I worked on bagging. There were two different sized bags they were using. They were using 100 lb bags and they were using 50 lb bags. We had to use those big bags when we ran out of the smaller ones and those big bags had asbestos fibres in them and they were a different type of fibres to what we were using. Some of the bags had brown fibres in them and some has real blue fibres and they were long fibres. I was instructed to turn the bags inside out and get rid of the old fibre.
>
> Some of those bags had holes in them and they could not use them and some of the Aboriginal people working in the mine used to bring those old bags home and they used to use them for doormats and carrying wood. I was one of them who used to bring those old bags home.[32]

The bags of fibre were then loaded onto semi-trailers for transport from the mine, the loading process another extremely dusty and dangerous one. J Winters who was an Industrial Hygiene Engineer with James Hardie provided this description in 1971:

> It is performed by six men each week and takes about one hour to complete. None of the men wear masks and as it is heavy physical work the men's breathing rate is very high, consequently their exposure is great. Probably the one redeeming feature during the testing period was the stiff breeze blowing which dispersed fibre away from the loading area. Without this, dust levels would have been many times greater than the 29.0 fibres c/c recorded.[33]

At this time the official standard was 4 fibres c/c.

---

31   1984 Inquiry, G F Burke manager, transcript of evidence, 184.
32   1984 Inquiry, transcript of evidence, 162-63
33   J Winters, Industrial Hygiene Survey Baryulgil 1971, 1984 Inquiry, transcript of evidence, 2923.

WORKING AND LIVING IN BARYULGIL

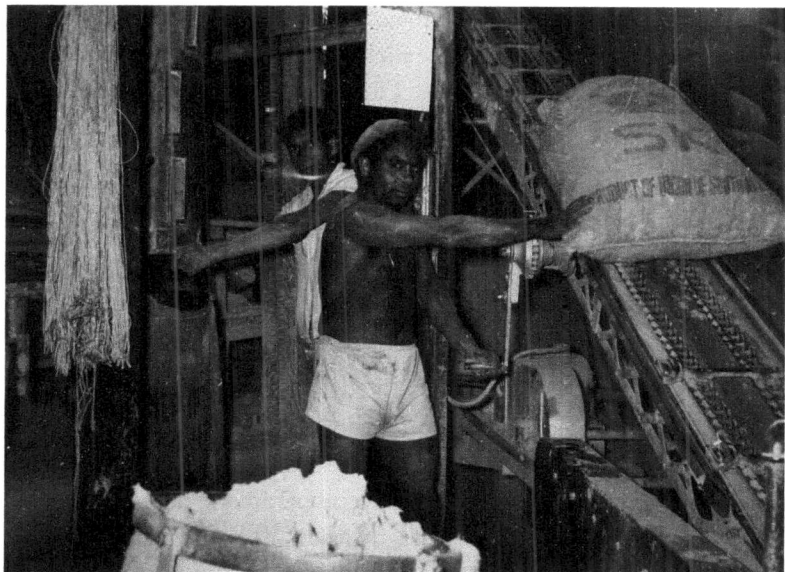

Figure 9.1: Workers bag asbestos fibre at Baryulgil mill
Courtesy: Darcy McFadden/*The Northern Star*

It is not therefore difficult to see where the dust that enveloped Baryulgil came from. The very worst source was the bag house, the dust collection building which James Hardie's Medical Officer, S F McCullagh, himself described in the following terms after a 1972 inspection.

> This is unquestionably the worst dust source. I inspected the mine on a quite still day after much recent rain. Nonetheless billowing clouds of fibre could be seen coming from this building and Mr Burke [manager] tells me he has, on occasion, seen such clouds from distances of several miles. We have, on previous occasions, obtained counts of about 1000 f. cc here and I have no doubt that the count was of that order when I made my inspection.[34]

This was an extraordinary 200–300 times above the official standard. The whole building was unenclosed and open to the wind, so the Medical Officer recommended enclosure.

No worker was stationed constantly in this building but the dust collector bags had to be regularly emptied manually, so someone had to enter the building and do the job as quickly as possible! Angus Cave recalled the procedure:

---

34   1984 Inquiry, 14 December 1983, document submission, 93.

We didn't wear masks or any protective gear...[you'd] take a lungful of air, walk in and you've got a stick...to beat the bag. You'd stand there and beat it like a carpet ... I'd be out of breath. I'd shoot outside, and breathe in, go back in, and it would take two or three times to change the bag.[35]

As at Wittenoom, working in the mill was dustier and therefore more hazardous than working in the mine itself. And the solutions applied by managements to tackle the dust problem were mostly "band-aids".[36]

Cleaning up the mill for inspections

Workers remember that government inspectors' visits were preceded by weekend clean ups on overtime. At the time many saw this as housekeeping by management wanting to present a favourable image of the mine; subsequently workers became angry at the misleading picture that had resulted. Neil Walker remembered the practice during the time he worked at the mine from 1970 to 1974.

There was suddenly a big clean up job, mainly in the mill itself. First of all he [the manager] would get all the hoses and jackhammers down in the quarry and he would run it up to the mill. They would pump the air through that way. They would go around with the air hose blowing to the ground all the dust that used to lie on the beams on top, and once it hit the ground they swept it up. That was a couple of days before the mines inspector was due, and while he was there they used to cut the feedback in the mill when they were processing the asbestos in the quarry. They cut it back so that it would go through the shaker screen very slowly so there was not much dust created at the time the inspector was there. As soon as he went through the gate the manager would instruct the engineer or anyone up there at the time to turn the feedback up to full production, which would create this dust in the mill again.[37]

Evidence elicited at the 1984 inquiry from government officials confirmed it as established practice to inform management of inspectors' impending

---

35 Matt Peacock, *Killer company. James Hardie exposed* (Sydney: ABC Books, 2009), 95.
36 1984 Inquiry, G F Burke Baryulgil manager, transcript of evidence, 187.
37 1984 Inquiry, transcript of evidence, 152–53. Confirmed by W H Hindle, mine fitter 1954–1979, 279–82; and by C R Sheather, mill production foreman 1969–1972, 299–301.

arrival. To these officials this was necessary to ensure that the mine was working and their trip to the bush was not wasted time and money.[38] The parallels with Mines Department inspections of Wittenoom's plant are striking: Australian Blue Asbestos management knew of departmental visits and were also accused of clean ups, temporary "breakdowns", and slow running of the mill plant to ensure reasonably acceptable dust counts.[39]

Signs of illness

Long-term workers at the mine found themselves constantly short of breath and susceptible to repeated bouts of bronchitis. Ken Gordon tells of walking up the hill to the quarry.

> I'd have to have three or four spells… well most of the men there now have to have two or three spells before they get to the top.[40]

Yet, as Neil Walker recalls, their symptoms were not recognised as asbestos related.

> Us chaps, when we get sick and go to the doctors, it's acute bronchitis…I cough all the time: phlegm, all the time.[41]

Neil died a painful death from asbestosis in 1998. His widow Linda recalled his suffering.

> In the end he couldn't walk, he couldn't talk. Sometimes he couldn't sleep because he couldn't breathe and I would sit on the verandah at 2 o'clock in the morning. When you would see him like this you would pray for death because it was so painful.[42]

Many Baryulgil people, both miners and residents, have experienced serious respiratory problems; a very few were diagnosed with asbestos related disease but most were not, and there remains a sharp contrast between official calculations of the number of those damaged or killed by asbestos related diseases at Baryulgil and the conclusions of Bandjalong people.

---

38   1984 Inquiry, transcript of evidence, 1059–67.
39   For instance, exchange of letters between WA District Inspector of Mines, Chief Inspector Mines and State Mining Engineer, 17 March–19 April 1958. Plaintiff's Exhibits WV-04034–04042. Motley Rice LLC exhibits list, 25 September 2006.
40   *Asbestos—work as a health hazard*, 112.
41   *Asbestos—work as a health hazard*, 110–11.
42   *The Saturday Paper*, 7 November 2015.

When the New South Wales parliament was debating the successful James Hardie Civil Liabilities Bill in 2005, the Attorney General, while complementing James Hardie for extending its civil liability to Baryulgil people, advised reassuringly that "the lung checks done by the New South Wales Dust Diseases Board suggest that there are very few cases of asbestos diseases in the Baryulgil community".[43] The community did not and does not agree.

Delayed knowledge of the danger

The Baryulgil community, including mineworkers, knew little of the risks of exposure to asbestos fibre until as late as 1977 when the death of Andy Donnelly, aged 45 and a millhand at the mine for 28 years,[44] alarmed everyone.[45] At the same time the ABC's media exposé by Matt Peacock warned the community about the danger and confirmed people's long-held worries about the continual ill health of family and neighbours, especially those working at the mine. Yet two cases of asbestosis in Baryulgil mineworkers had been diagnosed at Grafton as early as 1949 and 1952.[46] These diagnoses—and others that followed—seem to have remained personal knowledge, the wider community being regularly reassured by management and advised by authorities of the prevalence of bronchitis in the community but not of the risk of asbestos related disease. Even Andy Donnelly's cause of death was disputed, with doctors disagreeing on whether asbestosis was present or not.[47]

Thus the widespread ill health was attributed to chronic bronchitis, which undoubtedly some of it was because exposure to asbestos dust contributed to its development, whilst community members remained ignorant of the great danger they faced. To Pauline Gordon it was "just rubbish":

> We did not know it was dangerous stuff going down into your lungs. It was just rubbish. The same as in a dust storm; you put a handkerchief up to your face; you do not think the dust is poison.[48]

---

43 B Debus, NSW Legislative Assembly *Hansard*, 1 December 2005.
44 1984 Inquiry, document submission, 2191–91 and 2256.
45 Neil Walker, 1984 Inquiry, transcript of evidence, 2419.
46 C C Lawrence, Aboriginal Legal Service of NSW, 1984 Inquiry, transcript of evidence, 658-60.
47 1984 Inquiry, document submission, 2191–91.
48 1984 Inquiry, transcript of evidence, 159.

To Laurie Wilson it was "just a cough":

> We just thought it would make you cough all the time, you know I been cutting cane nearly all my life, for years—and I been a ganger for years—and every day you'd come out of there covered in soot, you were in amongst it all day, but it never affected anyone, but this is different—the potential, you know it is "potent" and [before the 1970s] I've never seen anybody even talking amongst ourselves.[49]

For Neil Walker the necessity for paid work was pressing:

> You are not going to question the hand that feeds you. A lot of us could not get work anywhere else and I suppose to a certain extent we were ignorant.[50]

Journalist Matt Peacock described the Baryulgil community's surprising lack of knowledge of the risks of asbestos exposure when he first visited in 1977.

> They were all coughing, but what struck me was when I spoke to them and asked them if they knew the dangers of asbestos. Nothing. "Has anybody ever mentioned that it can give you cancer?" I don't think anybody had ever been made aware of the dangers of it. They were virtually swimming in the dust and kids crawling around in it.[51]

Workers' struggles for compensation have been long drawn out, more so than those of others who have worked in the asbestos industry. The NSW Workers Compensation (Dust Diseases) Board granted workers' compensation to only one former Baryulgil miner in the years to 1984.[52] He worked at the mine from 1944 to 1966 as a labourer, jackhammer operator and leading hand in the open cut and was certified 40 per cent disabled in February 1969 before dying of asbestosis a few months later, aged 46.[53] This single application was the only one successful out of 28 Baryulgil

---

49   Uncle Laurie Wilson quoted in Peter Webster, *White dust black death* (Victoria BC: Trafford Publishing, 2005), 104.
50   1984 Inquiry, transcript of evidence, 159.
51   *The Saturday Paper*, 7 November 2015.
52   The former worker was Cyril Mundine. C C Lawrence Aboriginal Legal Service, 1984 Inquiry, transcript of evidence, 2474–75.
53   B Virgona Chairman Dust Diseases Board, 1984 Inquiry, transcript of evidence, 1135–36. Aboriginal Medical Service, 1984 Inquiry, document submission, 2188–89.

applications received in that time.⁵⁴ Between 2000 and 2015 only seven former Baryulgil mineworkers won compensation from the Board.⁵⁵

The failures of company, government, and union

There were multiple institutional failures to ensure that Baryulgil workers had a safe workplace. James Hardie's failure in its duty of care was the principal one; it was indefensible because it was the company's legal and moral responsibility as employer to ensure the health and safety of its workforce. Regular dust monitoring was begun only in 1970 and a medical monitoring scheme for workers established a year earlier,⁵⁶ but there seems to have been neither the interest nor will to tackle the dust problem effectively at any time. Critics accused the company of waging "a paper war" on workplace dust from the late 1960s without following through to actual implementation.⁵⁷ The 1984 government inquiry concluded that, for James Hardie, Baryulgil was always "a low priority". Nevertheless the dust hazard made it the company's most dangerous workplace.⁵⁸ Dust surveys conducted by government in 1969 and 1972 show a 67 per cent compliance in 1969 and only 17 per cent in 1972. Woodsreef did rather better as employer during the mine's last years, recording 80–100 per cent compliance with regulatory standards.⁵⁹

The Mines Inspectorate also failed. The inspectors visited two or three times a year but their reports did not reflect the seriousness of the dust hazard and were not critical of management. Indeed the Chief Inspector declared in 1984 that "as far as was practical, they [management] did meet the standards of the day, which were based on the medical evidence of the time".⁶⁰ In the mining industry "as far as was practical" has been commonly adopted to explain breaches of regulatory standards, but it is surprising to see the expression used with reference to Baryulgil's extensive non-compliance. Inspectors were overly optimistic about both existing conditions and foreshadowed improvements—any failings were about to disappear. It was not until 1978 as the mine was in its last throes that

---

54 B Virgona, 1984 Inquiry, transcript of evidence, 1140.
55 NSW Legislative Council parliamentary papers, *Questions and Answers*, 15, 11 August 2015, 417–18.
56 1984 Inquiry, *Report*, 57.
57 1984 Inquiry, transcript of evidence, 781.
58 1984 Inquiry, *Report*, 63.
59 1984 Inquiry, transcript of evidence, 715.
60 1984 Inquiry, transcript of evidence, 1059.

the Inspectorate directed that workers must wear respirators (except in rest areas) under threat of prosecution. It was far too late. In general, however, the Chief Inspector did not support prosecutions: "I believe it is going to make the job more difficult if we prosecute. I see my task is to try to improve the conditions, not to rush out and prove to people that I have so many prosecutions."[61] He regarded the regulatory role as one of guiding and encouraging not policing. As well, the Mines Inspectorate did not include informing and educating workers in its tasks—that was management's job.[62] So there was little communication with the workforce.

The Department of Health took a different attitude to the Baryulgil workplace, the Acting Chief Medical Officer telling the 1984 Inquiry that "we are very concerned about the whole episode at Baryulgil and our main hope is that the findings of this inquiry will add to our feeling that such an episode will never happen again".[63] The Industrial Hygiene Branch of the Division of Occupational Health in the Health Department carried out fibre and dust monitoring at the request of the Dust Diseases Board from the late 1950s until the mid-1970s, a task these staff could do effectively. The Chief Scientific Officer, Dr Eva Francis, who oversaw most of these tests, summarised their overall results thus: "the use of dust control measures and respiratory protection were extremely limited"; but she also noted that controls improved over time. When quizzed as to why governments were slow to act on the asbestos hazard in industry and why her Division hadn't done more, she reminded everyone of the political and administrative reality: "Our Division of Occupational Health was the tip of the tail in the Health Department. I do not think many people listen to our Director. We are a very tiny Division. We were just nothing."[64] As well as being small, the Division was established to service requests for investigation of possible workplace hazards; it was not tasked with an educational role. It provided explanations to individual workers in locations it was testing in order to fulfill its technical tasks but it did not play any wider educational role.

The Australian Workers Union, the trade union covering these mineworkers, also failed its responsibility as its members' representative for which union dues were paid. It had no effective workplace presence at Baryulgil.[65] As at Wittenoom the union did almost nothing to protect its

---

61 1984 Inquiry, transcript of evidence, 1122–23.
62 1984 Inquiry, *Report*, 56–7.
63 1984 Inquiry, transcript of evidence, 1059.
64 1984 Inquiry, transcript of evidence, 1084.
65 1984 Inquiry, *Report*, 43.

members, although an organiser, T Breen, making a passing visit in 1944 could easily identify some of the problems.

> Conditions are far from satisfactory. The men are housed in huts with dirt floors and cooking at open fires with no covering to keep weather out. The recreation room is a place in name only, as the water gushes through the dirt floor and it is impossible for men to go into it. The flume taking off the exhaust is too short and the dust blows back to the men in the open cut. The Quarry Award is being observed and it is my opinion, because of the hazard of this industry, that far shorter hours should be worked.[66]

Baryulgil miners and the local community were the victims of this network of systemic failures at the centre of which sat James Hardie. While there were many parallels with the experiences of Wittenoom workers and residents there can be no doubt that Baryulgil's Aboriginality added another dimension to the community's disadvantage and suffering.

This is our country

Baryulgil stands not just as an instance of unacceptable corporate practice and regulatory failure, for Aboriginal people it is more than that, as Chris Lawrence from the Aboriginal Legal Service explained:

> It is the belief of Aboriginal people in New South Wales and, in particular, the belief of the Baryulgil community that frequently over the last 200 years Aboriginal people have been mistreated and that nowhere is this disgraceful history better illustrated than at Baryulgil.[67]

Baryulgil's people have experienced a double tragedy and the anger and sense of injustice run deep. Linda Walker insists:

> It is our land, it is our country. They came along and said it is the living conditions that are causing all the problems, the smoking and alcohol. I don't believe that. A lot of people didn't drink or smoke, a lot of them worked very hard.[68]

---

66   *The Australian Worker* (Sydney), 26 July 1944, 11.
67   1984 Inquiry, 14 December 1983, transcript of evidence, 6.
68   *The Saturday Paper*, 7 November 2015.

Pauline Gordon's was a cry from the heart:

> We live here. We can't go away and live anywhere else or in town because this is where our people and our people's father and my great-grandmother and all our people lived. We're a part of this town... When we die we'll go back into the ground where we come from... This is our own home here.[69]

---

69 *Asbestos—work as a health hazard*, 117.

Part 4
Asbestos in the Courts: The Battles for Compensation

Chapter 10

THE HISTORY OF ASBESTOS LITIGATION

John Gordon

The legal story of the consequences of asbestos disease is a long one. It starts in the 1930s when the attorney for John Manville Asbestos Corporation noted the menace posed to the company by ambulance-chasing lawyers in combination with unscrupulous doctors. Even back in the eight years after asbestosis had been named in 1927 asbestos corporations were more worried about being exposed and paying for the dangers than they were in protecting their employees and the people in the community who were being exposed to their products. That was the attitude that prevailed and continued to prevail throughout the story of asbestos well into the 1980s and 1990s. In this chapter we explore the history of asbestos litigation over this period.

Knowledge of the risks and dangers of exposing people to asbestos developed from about 1898 and continued to grow throughout the 20th century. Landmarks included the naming of "asbestosis" in 1927, the Merewether and Price/UK government report of 1930 on the effect of asbestos on the lungs, and the recognition of carcinogenic consequences (1938-1955) until, on confirmation of the association of mesothelioma with asbestos in the late 1950s, all the relevant etiologies were established.

In 1976 the World Health Organisation (WHO) and the International Agency for Research in Cancer (IARC) issued their statement confirming that there was no safe level of exposure, that no asbestos fibre was free of carcinogenic risk, that there were multiplicative consequences of smoking and asbestos, and that risks extended beyond the asbestos factory to the surrounding neighbourhood. By this time knowledge of the nature and extent of the risk posed to workers and consumers from asbestos exposure was essentially complete.

The history of litigation begins in the US in 1927, just as knowledge was beginning to dawn about the link between asbestos exposure and disease.

Asbestos litigation: US

In 1927, the year W E Cooke named the disease "asbestosis", a foreman in the weaving department of a US asbestos factory filed a claim for workers' compensation, and the Massachusetts Industrial Accident Board awarded the man compensation for disability from occupational lung disease.

The first common law damages claims brought in the US appear to be those brought in 1929 by attorney Samuel Greenstone against Johns Manville Corporation on behalf of 11 employees of the Johns Manville's New Jersey plant, alleging disability from lung damage. A settlement of US$30,000 for all the cases was agreed in 1933, and Greenstone undertook not to bring any new actions. About 20 further suits were filed against Johns Manville in 1935, but the Courts in Illinois ruled that the state Workers Compensation statutes precluded employees in that state bringing common law damages claims.

It is worth observing that managers C W Powell, K O Brown, and M G King from the Australian Colonial Sugar Refining Company (CSR) commenced visits to Johns Manville in the 1930s as they sought to use Johns Manville as a model for its Building Materials Division, of which Australian Blue Asbestos at Wittenoom and product manufacturer Asbestos Products Ltd in Alexandria, NSW were the first manifestations.

As a result of insurance industry concerns with the growing incidence of asbestos disease, 50 US asbestos companies and their insurers met in January 1935. Johns Manville's attorney Vandiver Brown took notes and recorded that the meeting discussed "the menace of ambulance-chasing lawyers in combination with unscrupulous doctors". This menace was seen to be greatest where juries decided the facts in each case. One speaker called for properly drawn workers' compensation laws that would:

- "eliminate the jury", replacing it with an appointed medical board within the workers' compensation system;
- "eliminate the shyster lawyer and the quack doctor" by limiting their fees under law;
- "permit the correcting of initial mistakes in the making of awards" by setting up hearing procedures where new evidence could be offered to contest awards of compensation.[1]

---

1   B Castleman, S Berger, *Asbestos: medical and legal aspects* (New York: Law & Business, 1984; 5th edn, 2005), 154–55.

Deprecation of medical practitioners who were alert enough—and cared enough—to see the extent of the devastating consequences of asbestos became something of a theme with asbestos producers jealous of their profits. When, in 1955, the chief of the Environmental Cancer section of the National Cancer Institute, Wilhelm Hueper, urged that "[t]he available scientific evidence is adequate for recognizing asbestosis cancer of the lung for medicolegal reasons as an occupational disease" and gave evidence to that effect in asbestos lung cancer claims, an industry representative wrote:

> Out of every one hundred people employed in asbestos industries (or any other industry for that matter), three will die of lung cancer. With a "mad dog" like Dr Hueper loose on the subject of asbestos, future claim results can be alarming.[2]

The character assassination that was later directed at Professor Irving Selikoff of the Mt Sinai Hospital—whose ambition was nothing other than, as he said to the author in 1985, "let's save some lives"—was perhaps the nadir of the US asbestos industry's disgraceful misconduct.

The first asbestos product liability claim in the US appears to have been that of Bernard Dugan, a labourer with asbestosis, who mixed asbestos in repair and construction work and who sued Johns Manville subsidiary Aycock Corporation for negligence in 1933. Foretelling a problem that was to significantly impact similar litigation in Australia many years later, Mr Dugan died in 1934 before his claim could be heard.

A 30-year insulation worker with asbestosis, Frederick LeGrande, sued Johns Manville in 1957 for failing to warn him of dangers of breathing asbestos from its insulation products that he worked with. After their failure to answer interrogatories the company was ordered by the Court to file answers and the deponent falsely claimed on oath:

> This deponent has no knowledge of any case of asbestosis ever being contracted by an applicator. Asbestosis was first contracted by an employee of this defendant at one of its plants in 1946... Since this defendant never received notice of any claim of asbestosis resulting to any persons other than our employees who were engaged in the manufacture of products, we had no reason to issue any warnings, instructions or preventions to any other persons.[3]

---

2   Castleman, Berger, *Asbestos: medical and legal aspects*, 169.
3   Castleman, Berger, *Asbestos: medical and legal aspects*, 185.

Just as the trial jury was about to be selected in March 1959, the case settled for $35,000.

Another case by an insulation worker against Johns Manville (Wenham) was settled out of court in 1961 for $10,000, but a 1960 claim by the widow of insulator Clarence Faciane, who died of lung cancer, against Eagle Picher, ten other manufacturers, and Lorillard and R J Reynolds tobacco companies was dismissed because the widow could not prove whose asbestos products her husband had used.

The 1970s brought the landmark US product liability cases which, through revelations from the previously hidden documents of companies like Johns Manville, were to expose the sordid history of the industry's calculated misconduct and attempts to cover it up, recounted by Paul Brodeur in his book *Outrageous misconduct* (1985).[4] Those cases included *Borel v Fibreboard Paper Products* 493 F. 2d 1076 (1973); *Karjala v Johns Manville Products Corp* 523 F 2d 155 Minn 8th Circ. (1975); *Yandle et al v PPG Industries Inc et al*. Civil No Ty-74-3-CA, US District Court, ED Texas, Tyler Div (Dec. 1977).

The *Borel* case was commenced in 1961 by a 40-year-old insulator, asbestosis sufferer Claude Tomplait, and concluded in September 1973 when Wisdom J on the Fifth Circuit Court of Appeal stated:

> Under the law of torts, a person has long been liable for the foreseeable harm caused by his own negligence. This principle applies to the manufacture of products as it does to almost every other area of human endeavour. It implies a duty to warn of foreseeable dangers associated with those products. This duty to warn extends to all users and consumers, including the common worker in the shop or in the field. Where the law has imposed a duty, courts stand ready in proper cases to enforce the rights so created. Here there was a duty to speak, but the defendants remained silent. The district court's judgment does no more than hold the defendants liable for the foreseeable consequences of their own inaction.

In one case in 1982, *Jackson v Johns Manville*, brought by a shipyard insulator who had asbestosis, attorney Ron Motley delivered a memorable closing argument to the jury in Pascagoula Mississippi:

> Now ladies and gentlemen of the jury, I need to spend a moment on the defences raised by these asbestos companies. I call it the four-dog

---

4   P Brodeur, *Outrageous misconduct: The asbestos industry on trial* (New York: Pantheon, 1985).

defence, and let me tell you why. There was a case one time that I was told about that happened in Alabama. This little four-year-old girl was out in the street in front of her house and a neighbour's Doberman pinscher jumped over the fence and bit her. It caused her some serious injuries, and the father had to go to court because his little girl was hurt. They got up in the closing argument and the lawyer who represented the dog owner said "Here are our defences. Our first defence is my client doesn't own a dog". In this case, the asbestos companies are saying "James Jackson wasn't exposed to our product". The second defence of the dog owner was "well we own a dog, but another dog bit her". Asbestos companies want to shift responsibility to anyone they can – Ingalls shipyard, the Navy, the Union, other defendants, smoking, silicosis. The third defence of the dog owner was "I own a dog, the dog bit the child, but the child knew the dog was dangerous; or the child shouldn't have been in the street". In this case they are going to stand up here and have the gall to tell you "we didn't know asbestos could kill you, but James Jackson should have known". Contributory negligence. They say it was James' fault. He shouldn't have been in the street. The fourth defence is "While we own the dog, and we admit our dog bit the child, the child is not hurt because of the bite. The gangrene that is in her leg came from something other than the dog bite."

In the same case, another attorney Scott Baldwin referred to the 1933 Manville settlement with Samuel Greenstone and went on:

They settled eleven in 1933, but more important when they settled those eleven lawsuits in 1933, they bought the lawyer. They made him agree not to bring any more lawsuits against Johns Manville. To me that was a signal of things to come. It is like finding a dog's tooth in a bowl of chilli. It suggests something to you.

His concluding remarks are regarded as some of the most dramatic and compelling in asbestos litigation:

You know a famous jurist many years ago said—I think it was Learned Hand—"A corporation has no mind; it has no conscience; it has no heart; and it has no soul". You can't strike its heart; it has none. The only way you can get the attention of a corporation and talk to it is through its wallet.

The jury awarded $1,016,500, including punitive damages of $500,000 against Johns Manville and $125,000 in punitive damages against Raybestos Manhattan.

By 1982 when it filed for Chapter 11 Bankruptcy protection Johns Manville had 17,000 lawsuits pending against it, and with assets of nearly US$2 billion was the most financially healthy company ever to have done so.

Asbestos litigation: UK

In 1931, as a result of the Merewether and Price report, asbestosis was scheduled as a compensable industrial disease in the UK,[5] though it excluded workers who were already disabled but were no longer in the industry, and those who had left the industry three or more years before from filing a claim. These sorts of problems—and the relative ease with which common law claims could be brought—led to claims for inhalation injury and chemical carcinogenesis being routinely pursued in the UK: *Bonnington Castings v Wardlaw* [1956] AC 613; *Nicholson v Atlas Steel Foundry* [1957] 1 WLR 613; *Cartwright v GKN Sankey Ltd* [1972] 12 KIR 43; *Wright v Dunlop Rubber Co Ltd*. [1972] 13 KIR 255 (CA). *Bonnington Castings* and *Nicholson* were decisions of the UK's highest appeal court, the House of Lords, which established that, where it was impossible to determine the amount of harmful dust contributed by the Defendant's breach of duty to the total dust inhaled, the Plaintiff need only establish that the breach of the duty had made a material (more than minimal) contribution to the totality of the harmful dust (tortious and non-tortious) which had caused the injury.

One silicosis claim—*Cartledge v E Jopling & Sons Ltd* [1963] AC 758— where the statute of limitations had expired before the Plaintiff was aware of his disease led to changes to the UK statute of limitations in 1963, whereupon time ran only from awareness of the disease.

The first common law asbestos litigation in the UK appears to have been *Sales v Dicks Asbestos & Insulating Co Ltd* (unreported), 19 October 1967.

The first asbestos matter reported was S*kingsley v Cape Asbestos Co Ltd* [1968] 2 Lloyd's Rep 201, which was an *ex parte* application under the 1963 Limitation Act by a worker with asbestosis for leave to proceed with a damages claim, the relevant knowledge of his entitlement having been conveyed by "one of his colleagues in a public house". Leave was granted and upheld on appeal.

---

5   Asbestos Industry Regulations 1931 (UK).

Shortly after came *Newton v Cammell Laird & Co (Shipbuilders & Engineers) Ltd* [1969] 1 WLR 415, which was a claim brought by the widow of a worker exposed to asbestos in ship boiler rooms from 1943 to 1955. Although the case report talks of asbestosis and pneumoconiosis, there is an intriguing reference to the deceased being diagnosed by a chest consultant with a malignancy in 1965, and being told he had "pleurisy" due to asbestos. He died seven months later. A preliminary issue on the question whether the claim was statute-barred was heard, and it was held that, as it was reasonable for the worker to be more concerned with "fighting for his life" than going to lawyers in the twelve-month period from diagnosis (of which he survived seven), it was not barred. The company appealed, but the ruling was unanimously upheld.

Then came the *Smith v Central Asbestos* Co Ltd [1972] 1 QB 244 cases. The trials ran for twelve days on the issues of negligence, breach of statutory duty, and damages in this group of seven claimants with asbestosis. The Defendants ultimately admitted breach of the 1931 Regulations, but alleged contributory negligence against the workers for failing to wear masks. The workers were successful, contributory negligence being rejected on the basis that the danger from asbestos, "especially the danger from the tiny particles which were invisible", was not brought home to the men. On appeal the sole issue was interpretation of the 1963 Limitation Act. The Plaintiffs were successful in the Court of Appeal and their claims were upheld in the House of Lords (*Central Asbestos Co Ltd v. Dodd* [1973] AC 518).

In *Bryce v Swan Hunter Group plc* [1987] 2 Lloyd's Rep 426, Mr Bryce had died of mesothelioma after working in the shipyards for many years. Phillips J found that, although the additional exposure to asbestos dust attributable to breaches of duty by the Defendants was significant in itself, it was less in degree than the exposure that he would in any event have experienced during his working life. It was not possible for the Plaintiff to prove on the balance of probabilities that the additional fibres inhaled by Mr Bryce as the result of breaches of duty by either of the Defendants were a cause of his mesothelioma. It was equally impossible for either of them to prove on the balance of probabilities that their breaches of duty were not at least a contributory cause of Mr Bryce contacting that disease.

Phillips J held that in these circumstances the Plaintiff could successfully invoke "the principle in *McGhee v National Coal Board* as identified by the Court of Appeal in *Wilsher*". Whether the Defendants' breaches of duty merely added to the number of possible initiators of mesothelioma in Mr Bryce's lungs, or whether they also produced a cumulative effect on the reduction of his body's defence mechanism, they increased the risk of his developing mesothelioma. Because he did in fact develop mesothelioma, each of the Defendants must be taken to have caused the mesothelioma by its breach of duty.

On the foreseeability of injury in areas involving developing knowledge, two cases involving carcinogenic substances which had significant importance in determining the liability of asbestos Defendants were *Stokes v Guest, Keen and Nettlefold (Bolts and Nuts) Ltd* [1968] 1 WLR 1776 (scrotal epithelioma from mineral oil) and *Wright v Dunlop Rubber Co* (1971) 11 KIR 311 (bladder cancer from chemicals used in making rubber products). In *Stokes*, it was held at 1983:

> ... the overall test is still the conduct of the reasonable and prudent employer, taking positive thought for the safety of his workers in the light of what he knows or ought to know; where there is a recognised and general practice which has been followed for a substantial period in similar circumstances without mishap, he is entitled to follow it, unless in the light of common sense or newer knowledge it is clearly bad; but, where there is developing knowledge, he must keep reasonably abreast of it and not be too slow to apply it; and where he has in fact greater than average knowledge of the risks, he may be thereby obliged to take more than the average or standard precautions.

In Wright at 272:

> If the manufacturer discovers that the product is unsafe, or has reason to believe that it may be unsafe, his duty may be to cease forthwith to manufacture or supply the product in an unsafe form. It may be that in some circumstances the duty would be fulfilled by less drastic action; by, for example, giving proper warning to persons to whom the product is supplied of the relevant facts as known or suspected giving rise to the actual potential risk. Factors which would be relevant would be the gravity of the consequences if the risk should become a reality and the gravity of the consequences which would arise from the withdrawal of the product.

And:

> It is obvious also that the duty is not necessarily confined to the period before the product is first produced or put onto the market. Thus, if, when a product is first marketed there is no reason to suppose that it

is carcinogenic, but thereafter information shows or gives reason to suspect that it may be carcinogenic, the manufacturer has failed in its duty if he failed to do whatever may have been reasonable in the circumstances to keep up to date with knowledge of such developments and acting with whatever promptness fairly reflects the nature of the information and the seriousness of the possible consequences.

A claim by a widower whose wife had died from mesothelioma, having washed his asbestos-riddled work clothes until 1965, was unsuccessful on the grounds that his employer could not have foreseen any risk to his wife from such activity before 1965; *Gunn v Wallsend Shipway and Engineering Co Ltd* (unreported, QBD, Waterhouse J,. 7 November 1988; *The Times*, 23 January 1989), which concluded:

> The reality of the matter is that ... no-one in the industrial world before October 1965 directed his or her mind to the risk of physical injury from domestic exposure to asbestos dust, except in what I will call "the asbestos neighbourhood cases" ... It is unlikely that they [the defendants] would have become aware of the risk from domestic exposure to asbestos dust before about the end of 1965.

But a contrary conclusion was expressed in *Owen v IMI Yorkshire Copper Tube* (unreported, 15 June 1995) by Buxton J (as he then was). He could not agree with Waterhouse J 'that the literature justifies the conclusion until 1960, that asbestosis was attributable only to heavy and prolonged exposure". He expressed the view that from the beginning of Mr Owen's employment in 1951, "the difficulties related to and the threats posed by asbestos were sufficiently well-known, and sufficiently uncertain in their extent and effect, for employers to be under a duty to reduce exposure to the greatest extent possible". He did so "in the context of the absence of any means of knowledge of what constituted a safe level of exposure". He accepted the submission that "a reasonable employer, being necessarily ignorant of any future potential asbestos exposure, cannot safely assume that there will never be sufficient cumulative exposure". In an uncertain state of knowledge, the risk could not (in the words of Lord Upjohn in *Czarnikow Ltd v Koufos* [1969] 1 AC 350, at p 422C) be "brushed aside as far fetched".[6]

---

6 See also *Margereson v J W Roberts Ltd.* (unreported) 27 October 1995 (Holland J), Court of Appeal, UK, [1996] PIQR P358 2 April 1996; summarised at *1996 TLR 238*, 17 April 1996; and see Steele and Wikely "Dust on the streets and liability for environmental cancers", *Modern Law Review*, 60, 1997, 265.

Asbestos litigation: Australia

In Australia the Commonwealth Government Health Department identified asbestos as a serious hazard in industry in 1922,[7] and the *Merewether and Price Report* arrived shortly after its publication. The information in it led directly to the WA Health Department and Factories Inspectorate conducting inspections of James Hardie's Rivervale asbestos product manufacturing plant and medical examinations of employees working there in 1935. Similar inspections were made of Hardie plants at Camellia, New South Wales, and at Brooklyn, Victoria, in 1938.

In 1943 Dr D O Shiels of the Victorian Health Department warned the Commonwealth Government of asbestos disease risks to workers cutting asbestos panels at the Williamstown Naval dockyards, and the Victorian Government of risks to workers using asbestos lagging in the power stations in the Latrobe Valley in November 1944. His efforts led to the enactment in 1945 in Victoria of Regulations limiting any exposure to materials containing asbestos to 5 million particles per cubic foot,[8] a limit known at the time by industry to be "a very small concentration, so small in fact that the conditions may look good even to a critical eye and still present an exposure greater than this low limit" [necessitating that] "the only safe procedure is to have recourse to actual dust determinations".[9]

In 1948, Dr Eric Saint presciently warned CSR of the potential for the Wittenoom blue asbestos mill to produce "the richest and most lethal crop of cases of asbestosis in the world's literature". Dr Jim McNulty warned against exposing workers to asbestos tailings in the town in 1958 and diagnosed the first Australian mesothelioma in 1960, publishing the case in 1962 with a warning about the mesothelioma risk from "transitory exposure to crocidolite in susceptible persons". [10]

James Hardie's safety officer Peter Russell told the James Hardie management in April 1961 that asbestos was regarded as "one of the most dangerous of industrial poisons" and by 1964 that the company had a "moral obligation" to asbestos product users to provide warnings of the dangers in using their products.

---

7   *An Index to health hazards in industry*, Commonwealth Department of Health, 1922.
8   Victoria, *Health (Harmful Gases, Vapours, Fumes, Mists, Smokes and Dusts) Regulations1945 (Vic)*.
9   Warren Cook "The occupational disease hazard", *Industrial Medicine*, 11, 4, April 1942, 193–97.
10 J C McNulty, "Malignant pleural mesothelioma in an asbestos worker", *Medical Journal of Australia*, 2, 1962, 953–54.

Thirteen years later, with its asbestos product sales booming and still with no warnings on its products, the committee at James Hardie responsible for occupational and consumer safety dismissed the 1976 WHO/IARC statement as "quite irresponsible".

The history of litigation in Australia shows the extent to which local asbestos companies sought to evade their responsibilities towards their workers. The following sections detail the Australian workers compensation and common law cases.

Australian workers compensation cases

Jones v James Hardie & Co Ltd [1939] NSWCR 129

This case may never have come to light had the author not, on a hunch, looked up some old NSW law reports in the early 1990s. James Hardie had never mentioned it in litigation before then.

Samuel Jones worked for James Hardie from 1919 until 1937. He had previously worked as an anthracite miner and a labourer. At the age of 53 he developed shortness of breath and weight loss. He died in 1939. His widow brought a claim for compensation, alleging her husband's lung fibrosis had been an injury arising out of or in the course of his employment with James Hardie. The company denied this and, for good measure, argued that proper notice of the claim had not been given which caused it to be prejudiced. Evidence from co-workers was given of the work Samuel did, raking out asbestos from rooms and bins, and of how it would get in one's nose and throat. James Hardie's works manager claimed that "the asbestos was milled and the dust was taken out of it before it was received". The dust in the mixing room was cement dust, and in any event, no complaints had been received from the workers.

A Dr Tymms was said to have investigated the factory and stated there was a "possibility of an asbestos hazard". The deceased's doctor, Dr Stanton, said he had attended Mr Jones in 1937 for "silicosis of the lungs". Three learned physicians had looked at the X-rays and interpreted the fibrosis as silicosis, and opined it was "impossible to say whether asbestos had or had not played a part". No asbestos bodies were found in eight sputum samples. Dr W E Fisher, called for the applicant, argued that, on the basis of the asbestos exposure, the terminal clinical picture could be accounted for by asbestos dust, but Drs W T Nelson and G C Willcocks felt that the death could be accounted for entirely by reference to silicosis.

Despite the dissemination of the *Merewether and Price Report* in Australia (and its role in causing the examinations of the Hardie plant and its workers in 1935 in Western Australia), no medical literature seems to have been referred to and the Court concluded that "There is nothing known as to what degree of exposure is necessary to cause asbestosis". The Court found that a conclusion that asbestos had caused or accelerated Mr Jones' death was "entirely conjectural" and that a "completely satisfying explanation for the death of the deceased is found in a ... condition of silicosis complicated by a super-added infection". It is not recorded if that explanation was completely satisfying to Mrs Jones, nor how she coped having lost her husband and the family income earner at age 53, but it is not hard to imagine.

Ian Dignam

Having heard about asbestosis in the 1930s from Johns Manville, as noted above, CSR learnt a bit more about it in September 1946 when the first case of asbestosis in a Wittenoom mill worker was picked up. Ian Dignam had been at the mill since it started in 1943, and the short period of three years' exposure should have set alarm bells ringing at CSR's Building Materials Division two years before Eric Saint issued his stunningly accurate prophesy, especially as CSR officers, apparently, believed that one had to be exposed for 10 to 15 years before asbestosis manifested.[11] It is not known whether Australian Blue Asbestos compensated Mr Dignam for his asbestosis.

Kemp v EMF Electric Co. Pty Ltd (5934/1956) (Stretton J. & Wood M) 11 September 1957) Vol III (Decisions Workers Compensation Board (Victoria) (1951-1966)

The widow of Mr Kemp brought this claim for compensation arising from the death of her husband who died of lung cancer and asbestosis. He had been "substantially exposed to inhalation of asbestos particles in the course of his employment". The Board found the death from lung cancer to have been materially contributed to by the asbestosis which had been caused or aggravated in each employment.

Murdoch v SG Sayer Pty Ltd [1961] WCR 182

The applicant, Murdoch, became disabled from asbestosis and sought compensation from the Respondent, which was the last employer who employed the worker in any employment to the nature of which the disease was due. The Respondent argued that the disease was fully established prior to its

---

11   See *Barrow & Heys v CSR Ltd* (unreported) SCWA Rowland J., 4 August 1988 (BC 8801016 at 1330).

employing Murdoch and was caused by other employers whom it joined in the proceeding. Of these, only McDonald Constructions is named in the report.

Dr John Raftos, a physician, opined that given the history of exposure over 35 years, the latest (Sayer) exposure was a contributing cause. Dr Raftos gave evidence of how asbestosis developed and progressed. The Court considered the issue of the distinction between disease and injury and when a disease commences, as well as when one is disabled by a disease. The Court had no difficulty concluding that the applicant's work with the Respondent had aggravated the asbestosis and awarded compensation accordingly.

Murray v Wunderlich Ltd WCC NSW **Wall J., 8 August 1961**
The worker was employed at Wunderlich's NSW factory and developed asbestosis. The claim was opposed but upheld.

Sarna v Wunderlich Ltd WCC NSW **McClemans J. & jury, March 1967**
Mr Sarna was employed at Wunderlich from 1949 and contracted fibrosis. Dr Raftos gave evidence of the disease, its clinical signs, its onset, and its progression. He indicated that asbestos exposure led to significant increases in the incidence of cancer of the lung and the pleura. He said the association between asbestosis and cancer was more definite than that between smoking and cancer. The claim was settled during hearing.

Burrows v WA Government Railways Commission **(1982) 1 WCR WA 177**
The 59-year-old applicant had been a mechanical fitter at the Midland Railway Workshops, commencing in 1938 (after the WA Government had received the Merewether and Price report). He developed lung cancer and, in 1980, claimed compensation on the basis that the cancer had been caused by inhalation of asbestos fibres. The Respondent blamed the cancer on smoking and "causes unknown". In the absence of a finding of asbestosis, it argued, there was no "personal injury by accident" (which the Act required at that time).

Mr Burrows had been involved in the overhaul and maintenance of locomotive boilers which were covered with asbestos insulation blocks, asbestos blankets and asbestos rope. Cutting free the asbestos blocks generated dust so thick that the men could not see for thirty minutes. By 1943 Mr Burrows was working in the drawing office and from 1949 he was a mechanical inspector, but still visiting the depots. In 1964 the applicant inspected the first batch of rail cars which had just been sprayed with asbestos. Exposure was minimal after 1965. The applicant had smoked since 1944, about two ounces of tobacco a week until 1956 and then up to six cigarettes a day. He quit from 1964 to 1968 and, after suffering a nervous condition in 1968, his psychiatrist told him to take up smoking again, which he did until 1979. He developed bronchogenic carcinoma in June 1980. He had extensive fibrous thickening of the pleura. A biopsy found asbestos bodies in the lung and pleural plaques.

The Court accepted Dr A W Musk's evidence that smoking caused 80 per cent of lung cancers and of the multiplicative interaction between smoking and asbestos. It found on the balance of probabilities that both smoking and asbestos would contribute to the cancer—and the two together were more likely to do so. The Court accepted Dr Musk's evidence that the incidence of lung cancer from the interaction of smoking and asbestos was established.

The Court found that the evidence was inadequate to show that the applicant's cancer was caused by the asbestos alone but found on the balance of probabilities that it could have contributed to the cancer, it materially (and substantially) increased the risk of cancer and on balance did contribute to it. It accepted the proposition derived from the House of Lords decision in *McGhee v National Coal Board* (1972) 3 All ER 1008 that, if the work incident materially increased the risk of injury, then it had materially contributed to it, in the absence of proof to the contrary.

Further, applying its decision in *Rees v Australian Blue Asbestos* (see Full Court decision below) the Board found that inhalation of asbestos fibres was "injury by accident" within the meaning in the *Workers Compensation Act 1971*.

Australian Blue Asbestos Pty Ltd v Rees (unreported) SCWA Full Court, Heard September 1981.

The deceased Rees had, in 1966, contracted asbestosis from his work at Wittenoom for ABA and (asbestos cartage contractor) Brian O'Neill between 1955 and 1957. He was "continuously surrounded by thick asbestos dust and fibre". He had contracted lung cancer which metastasised to the brain. He also had cardiac failure, and in November 1977 he died. His widow sought compensation, but had to establish that the death was caused by a work-related injury or disease, namely, asbestosis. The Workers Compensation Board found that the asbestosis had contributed to the death and that the inhalation of asbestos fibres which contributed to the death was personal injury by accident. The State Government Insurance Organisation (SGIO),

ABA's insurer, appealed the decision to the Full Court of the WA Supreme Court. It accepted that the asbestos could have caused the cancer because of the statistical evidence that the asbestos increased by five times the chances of developing cancer, but argued that the widow had not proved that the asbestosis had caused the cancer and death.

Burt CJ cited the High Court decision in *Adelaide Stevedoring Co Ltd v Forst* (1940) 64 CLR 538 at 564 (Rich ACJ) for the approach that a court should adopt where medical science could not fully explain cause and effect and common-sense presumptions were available to do so. He referred to the evidence of Dr Janet Elder as to what might precipitate death in a patient with asbestosis, lung cancer, and metastases, and as to the further increase in risk of cancer precipitated by the occurrence of asbestosis. Thus, applying the judgment of Dixon J (at 569) from *Forst*, if medical science could not give a certain affirmative answer to the relevant question, the Court was entitled to accept Dr Elder's evidence as providing an accepted hypothesis and a probable inference connecting the asbestosis and the death, thus discharging the burden of proof. His Honour concluded that the recent decision of the Full Court of the Victorian Supreme Court in *Dahl v Grice (1981)* VR 513 confirmed the conclusion that there was sufficient evidence to sustain a finding in law in this case that there was a causal rather than a merely temporal or coincidental connection between the asbestosis and the death.

Wallace J recounted the opinion of Dr Elder that Mr Rees had died of respiratory failure and heart failure secondary to asbestosis, with the cancer, which was caused by the asbestosis, a contributory factor. He noted the increase in risk of cancer associated with asbestosis. The certified cause of death however was "carcinoma of the lung (stroke) right hemiplegia and cerebral metastases". However, he felt it would be extraordinary if mesothelioma was compensable, but lung cancer was not. Relying on the High Court decision in *Favelle Mort Ltd v Murray* 133 CLR 580, his Honour accepted that entry of asbestos fibre into the lung constituted personal injury by accident, and that Dr Elder's evidence was sufficient to find that the lung cancer and brain cancer were secondary to the heavy asbestos exposure and its traumatic effect on the lung tissue, including the fibrosis, occasioned by the asbestos exposure.

Brinsden J found that there was a clear line of causation between the exposure, the asbestosis, the cancer, and the death and upheld the finding. He saw no inconsistency with the alternate finding that the deceased had suffered personal injury by accident.

Van-Zyl v State Energy Commission (1983) 2WCR WA pt 1 68; Workers Compensation Board and Full Court, SCWA.

Theodorus Van-Zyl worked as an instrument fitter in State Electricity Commission power stations, where he was exposed to substantial amounts of asbestos lagging between 1954 and 1977. He had contracted lung cancer and died. His widow sought compensation on the basis that the deceased had suffered personal injury by accident by inhalation of asbestos and that the death was caused by the asbestosis. Mr Van-Zyl had been found to have pleural plaques and asbestos bodies in his lungs. He had smoked 10 to 15 cigarettes a day from 1954 until 1967 and then smoked an occasional cigar until he ceased smoking in 1970.

Dr A W Musk gave evidence that the actual molecular mechanism by which asbestos caused cancer was unknown, but that animal experiments and disease observed in working populations exposed to asbestos demonstrated that asbestos caused cancer, and that was generally accepted. Dr Musk said that the risk of cancer from asbestos exposure related to the intensity of the exposure and also time from first exposure. The Board was impressed by Dr Musk's evidence.

The Board found, on the balance of probabilities, that the cancer resulted from the asbestos exposure in the deceased's employment. Further, relying on the finding in the Board and the Full Court in *Rees*, it found that the deceased's inhalation of asbestos was a personal injury by accident which resulted in the death of the deceased.

The State Electricity Commission appealed by way that a case be stated for the Full Court of the Supreme Court on the questions whether there was any evidence upon which the Board could find that by exposure of the deceased to asbestos there was an inhalation of asbestos and that this was a personal injury by accident which resulted in his death, and whether the Board had erred in law in awarding compensation. The Full Court (Wallace, Brinsden and Smith JJ) answered the first question affirmatively and dismissed the appeal.

Asbestos Common Law litigation

Cunningham v Wunderlich Pty Ltd (May 1972)

Agnes Cunningham was the wife of a Wunderlich factory worker who had worked at the Rosehill, NSW factory as an electrician from 1957. She contracted mesothelioma as a consequence of having laundered her husband's asbestos-covered work clothes. Mrs Cunningham died in May 1972, aged 57, and her husband and their two young sons brought a common law claim against Wunderlich, and opted for trial by judge and jury. At that stage, Wunderlich was a wholly owned subsidiary of CSR Ltd. After taking advice that the case was unlikely to succeed, CSR/Wunderlich settled, in 1975, for about $30,000.

Benson v James Hardie & Co Pty Ltd (Supreme Court of South Australia No. 1365 of 1975)

This would seem to have been the first common law claim against James Hardie issued in Australia for asbestos disease damages. Tom Benson had worked at Port Adelaide from 1958 to 1962 and had contracted asbestosis in January 1975. He sought an extension of time in which to bring his claim. It is not known what happened to this claim.

Maas v Midalco Ltd (Supreme Court of WA, 1977)

In 1977 a former worker from the Wittenoom mine, Cornelius Maas, aged 42, married with three children, aged 11, 15, and 16, and suffering from asbestosis and mesothelioma, issued proceedings against Midalco (formerly Australian Blue Asbestos). He had worked at Wittenoom from October 1957 until November 1959. He died before the case came on leaving his family devastated and destitute, and, to CSR's considerable relief, his widow did not continue with the claim. We know that in June 1977 Robert Darge of the SGIO had urged CSR not to offer to settle the claim—"the precedent is too dangerous and too expensive to be generous". N E Irving from CSR personnel, who had been to Wittenoom in the early 1960s, agreed. He thought the company should rely on ABA's limited liability and the "corporate veil" between it and CSR which had controlled it. "Even if the workers die like flies they will never be able to pin anything on CSR", wrote Irving in 1977.[12] In 1989, widow Reike Maas was paid damages as part of the Wittenoom group settlement.

Thomas v Gas & Fuel Corporation of Victoria (Supreme Court of Victoria, May 1978)

This was the first common law claim brought in Victoria, issued by Slater & Gordon in May 1978. The Plaintiff had developed asbestosis after three and a half years placing asbestos sheets between the outer and inner coatings of

---

12 See R Vojakovic and J Gordon "The victim's perspective", in G A Peters and B J Peters, *Sourcebook on asbestos disease*, 13 (Charlottesville VA: Michie, 1996).

cooking utensils. There was an application before Gray J., to extend time under the *Limitation of Actions Act*. This was successful and shortly afterwards the statutory corporation settled.

Meletis v James Hardie

This claim was brought by Theo Meletis who had worked at the James Hardie plant in Brooklyn from 1956 to 1974 and had developed asbestosis. The claim was issued by Slater & Gordon in November 1978 and an extension of time under the statute of limitations was granted by Menhennitt J. After an argument about document discovery in August 1979, James Hardie produced 117 documents. After an attempt by Hardie and its legal officer Lionel Denmead to involve Mr Meletis' priest to have him settle the claim at St Nicholaos Church, Yarraville, in February 1980, the claim eventually settled in October 1982 just before the trial.

Joosten v Midalco Pty Ltd (unreported) SCWA (Wallace J) 9 October 1979 (1989) AILR 499

Joan Joosten had been a stenographer employed by Australian Blue Asbestos working in the office adjacent to the old mill at Wittenoom between 1950 and 1953. This was two years after Dr Eric Saint's warning to CSR. In February 1977, shortly before Irving from CSR had observed that the workers could die like flies without pinning anything on CSR, Joan developed mesothelioma and brought a claim for damages in the WA Supreme Court. CSR denied everything, including that she had mesothelioma or, if she did, that it was caused by three years in the atrocious blue asbestos-contaminated office at Wittenoom. And it maintained this defence even after the evidence of the three respiratory specialists, Dr Elder, Dr Musk, and Dr Elphick, that it was 99 per cent likely that Mrs Joosten contracted the disease from her exposure at Wittenoom. CSR also pleaded the statute of limitations, but on this point the judge found for Mrs Joosten, holding that she had suffered no injury in respect of which time could have run until the disease was diagnosed in 1978, there having been no indication on a 1975 X-ray.

Despite holding many thousands of documents that would later be crucial in demonstrating CSR's negligence at Wittenoom, ABA's list of discovered documents comprised about 100 records. The trial in June 1979 ran for seven days. Judgment was delivered on 9 October 1979.

Wallace J found the CSR witnesses to be "impressive, well trained, technical experts". He doubted the Plaintiff's evidence that the office was never cleaned due to "the quality of its officers". None of them, except Ozzie Allan, had apparently heard of asbestosis. One of them, Malcolm King, later gave sworn evidence that he had not heard about asbestosis until the 1960s. Documents in CSR's head office, which King had written, told a different story. Presumably he had known about Ian Dignam and the things Dr Eric Saint had said, but he must have forgotten. He and K O Brown must have missed the UK Chief Inspector of Factories Reports in the CSR Library. Dr H M Rennie, who claimed he didn't learn about asbestosis until a trip to Johannesburg "some years after 1953" must have missed the sessions at the ILO Conference in Sydney he had attended in 1950 where Dr Gordon Smith outlined the causes and consequences of asbestosis and the association between asbestos and lung cancer, as well as Dr Merewether's session describing the asbestos lung and pleural cancers the UK Inspectors were seeing in asbestos workers.

Wallace J found that the office in which Joan Joosten had worked at Wittenoom was "subjected to considerable dust fallout from the mill" but that CSR had "made every endeavour to reduce the dust incidence".

C H Broadhurst, who had been the CSR officer who was informed about Dignam's asbestosis in 1946 after three years at the mill, and to whom Dr Eric Saint had directed his warning, told the court he didn't think there was any particular risk because silicosis required "long term exposure to pollute a worker's lungs and the company intended to have the dust incidence well under control before such a period of time should expire".

In Mines Inspector Lloyd's report in October 1950 (two years after Dr Saint's warning and five years after Victoria had set a statutory limit of 176p/cc (5mppcf) for any exposure to dust containing asbestos), all dust readings in the mill exceeded 300p/cc and most exceeded 1000p/cc. At the powerhouse next to the mill the count was 210, and in the men's dining room 1000 p/cc. Evidence in later cases (and documents from CSR's own records) showed that the mill was cleaned up and run more slowly when it was known that the Mines Inspectors were coming to town.

In the absence of any evidence about Ian Dignam, or any evidence from Dr Saint whose reports lay in government records that health minister Ray Young had told the parliament before Mrs Joosten's trial "had been destroyed", Mrs Joosten struggled to prove that CSR should have been aware of a risk to her health. Mrs Joosten relied on the UK case of *Wright v Dunlop Rubber* to make good her argument that the failure by CSR to have apprehended any risk from asbestos exposure led to its failure to take any step to reduce the dust which might have meant she avoided contracting mesothelioma. It was a sound argument, to be upheld in later cases of Wittenoom workers (*Heys/Barrow v CSR*) as well as children exposed in the township (*Young/Olsen v CSR*). But it did not succeed here, the judge not being prepared to attribute "culpa" to "such responsible officers". He was not prepared to condemn as negligence that which, in his opinion, "was sad misadventure". He distinguished *Wright* because there the Defendant did know the carcinogenic qualities of the Nonox S. That leads to the conclusion that, if the "responsible officers" had been honest in their evidence, Mrs Joosten was likely to have won.

With Joan Joosten's health deteriorating, an appeal was lodged and pursued expeditiously. Rowland QC thought it should succeed. CSR debated the merits of offering Bert Joosten a loan through the Wittenoom Trust. The appeal was listed for hearing on 10 March 1980 but, despite a brave fight, Joan Joosten died half an hour before the appeal was heard, and the hearing did not proceed.

It was only in 1989 that Mrs Joosten's estate and dependents, along with that of Cornelius Maas and his widow Reike, were awarded damages as part of the Wittenoom Group settlement.

James Hardie Common Law claims referred to in the QBE claim

In 1983, James Hardie's public liability and product liability insurer, QBE, anticipating an onslaught of asbestos claims, sought to cancel the policies for a wilful failure to disclose material facts concerning the insured risk. James Hardie issued proceedings seeking to enforce the insurance policies. In the Statement of Claim dated July 1983 in the proceedings in the NSW Supreme Court (14093) brought by James Hardie Industries and James Hardie & Coy Pty Ltd against QBE, seeking to enforce the policies for the asbestos disease claims brought against it, it is revealed that by July 1983 there had been numerous asbestos disease claim proceedings brought against James Hardie.[13]

---

13   *Ronald Said* (mesothelioma from environmental exposure as a worker at the Goodyear factory adjacent to the James Hardie factory); *Ronald Baker* (died 25 May 1982) (mesothelioma product liability claim from use of James Hardie building and insulation products); see *Baker v Australian Asbestos* (1984) 3 NSWLR 595; *Francis Raymond Spring* (asbestosis from environmental exposure as a worker at the Goodyear factory adjacent to the James Hardie factory); *Goodyear Pty Ltd* (nuisance claim by owner of premises adjacent to James Hardie re asbestos dust contamination – paid $20,000 in partial settlement); *James McClymont* (died 23 February 1983) (mesothelioma product liability from use of James Hardie products); *Maxwell Funston* (died 26 November 1980) (builder – mesothelioma product liability claim from using James Hardie building products); US claims arising from Johns Manville and other product

Footner v Broken Hill Associated Smelters Pty Ltd (1983) 33SASR 58

Thomas Footner was exposed to asbestos from the use of millboard between 1944 and 1952 working at the Defendant's smelter. In 1982 he developed mesothelioma. Jacobs J, in the Supreme Court of South Australia, found that there was no statute of limitations defence because there had been no damage that was more than minimal until the tumour developed and manifested. The Defendant's officers, incredibly, felt, in answers to interrogatories, that they couldn't confirm that millboard contained asbestos. However, again, giving significant weight to the evidence that mesothelioma had not been conclusively connected with asbestos until after Mr Footner's exposure, the judge found that the Defendant had not been in breach of its duty of care.

Pedrotti v Midalco

Rino Pedrotti had mesothelioma as a result of working at Wittenoom in the early 1960s. His claim had been commenced by Lavan Solomon lawyers in 1984 and then nothing much had happened. The Asbestos Diseases Society eventually called in Joan Joosten's lawyers, Taylor Smart, and the matter was hurriedly listed for a bedside hearing at Sir Charles Gairdner Hospital in February 1986. Three days before the hearing Rino was shifted out to Swan Districts Hospital, where, on the morning of the hearing, he died. His widow Maria also had to await the Group Settlement negotiated by Slater & Gordon in 1989 to obtain compensation.

Pilmer v Mcphersons LTD (SCV) (Gobbo J and a jury) (September 1985)

This was the first common law damages claim to go to verdict. Harold Pilmer suffered from malignant mesothelioma as a consequence of his asbestos exposure selling various asbestos products and loose asbestos at the hardware store and warehouse where he worked in the 1940s and 1950s. He developed mesothelioma in 1983. Peter Gordon of Slater & Gordon decided that he could pursue a damages claim, and this was successful in the Supreme Court of Victoria before a judge and jury in his claim for damages. Mr Pilmer received damages of $270,000. The case demonstrated that such cases could be won, even though the exposures which caused the disease had occurred 30 to 40 years earlier.

---

liability litigation eg; *Walters v Johns Manville Sales Corp., James Hardie & Co. Pty Ltd and others* (Superior Court of California, County of Los Angeles), (WECO72944) Filed 12 March 1984.

Hyslop v Australian Paper Manufacturers (SCV) (September 1986)
Bill Hyslop developed lung cancer and brain metastases in July 1985. A writ claiming damages against his employer Australian Paper Manufacturers Ltd was issued in June 1986. Mr Hyslop had worked in the powerhouse of its processing mill at Fairfield where he was exposed, mixing, applying and removing asbestos lagging between 1953 and 1982.

For the first time in Australia, Nicholson J, on 3 September 1986 ordered that the evidence to be taken *de bene esse* at Mr Hyslop's bedside be videotaped. The case began in the Victorian Supreme Court before a judge and jury on 17 September, but settled for $120,000 shortly after the jury saw the videotaped evidence.

Adam v Midalco Pty Ltd (SCV) (1986)
Ray Adam had worked at Wittenoom in 1948, exposed to asbestos in the mine and mill and sleeping nearby in the tents then provided as worker accommodation. He developed mesothelioma and lung cancer in October 1986. He gave evidence *de bene esse* on 30 December 1986 but died shortly after. His widow received $60,000 damages in the Wittenoom Group Settlement in 1989.

Henderson v State Electricity Commission of Victoria (SCV) October 1987, Murphy J and jury.
Tony Henderson worked as a pipe fitter at State Electricity Commission of Victoria (SECV) power stations in the Latrobe Valley between 1970 and 1979. He was exposed to substantial amounts of asbestos lagging. He had been a smoker and developed lung cancer in 1987. Slater & Gordon issued the claim which came on for trial before P Murphy J and a jury in October 1987. One witness described the lagging in the air as like "fine flakes of snow". Dr Julian Lee gave evidence for the SECV telling Melbourne how much better the Sydney hospitals and medical researchers were than those in Melbourne.

This was the first asbestos/smoking lung cancer claim to reach a verdict, and the first of hundreds against the SECV. The jury found the SECV negligent and awarded $180,000 reduced by $83,000 for contributory negligence from smoking.

Simpson v Midalco Pty Ltd (unreported) WASC Brinsden J., (20 November 1987) (on appeal) WASC Full Court Wallace, Franklyn, Walsh JJ. (7 December 1988).
Walter Simpson had diffuse interstitial fibrosis, finger clubbing, numerous asbestos bodies on lung tissue sections, and, shortly before his case came

to trial, an asbestos related pleural effusion. He had worked at Wittenoom between July 1962 and March 1964, which, it was common ground between the witnesses, constituted a significant occupational exposure. He brought a claim for damages against ABA/Midalco claiming the respiratory injuries he suffered were caused by breach of its duty of care. The trial ran for 40 days, contested on all issues.

Most seriously contested was the issue of the cause of the lung fibrosis. No other cause for the interstitial fibrosis than asbestos was seriously suggested although nearly every other possible cause was speculated by the Defendant's medical witnesses (Dr J Lee, Dr B Gandevia, Dr P Breidahl, and Professor B Warren). Such causes and other diagnoses had been considered by the Plaintiff's medical advisors (Professor D Henderson, Professor A W Musk, Professor K Shilkin, Professor B Robinson, Dr K Finucane, Dr J Papadimitriou, and Dr C Minty) and rejected.

The "company line" relied upon by the Defendant was that the Plaintiff was not suffering from "classical asbestosis" by radiological or pathological definition (properly diagnosable only on autopsy), and thus there must be some other cause for the fibrosis, or the cause was unknown. It was suggested that the Plaintiff might have had pneumonia and that might account for the fibrosis. There seemed little dispute that Mr Simpson's pleural effusions were asbestos-caused.

The trial judge preferred the evidence of the Defendant's medical witnesses. He concluded that the lung biopsy demonstrated interstitial fibrosis and asbestos exposure and the possibility of early asbestosis. He thought the pleural effusion must have been caused by a pneumonia.

Astonishingly, despite the 11 weeks of evidence, the Judge made no provisional finding on the question of the negligence of the Defendant, against the possibility that an appeal court might come to a different conclusion on the question of whether Simpson suffered from asbestosis or asbestos related pleural effusion.

On appeal, in a unanimous judgment, the Full Court overturned the trial judgment and ordered a new trial. The Appeal Court pointed out that the suggestion that Mr Simpson might have had pneumonia came from senior counsel for Midalco, not from any medical evidence or record. It followed that pneumonia had to be rejected as the explanation for the lung changes and for the pleural effusion.

Their Honours considered the trial judge had posed the wrong test when he asked if the Plaintiff had negatived all other possible explanations, when most were conjectural, speculative or theoretical. His Honour had not properly had regard to the standard of proof enunciated by the High Court in *Adelaide Stevedoring v Forst* (1940) 64 CLR 538.

The appeal judges thought particularly telling Dr A W Musk's unchallenged evidence for the Plaintiff (supported by Dr B Robinson) that, in the general population, one person in a thousand suffered interstitial fibrosis, whereas in those exposed to asbestos at Wittenoom, the figure was 10 to 15 per cent; "That factor alone, one would have thought, would have gone a long way towards, if not on its own, justifying a finding on the balance of probabilities". His Honour's finding that the effusion was not asbestos related was "unsafe and unsatisfactory, based on a misconception of the evidence". A retrial was ordered on the negligence question, but the claim was settled for $220,000.

Rabenault v Midalco Pty Ltd (unreported SCV April-23 May 1988); (on appeal) *Midalco Pty Ltd v Rabenault* [1989] VR 461 (August-September 1988).

Klaus Rabenault worked at Wittenoom in 1960 and 1961, for three months in the Colonial Mill and then in the mine. In the mill he worked in the bagging section and had cleared away by hand asbestos fibre which got clogged in the chutes. Hessian plugged holes in machinery, pipes, and ducts through which asbestos escaped into the mill environment. In October 1987 Klaus developed mesothelioma.

Klaus Rabenault instructed Slater & Gordon and his claim proceeded to trial before Hampel J and a jury in the Supreme Court of Victoria in April and May 1988, whilst the Barrow and Heys trial reached its sixth month of hearing in the WA Supreme Court. *Rabenault* ran for 32 days.

Kaye J., in the Full Court (at 464–5) recounted the evidence at trial including that CSR had had access to relevant asbestos literature in its own extensive library in Sydney, in addition to being alerted to asbestos risks to workers from Dr E G Saint in 1948 and Dr J McNulty in 1959. It was also informed of the link with mesothelioma by the then manager of the mine and mill in 1960.

At the conclusion of the trial, the jury found that the Defendant's negligence had caused the Plaintiff's mesothelioma and awarded him compensatory damages of $426,000. But, for the first time ever in Australia in a negligence claim, the jury also found that the Defendant had been guilty of reckless misconduct and awarded punitive and exemplary damages of $250,000 for exposing Klaus Rabenault to the massive amounts of asbestos in which he had worked at Wittenoom.

CSR appealed against the punitive damages award. The Full Court unanimously dismissed the appeal. This included the comment from Kaye J. (at 473) that "I consider that a strong case supporting a finding of recklessness—indeed of continuing, conscious and contumelious disregard by the defendant for the Plaintiff's right to be free from the risk of injury or disease—was made out".

Barrow and Heys v CSR LTD and Midalco Pty Ltd (unreported) SCWA Rowland J. (4 August 1988) (BC 8801016)

CSR had finally discovered a lot of its records and documents relating to Wittenoom and, upon the change of the Western Australian state government in 1983, the *Limitation Act* had been changed and the state records that the Minister had told parliament had been destroyed had been found. For the first time the question of CSR's responsibility for the death and suffering of Wittenoom was to be tested. This was necessary, Slater & Gordon had assumed, because ABA had been stripped of its assets and, for claims arising from exposure before 1959, had insurance coverage with the SGIO of only $2,000.

Peter Heys and Tim Barrow had been exposed before 1959. Mr Barrow had worked in and around the mill about the same time as Joan Joosten between 1948 and 1951, and Mr Heys had spent three months as a bagger in late 1955.

Mr Barrow developed mesothelioma in January 1986 and also had pleural plaques and asbestosis. Mr Heys contracted mesothelioma in 1987. Their trial before Rowland J in the Supreme Court of WA commenced in November 1987, the day before judgment in Wally Simpson's trial was handed down.

The trial occupied 131 sitting days. There were 69 witnesses, 730 exhibits, and 11,000 pages of transcript. Judgment was given on 4 August 1988 in favour of Tim Barrow in the sum of $216,000 and for the estate and dependents of Peter Heys in the sum of $155,000. He had died on Good Friday 1988 during the trial.

Justice Rowland had found CSR owed a duty of care directly to the workers at Wittenoom: 'It would be completely unrealistic to suggest that ABA controlled its destiny in any real sense. CSR exercised hands-on management'.

He found as a fact "that at most times the dust in the mill was excessive and in fact excessive to a marked degree. I also find that dust in the immediate vicinity of the mill was excessive to a marked degree". As to the CSR officers K O Brown and M G King, they should have been aware prior to [1956] that unacceptable and dangerous quantities of dust were not being captured and that existing equipment was not coping, and, as I find, had never adequately coped... It is my finding that their claimed knowledge [of dust suppression techniques] was not implemented or they were unable to implement it for reasons not apparent... dust suppression was given little priority.

As to the hazards of asbestos, he summarised the evidence: "Brown made no enquiries and King may have had discussions of dust hazards but he cannot recall".

Rowland J found, after hearing evidence from Professor Eric Saint, that in 1948 he had expressed his concern to mine personnel in graphic terms, and that they would have been conveyed to Sydney in the manager's monthly reports (which couldn't be found). He found that there was a foreseeable risk of workers at the mill contracting asbestosis from short periods at the mill. He found that CSR and ABA did not do enough to understand the hazards and the available means of avoiding them or minimising them. He found that the workers had not been warned of the dangers. He found taking steps to reduce exposure would have materially reduced the risk of all asbestos diseases, and the failure to do so constituted negligence which had caused or made a material contribution to the mesothelioma contracted by each of Peter Heys and Tim Barrow. CSR filed an appeal against the judgment but later abandoned the appeal before it was heard.

Watson v State of Western Australia (unreported SCWA) (27 May 1988) (on appeal); *Western Australia v Watson* (1990) WAR 248

Colin Watson claimed damages against the state for his asbestosis and pleural disease which arose as a result of his exposure to Wittenoom-mined asbestos whilst working in 1958-59 as a tally clerk and wharf lumper for the State Harbour and Lights Department at Point Samson in northern Western Australia. This was the port where the asbestos was shipped to Fremantle. As a tally clerk Colin counted the bags coming off the trucks from Wittenoom into the sheds and then from the sheds onto the boats. Bags of blue asbestos thrown off trucks burst open, filling the shed with dust and fibre. Then he worked loading the bags into the airless holds of ships. Again, he would be covered with asbestos.

Colin went on to become a stage compère, comedian, and singer and, according to former football and media star John K Watts who gave evidence at the trial, a very good one. He developed asbestosis and pleural disease in 1982 and by 1987 when he consulted Dr Musk he was totally disabled, confined to a wheelchair with oxygen.

Pidgeon J ruled in favour of Mr Watson and awarded him over $400,000 in damages. The state of Western Australia appealed, but the Appeal Court dismissed the appeal and awarded Mr Watson further damages up to $600,000. All matters had been fiercely contested by the state, including the diagnosis of asbestosis.

Taylor v CSR & Midalco (SCWA)(December 1992) Olsen (Young) v CSR Ltd **(unreported) DDT NSW judgment 24 December 1994) (on appeal);** *CSR Ltd v Young* **(1998) Aust Torts Rep 81-468**

Brent Taylor had spent the first five years of his life in Wittenoom in the early 1960s. Aged 32 with a wife and two small children he contracted mesothelioma in 1992 and Slater & Gordon issued proceedings against CSR & Midalco alleging a breach of duty of care to the children of employees who lived in the Wittenoom township, where tailings had been spread over all public areas and had been sold to employees to spread on their gardens and lawns. On the morning of his trial in the Supreme Court of WA in December 1992, CSR settled the claim for $450,000. That did not resolve the issue however and CSR forced another child of Wittenoom, Vivien Olson, to run her claim in the NSW Dust Diseases Tribunal. She won the trial on Christmas eve 1994 (*Olson v CSR Ltd* (unreported) DDT NSW judgment 24 December 1994.). CSR appealed and the estate and dependents of Mrs Olson were again successful: *CSR Ltd v Young* (1998) Aust Torts Rep 81-468.

Wittenoom Group Settlement September/November 1989

CSR paid $18,266,000 (with damages ranging from $30,000 to $600,000) to 200 Wittenoom claimants in this group settlement agreed between Slater & Gordon and CSR on 28 September 1989, signed 30 November 1989 and paid December 1989. This included settlement of the claims brought by Cornelius Maas, Joan Joosten, Rino Pedrotti and Ray Adam.

Conclusions and Consequences

This chapter has provided an historical review of the progress of asbestos litigation through the courts up to the late 1990s. Australian cases have been seen in the context of landmark cases in the UK and the US.

However, asbestos litigation continues to this day, and in Australia the lawyers and doctors involved in these early days are still being called upon to represent ill and dying patients in courts across the country. But with each new case, each new precedent, the sufferers of asbestos disease who come after the early litigators benefit by not having to fight the same battle.

Thus one most important consequence of the litigation recounted above—and that which has occurred since—is that many thousands of people who contracted asbestos disease have received compensation. Their lives and the lives of those they love have been made a little better. They have been able to do things they might not have been able to do earlier in their lives. They may have bought a home (perhaps for the first time). They have been able to live—and perhaps to die—in a bit more comfort. And that is something that thirty years ago seemed a remote and unlikely ambition.

The success story that is the history of Australian asbestos litigation would not have been written without the dedication and determination of the many dedicated lawyers who have taken on the asbestos industry and brought it to account in the courts. They have been assisted by campaigners like Robert and Rose Marie Vojakovic at the Asbestos Diseases Society of Australia who would not accept defeat, who got the laws in WA changed and the lost documents found, and who have benefited so many with their tireless work over three decades. Tribute must also be paid to the members of the medical profession who have done so much to help their patients achieve justice and compensation. They are truly heroes who have endured much for no other purpose than that they cared enough to help those who turned to them in their darkest hours.

Part 5
Asbestos Today:
The Lingering Legacy

Chapter 11

THE ONGOING PROBLEM OF ASBESTOS *IN SITU*

Peter Franklin & Alison Reid

Australia was a large producer and consumer of all types of asbestos, ranking first, on a per capita basis, in the world for gross consumption of asbestos cement products during the 1950s. Both crocidolite (blue asbestos) and chrysotile (white asbestos) were mined in Australia, while from the period just prior to 1930 until 1983 over 1.5 million tons of raw chrysotile and amosite (brown asbestos) were imported. Asbestos was used in over 3000 products including asbestos cement sheets, guttering, gables, eaves, carpet and tile underlays, thermal insulation, textile and cloth products, anti-friction materials (for example, brakes and clutches), gaskets and packings, and patching and taping compounds. Its use was slowly phased out in the 1970s and 1980s, but it is still found in structures built in the late 1980s. A total ban on the manufacture, use, reuse, import, transport, storage, or sale of all forms of asbestos did not come into effect until the end of 2003. Although asbestos is banned it remains ubiquitous in the built environment and many of the asbestos products installed in earlier decades remain in situ around Australia. This chapter explores asbestos in the built environment today, including the potential pathways of exposure for the general community, and the potential risk these exposures pose. Because of the extensive use of asbestos the risk of potential exposure in both the indoor and outdoor environments remains high, even while the actual exposure levels are mostly very low.

Asbestos in the built environment

Asbestos has become a ubiquitous contaminant of ambient air with very low concentrations of asbestos measured in most urban centres in industrialised countries.[1] Asbestos fibres can be found in the lungs of many people who have

---

1   Australian Safety and Compensation Council, *Literature review of asbestos fibre release from building materials following weathering and/or corrosion* (Canberra: Australian Safety and Compensation Council, 2008).

not had any occupational exposure.[2] The potential non-occupational exposure pathways for individuals are wide and varied. Historically, the most important non-occupational exposures were obtained from living with an asbestos worker or living in close proximity to an asbestos mine or factory. These exposures have consistently been associated with disease.[3] However, after the ban on the mining and manufacturing of asbestos and asbestos products in countries like Australia, these exposures have been less common. Of increasing importance today, which is anticipated to continue well into the future, is non-occupational exposure resulting from fibres released from asbestos-containing materials (ACM) in the built environment, during activities such as renovation, demolition and removal.[4] Asbestos fibres are also released as a result of general degradation (weathering) and damage to ACM, as well as damage from disasters such as fires, storms, cyclones and floods. All of these scenarios can cause both short-term increases in airborne fibres and long-term contamination of land with asbestos fragments and fibre bundles.

1. Asbestos products *in situ*

In situ asbestos products in buildings are now at least 30 years old, with most being much older. Like any building material, as they age they will deteriorate. The level of degradation caused by general ageing is not well understood and will depend on how well the products are maintained. Well-maintained ACM are unlikely to spontaneously release or shed respirable asbestos fibres, but damaged products can do so.[5]

Indoor products are less likely to weather than outdoor products, although there may be some degradation as a result of physical contact and movement of the building (for example, vibration). Airborne asbestos fibre concentrations in buildings are generally very low and not much greater than outdoor

---

2   M Casali, M Carugno, A Cattaneo, D Consonni, C Mensi, U Genovese, D M Cavallo, A Somigliana and A C Pesatori, "Asbestos lung burden in necroscopic samples from the general population of Milan, Italy", *Annals of Occupational Hygiene*, 59, 7, 2015, 909–21. doi: 10.1093/annhyg/mev028. C Gilham, C Rake, G Burdett, A G Nicholson, L Davison, A Franchini, J Carpenter, J Hodgson, A Darnton and J Peto, "Pleural mesothelioma and lung cancer risks in relation to occupational history and asbestos lung burden", *Occupational and Environmental Medicine*, 73, 5, 2016, 290–99. doi: 10.1136/oemed-2015-103074.

3   C W Noonan, "Environmental asbestos exposure and risk of mesothelioma", *Annals of Translational Medicine*, 5, 11, 2017, 234. doi: 10.21037/atm.2017.03.74.

4   P J Landrigan, "The third wave of asbestos disease: exposure to asbestos in place. Public health control. Introduction", *Annals of the New York Academy of Sciences*, 643, 1991, xv–xvi.

5   R J Lee and D R Van Orden, "Airborne asbestos in buildings", Regulatory Toxicology and Pharmacology 50, 2, 2008, 218–25. doi: 10.1016/j.yrtph.2007.10.005.

WHERE ASBESTOS MAY BE FOUND IN A TYPICAL HOME

- Insulation for hot water pipes and tank
- Dog kennel & animal enclosures
- Sheds & external toilets
- Splashback
- Internal angle mouldings
- Backing of vinyl floor sheeting & lino tiles
- Flues to fireplaces
- Insulation below wood heater
- Backing for electrical meter boards

- Fence
- Loose fill insulation in roof cavity
- Corrugated asbestos-cement roofing
- Ridge capping
- Eaves and gables ends
- Garage
- Internal & external ventilators
- Downpipes
- Gutters
- "Tilux" marble finish wall panel
- Compressed asbestos sheet cement flooring
- External angle mouldings
- Internal walls & ceilings & behind wall paper
- Carpet underlay and adhesives
- Wall sheeting exterior (potentially under cladding)

OTHER
- Brake and clutch linings
- Buried and dumped waste materials
- Naturally occurring asbestos in certain regions

Figure 11.1: Asbestos Awareness Healthy House Checklist. A homeowner's guide to identifying asbestos-containing material to manage it safely

Courtesy: Asbestosawareness.com.au.

levels.[6] In a 2008 study of 752 buildings, including schools, universities, public buildings, and homes, conducted over a ten-year period, Lee and Van Orden found that although indoor concentrations were greater than outdoors

> ...in-place ACM does not result in elevated airborne asbestos in building atmospheres approaching regulatory levels and that it does not result in a significantly increased risk to building occupants.

Of concern was that the highest indoor concentrations, on average, were found in schools, which was probably owing to a greater level of activity in these buildings.[7] Figure 11.1 shows where asbestos may be found in the average home.

---

6   A Bardsley, *Asbestos exposure in New Zealand: Review of the scientific evidence of non-occupational risks. A report on behalf of the Royal Society of New Zealand and the Office of the Prime Minister's Chief Science Advisor*, 2015. https://royalsociety.org.nz/assets/documents/Asbestos-exposure-in-New-Zealand-April-2015.pdf. Accessed 11 October 2018. S K Brown, "Asbestos", in *Indoor air quality handbook*, eds J D Spengler, J M Samet and J F McCarthy (New York: McGraw-Hill Professional, 2001), 38.1–38.17. Lee and Van Orden, "Airborne asbestos in buildings".

7   Lee and Van Orden, "Airborne asbestos in buildings". Brown, "Asbestos".

Asbestos products that are located outdoors (for instance, external cladding, fences, roofs) are more likely to be subject to weathering and deterioration. The damage to these products can be highly visible. Cracked and broken ACM fences and wall sheets are common in areas where these products were used extensively. General deterioration is less obvious, but erosion of ACM can remove cement particles and result in the release of asbestos fibres. The contribution of damaged and weathered materials to urban asbestos pollution is very difficult to determine. However, typical ambient air levels of asbestos fibres in cities are about 0.0001 f/mL, ten-fold higher than rural areas (remote from any special sources of asbestos).[8] The sources of increased concentrations in cities are varied and although fibre release from individual products, even if highly degraded, will be small there are very many of these products in the built environment.

There are two main approaches to the management of asbestos in the built environment.[9] The first is risk-based, which advocates action based on the potential risk. This is the current strategy in most jurisdictions. Under this approach duty holders are required to identify asbestos, assess the risk it poses, and implement control measures to eliminate those risks. This includes management *in situ* as this may pose a lower risk than removal, because removal can cause the release of fibres if not done carefully (see below). Removal is based on the condition of the product and is recommended for badly damaged or deteriorating material, although determining the level of degradation when removal is required can be difficult. Removal of ACM, even if in good condition, during renovation or other building works (opportunistic removal) is also encouraged under this approach. This is the most common approach as it is regarded as striking a balance between recognising the dangers posed by asbestos but weighing these against the logistical issues and costs associated with a wholesale removal program. The second approach advocates a prioritised removal of all asbestos products from buildings. This is based on the premise that all asbestos products pose a potential health risk over time, either by degradation or physical damage. Incidents such as fires and storms can damage ACM even if it is in good condition, so asbestos products can never be considered "safe". Although the removal of all asbestos from buildings would be the ideal, it is a huge task and would be extremely costly.

---

8   Brown, "Asbestos".
9   Asbestos Safety and Eradication Agency, *Asbestos management review report June 2012* (Canberra: Employment and Workplace Relations Department of Education, 2012) www.asbestossafety.gov.au/sites/asea/files/documents/2017-10/asbestos_management_review_report_june_2012_0.pdf. Accessed 11 October 2018.

Case study: Asbestos roofs

Asbestos cement roofs are of particular concern as a potential source of exposure as these are much harder to maintain and are more exposed to the weather than some of the other outdoor products. Roofs have been subject to weathering by rain, sun, wind, hail, air pollution, moss/lichen growth, and salt (for coastal properties). These products undergo surface degradation of the weather-exposed surface, exposing an asbestos-enriched layer underneath. The loss of sheet thickness is of the order of 0.01 to 0.02 mm per year and the degradation generally becomes visible 15 to 20 years after roof installation.[10] The degradation has been associated with fibre release in the range of 10^6 to 10^8 fibres/$m^2 \cdot hr$.[11] These fibres not only become airborne, they can also be washed onto the soil leading to significant soil contamination over time. Roofs are also a particular risk in a natural disaster. For example, in a fire, roofs can "explode" and fibres and fragments scattered far from the source. (See "Natural Disasters" below).

As with all ACM products, the management of roofs is based on maintenance *in situ* and removal when degradation is severe. However, these products are getting very old and often have not been maintained adequately. Encapsulation (for example, painting or sealing) will afford some protection, but as the products become more damaged removal becomes the preferred option. However, the cost of removal and disposal can be high, which, unfortunately, is a disincentive for eliminating these products from the community.[12] Furthermore, removalists are sometimes reluctant to remove these products because of the potential dangers these jobs posed.[13]

2. Renovation and removal

Renovation and removal are the activities that, if done poorly, probably present the greatest contemporary risk of exposure to asbestos fibres. Indeed, of all the current exposures, renovation and removal are the most likely to be associated with disease.[14] These activities are a major source

---

10   Brown, "Asbestos".

11   K R Spurny, "On the release of asbestos fibers from weathered and corroded asbestos cement products", *Environmental Research*, 48 (1) 1989: 100-16. doi: 10.1016/S0013-9351(89)80089-1.

12   Asbestos Safety and Eradication Agency, *Asbestos management review report June 2012*.

13   C Gray, R N Carey and A Reid, "Current and future risks of asbestos exposure in the Australian community", *International Journal of Occupational and Environmental Health*, 22, 4, 2016, 292-99. doi: 10.1080/10773525.2016.1227037.

14   N J Olsen, P J. Franklin, A Reid, N H de Klerk, T J Threlfall, K Shilkin and B Musk, "Increasing incidence of malignant mesothelioma after exposure to asbestos during home maintenance and renovation", *Medical Journal of Australia*, 195, 5, 2011, 271-74. doi: 10.5694/mja11.10125.

of non-occupational exposure because of the large number of homes that are renovated, particularly older homes that are likely to contain ACM. Renovation and removal of asbestos from commercial, public, and residential buildings are also important sources of occupational exposure. Exposure can either be accidental (for example, a tradesman unaware of existing asbestos in a building) or result from professional asbestos removal.

Home renovation has been, and remains, a common activity in Australia.[15] In a survey of home owners in Adelaide, major renovations were undertaken in about 34 per cent of homes over a five-year period (1986–1991),[16] while over 44 per cent of respondents to a 2012 survey in NSW reported having home renovations.[17] Most home renovations are done by Do-It-Yourself (DIY) renovators rather than professionals,[18] and many of these DIY renovations involve asbestos.[19] For example, Park *et al.* reported in 2013 that over 60 per cent of DIY renovators in NSW were exposed to asbestos during renovation, while nearly a quarter of all renovations across Australia in 2015/16 involved asbestos.[20]

There are two main areas of concern with home renovation involving asbestos: poor awareness of asbestos products, and a lack of precautions/protection taken by many home owners who report doing DIY renovations involving asbestos. In a 2016 Australian-wide survey of home owners doing DIY renovation, approximately half felt knowledgeable about asbestos. There was an inverse relationship between asbestos awareness and age, with 62 per cent of DIYers over the age of 50 feeling knowledgeable about asbestos compared to 40 per cent of those under 50 years.[21] With regards to taking precautions, in the 2013 study by Park *et al.* only 12 per cent of those

---

15 Australian Bureau of Statistics. *Australian social trends 2002* (Canberra: Australian Bureau of Statistics, 2002). S Baum and R Hassan, "Home owners, home renovation and residential mobility", *Journal of Sociology*, 35, 1, 1999, 23–41.

16 Baum and Hassan, "Home owners, home renovation and residential mobility".

17 E K Park, D H Yates, R A Hyland and A R Johnson, "Asbestos exposure during home renovation in New South Wales", *Medical Journal of Australia*, 199, 6, 2013, 410–13.

18 Colmar Brunton, *National benchmark asbestos awareness survey 2014* (Asbestos Safety and Eradication Agency, 2014). www.asbestossafety.gov.au/research-publications/asbestos_safety_research. Accessed 11 October 2018. Park *et al.*, "Asbestos exposure during home renovation in New South Wales".

19 EY Sweeney, *National benchmark survey of awareness of and attitudes to asbestos 2016* (Asbestos Safety and Eradication Agency, 2016). https://www.asbestossafety.gov.au/sites/asea/files/documents/2018-02/Executive%20Summary%20from%20report.pdf. Accessed 11 October 2018. Park *et al.*, "Asbestos exposure during home renovation in NSW".

20 E Y Sweeney, *National benchmark survey of awareness of and attitudes to asbestos 2016*.

21 E Y Sweeney, *National benchmark survey of awareness of and attitudes to asbestos 2016*.

doing home renovation involving asbestos always wore respiratory protection, while over 30 per cent never wore protection of any sort. In that study bystander exposure was also an issue with nearly 40 per cent of partners and over 20 per cent of children reportedly exposed to asbestos during DIY home renovation.[22]

For professional removalists, rules and regulations for the safe removal of asbestos are well established. In Australia, most state Occupational Health and Safety regulations call up the National Occupational Health and Safety Council (NOHSC) Code of Practice for the Safe Removal of Asbestos.[23] There are no national codes of practice for home renovators and most Australian states and territories do not specifically regulate the removal of asbestos by homeowners.[24] Most states provide extensive advice to home/building owners about asbestos and the national environmental health body has published a document to assist home owners who may be doing renovations.[25] Most states or territories do not regulate the amount of bonded asbestos that can be removed by a home owner. The ACT, however, requires a qualified asbestos removalist for any removal of asbestos from homes, while home owners are only allowed to remove up to 10 m2 of ACM.

Renovation activities, particularly those involving the use of power tools, can produce short-term high concentrations of asbestos fibres, and major renovation works may increase background fibre concentrations in the medium term, contributing to increased cumulative exposure.[26] A number of studies have simulated renovation/removal activities and measured airborne fibre concentrations.[27] Some of the results are presented in Table 11.2. These studies demonstrate that fibre concentrations can be very high,

---

22   Park *et al.*, "Asbestos exposure during home renovation in NSW".

23   National Occupational Health and Safety Commission, *Code of Practice for the safe removal of asbestos* (2nd Edn. Canberra: National Occupational Health and Safety Commission, 2005).

24   As of 2017, Western Australia and Queensland were the only two states with public health regulations for the removal by the public of asbestos.

25   Environmental Health Standing Committee (enHealth), *Asbestos: A guide for householders and the general public* (Canberra: Australian Health Protection Principal Committee, 2013).

26   Brown, "Asbestos", 38.1–38.17.

27   G Benke, *Measurement of asbestos fibre release during removal works in a variety of DIY scenarios* (Asbestos Safety and Eradication Agency, 2016). www.asbestossafety.gov.au/sites/asea/files/documents/2017-10/ASEA_Report_fibre_release_in_DIY_scenarios_ACC_JULY16.pdf. Accessed 11 October 2018. Brown, "Asbestos".

exceeding, in the short term at least, the Australian workplace exposure standard (WES) for asbestos exposure of 0.1 f/ml (8-hour time weighted average). It is difficult, however, to compare the result directly with the WES as the sampling periods used in these studies are much shorter than the 8-hour occupational limit. However, these short-term exposures seem to be sufficient to cause disease. (See below, "*In situ* asbestos and asbestos related disease").

Activity	Concentration (f/mL)	Time
Occupational exposure limit	0.1*	8 hour (time-weighted average)
Removal of vinyl tiles by scraping	0.004 – 0.014	Short-term‡
Asbestos-cement sheet Hand saw Jigsaw Circular saw	1 – 4 2 – 100 10 – 20	Short-term‡
Removal of AC corrugated external roof sheeting in dry conditions	0.215†	18 min
Removal of AC flat external wall sheeting in dry conditions	0.213†	31 min
Removal of small sections of AC flat sheet to create penetrations	13.231†	5 min
Drilling and screwing into AC sheet	0.062†	15 min
Removal of AC wall panels in bathrooms	0.663†	15 min
Clean-up after task	0.898†	35 min
Removal of a small outdoor shed constructed of flat and corrugated AC sheeting	0.124†	108 min

Figure 11.2: Airborne asbestos fibre concentrations (fibres/mL) measured during selected renovation activities.
SOURCES: Brown, 2001; Benke, 2016.

‡ Time was not specified but "short-term" monitoring is usually 30 minutes (but can be shorter).

† These were personal samplers. All results from personal sampling were considerably greater than area sampling.

* A licenced removalist must stop asbestos removal work when the recorded respirable asbestos fibre level exceeds 0.02 fibres/ml. The removalist cannot resume removal work until air monitoring shows that the recorded respirable asbestos fibre level is below 0.01 fibres/ml.

3. Demolition

Demolition of buildings containing asbestos is a potential source of both short-term elevated airborne fibres and long-term contamination of the soil. Although there are established processes for the demolition of buildings containing asbestos, including prior removal of asbestos and dust minimisation during demolition, poor demolition remains an ongoing problem.[28] This is likely to remain a potential problem for some time to come owing to the large number of buildings that still contain asbestos materials.

There are few published data on airborne asbestos fibres generated by demolition. Perkins *et al.* in 2007 found very low levels of airborne asbestos fibres in the demolition of whole buildings when proper practices were observed, even in buildings that still contained significant amounts of asbestos.[29] However, when there are no attempts to reduce dust levels during demolition, airborne asbestos fibre levels can be high, often exceeding current occupational standards.[30]

Poor demolition and removal can also lead to soil contamination and expensive clean ups. The cost of remediation of contaminated soil can be hundreds of thousands of dollars,[31] can take many months to complete, and unnecessarily creates tonnes of hazardous waste that needs to be disposed of at specialised waste sites. The cost of remediation is often far greater than the cost of the initial demolition.

4. Illegal dumping

Illegal dumping of asbestos is a problem across Australia.[32] Although illegal dumping poses a potential health risk, the biggest impact is probably in the cost of clean up and site remediation. In a 2016 review it was estimated that, across Australia, about 6,300 tonnes of ACM is dumped each year

---

28 Poor demolition accounted for 25 per cent of asbestos complaints received by Western Australian local governments in 2011. (*WA Local Government Asbestos Survey*, 2011).

29 R A Perkins, J Hargesheimer and W Fourie, "Asbestos release from whole-building demolition of buildings with asbestos-containing material", *Journal of Occupational and Environmental Hygiene*, 4, 12, 2007, 889–94. doi: 10.1080/15459620701691023.

30 S K Brown, "Asbestos exposure during renovation and demolition of asbestos-cement clad buildings", *American Industrial Hygiene Association Journal*, 48, 5, 1987 478–86. H Kakooei, M Meshkani and K Azam, "Ambient monitoring of airborne asbestos in non-occupational environments in Tehran, Iran", *Atmospheric Environment*, 81, 2013, 671–75. doi: 10.1016/j.atmosenv.2013.09.022.

31 An example is provided by the WA Department of Health in the *Local Government Asbestos Survey*, 2011, of a poorly-done demolition that caused a twelve-month delay in the development of the site and cost an extra $200,000 in clean up and site preparation.

32 Asbestos Safety and Eradication Agency, *Asbestos management review report June 2012*.

and the cost of clean up is around $A11.2 million per annum.[33] These were crude estimates as the volumes or weight of illegally dumped ACMs or the costs of cleaning up these materials are not systematically recorded by local or state governments.

Asbestos material is often dumped in urban bushland or vacant blocks of land, but there have been numerous press reports of dumping in public open spaces and next to school grounds. Most dumped asbestos is ACM sheeting but can also include other asbestos-containing building materials, including friable material, and contaminated soils. Household renovators, building contractors, and asbestos removalists are considered the main culprits responsible for most incidents of illegally dumped ACMs.[34]

The primary motivations to dump ACMs illegally appear to be cost and convenience.[35] The disposal costs of asbestos at specialised waste sites can be high and licensed disposal sites are often sparse and not easily accessible.[36] Other reasons include:

- the opportunity for commercial operators to make higher profits (for example, by dumping illegally even when their client has been charged the full cost of legal disposal), and
- apathy and/or a perception that dealing with ACMs properly is too difficult.[37]

Dumped asbestos can cause significant community concern, particularly if found in public open space or on vacant blocks in residential areas. However, most dumped material is bonded ACM and, even though it can include broken and/or weathered fragments, there is not likely to be a large release of fibres. Problems may occur when the land where asbestos has been dumped is being developed. If the ACM is not adequately removed it

---

33   ACIL Allen Consultant, *Illegal asbestos dumping: review of issues and initiatives* (Asbestos Safety and Eradication Agency, 2016). https://www.asbestossafety.gov.au/sites/asea/files/documents/2017-10/ASEA_Report_Illegal_Asbestos_Dumping_Issues_and_Initiatives_final_ACC.pdf. Accessed 11 October 2018.

34   ACIL Allen Consultant, *Illegal asbestos dumping: review of issues and initiatives*.

35   ACIL Allen Consultant, *Illegal asbestos dumping: review of issues and initiatives*. Western Australian Department of Health, *Survey of local government and other regulators experience with asbestos incidents in the public sector* (Western Australian Department of Health, 2011). http://ww2.health.wa.gov.au/~/media/Files/Corporate/general%20documents/Asbestos/PDF/Local-Council-Asbestos-Survey-Report.pdf. Accessed 11 October 2018.

36   Gray, Carey and Reid, "Current and future risks of asbestos exposure in the Australian community", 292–99.

37   ACIL Allen Consultant, *Illegal asbestos dumping: review of issues and initiatives*.

can be crushed by heavy equipment or mixed with cleared vegetation and mulched, allowing fibres to become airborne. Again, the amount of fibres released into the air will not be high and the subsequent risk of disease will be extremely low, although it will not be zero.

5. Natural disasters (fires, cyclones and floods)

Asbestos that remains in the urban environment can release fibres as a result of natural disasters such as fire, cyclone, or flood. The main concern is the contamination that is caused after the event and the risk of exposure during clean up. There is little evidence that natural disasters involving damage to asbestos products cause significant public exposures during the event. [38] However, each of these events has the capacity to create considerable asbestos contamination that can lead to significant community disquiet, costly clean ups, and the potential for future exposure.

Fires are a particular concern as they occur more regularly than the other disaster events and can cause considerable release and dispersion of asbestos fibres.[39] Fires can involve a single dwelling/building or many structures, some or all of which may contain ACM. The emergency response to these events will depend on the extent of the damage and potential contamination.

Compared to other natural disasters, fires are more likely to liberate asbestos fibres from bonded asbestos products. Fires can cause the cement matrix of ACM to break and "spall". Spalls are flakes of material that are broken off the larger body as a result of a surface failure of that material. For asbestos cement products, water held within the matrix expands under heat causing a differential pressure build-up within the cement matrix that results in spalling, sometimes explosively.[40] The dominant (free) fibre emissions during a fire are associated with the spalling process.[41]

Despite the spalling that occurs during fires, airborne asbestos fibre concentrations are generally quite low during and immediately after a

---

38 Environmental Health Standing Committee (enHealth), *Management of asbestos in the non-occupational environment* (Canberra: Environmental Health Standing Committee, 2005).

39 Western Australian Department of Health, *Guidance note on the management of fire damaged asbestos*. (Perth: Western Australian Department of Health, 2015). http://ww2.health.wa.gov.au/~/media/Files/Corporate/general%20documents/Asbestos/PDF/Guidance-note-Management-of-fire-damaged-asbestos.pdf. Accessed 11 October 2018.

40 WA Department of Health, *Guidance note on the management of fire damaged asbestos*.

41 Noel Arnold & Associates, *Report on the investigation of the effect of fire on asbestos fibre contamination*, 2006. https://www2.health.vic.gov.au/about/publications/researchandreports/Report%20on%20the%20Investigation%20of%20the%20Effect%20of%20Fire%20on%20Asbestos%20Fibre%20Contamination. Accessed 11 October 2018.

fire event.[42] The reason is likely to be that high volumes of air drawn into the fire area would significantly dilute fibre concentrations. However, the free fibres and fibre bundles can travel long distances and be deposited well beyond the fire site.[43]

As with other instances of damage to asbestos products, subsequent ongoing contamination is a major problem. Soil, vegetation, and hard surfaces in and around the fire scene can be contaminated with fibres, fibre bundles and ACM fragments. Most asbestos will be deposited as large pieces or fragments of ACM, predominantly within or immediately about the area of the fire scene. Smaller quantities of asbestos fibre bundles and free asbestos fibre are liberated from their bonded form as a result of spalling and are deposited in measurable concentrations within the immediate vicinity of, and to a lesser extent beyond, the fire scene.[44]

Cyclones and floods will also lead to the damage and spread of asbestos material. The main concern with these disasters, however, is the contamination that will occur in the aftermath of the event and the risk of exposures during clean up.[45]

6. Contaminated sites

A site is considered contaminated "... if a substance present in or on that site is above background concentrations and presents, or has the potential to present, a risk of harm to human health, the environment or any environmental value". Asbestos is a common reason for a site to be officially classified as contaminated. For example, in Western Australia there were 2,346 classified contaminated sites. In over 50 per cent of sites, asbestos was present.[46]

Contamination of soil with asbestos-containing material occurs for many reasons, including illegal burial, incorrect demolition or removal procedures, fire or storm damage, or from historical waste sites. As discussed above, the ongoing asbestos contamination often presents a greater exposure risk than the initial activity.

---

42   Noel Arnold & Associates, *Report on the investigation of the effect of fire on asbestos fibre contamination.*

43   S Bridgman, "Community health risk assessment after a fire with asbestos containing fallout", *Journal of Epidemiology & Community Health*, 55, 12, 2002, 921–27.

44   WA Department of Health, *Guidance note on the management of fire damaged asbestos.*

45   Environmental Health Standing Committee (enHealth), *Management of asbestos in the non-occupational environment.*

46   Pierina Ottness, Senior Scientific Officer, Environmental Health Directorate, WA Department of Health, personal conversation with P Franklin.

The human health risk from asbestos-contaminated soil varies considerably depending on the form of asbestos (friable or bonded), its quantity, and the exposure situation, for example, the level of activity on the contaminated land. Contaminant asbestos can be in a range of forms, sizes, and degrees of deterioration and includes: ACM that may be in sound condition, although possibly broken or fragmented; fibrous asbestos (FA), which is friable asbestos material; and asbestos fines (AF), which includes free fibres of asbestos and small fibre bundles.[47]

The management of asbestos-contaminated sites focuses on ensuring airborne fibre levels are kept below 0.01 f/mL.[48] Current national guidelines for investigation of asbestos soil contamination are;

> 0.001 % w/w asbestos for FA and AF – All site uses
> 0.01 % w/w asbestos for ACM – Residential use, day care centres, preschools, etc.
> 0.04 % w/w asbestos for ACM – Residential, minimal soil access
> 0.02 % w/w asbestos for ACM – Parks, public open spaces, playing fields, etc.
> 0.05 % w/w asbestos for ACM – Commercial/Industrial

Remediation is based on the likelihood of exposure, not just soil concentrations, and may involve *in situ* management or removal of the soil, depending on where the contamination is, the sources of exposure and the land-uses.

In situ asbestos and asbestos related disease

In 1991 Landrigan suggested that industrialised countries were at the beginning of the third wave of asbestos related disease, which would occur in people repairing, renovating, or demolishing asbestos-containing buildings. The first wave occurred in those who mined, milled, or transported raw asbestos, or worked in the manufacture of asbestos products, and the second in workers who used those asbestos products.[49] There is no hard

---

47   Western Australian Department of Health, *Guidelines for the assessment, remediation and management of asbestos-contaminated sites in Western Australia*, (WA Department of Health, 2009). http://ww2.health.wa.gov.au/~/media/Files/Corporate/general%20documents/Asbestos/PDF/Guidelines-Asbestos-Contaminated%20Sites-May2009.pdf. Accessed 11 October 2018.

48   Environmental Health Standing Committee (enHealth), *Management of asbestos in the non-occupational environment*

49   Landrigan, "The third wave of asbestos disease: exposure to asbestos in place. Public health control. Introduction."

definition of third-wave exposure, and Landrigan most likely referred to third-wave occupational exposures (professional removalists and tradespeople who are inadvertently exposed), but it broadly could include any accidental, or intentional exposure to asbestos *in situ*, and incorporates occupational and non-occupational exposures. These exposures will vary from short-term high exposures that can occur during activities such as renovation and demolition, to long-term low level exposures from ACM degradation and ongoing contamination.

The existence of a "third-wave" of disease is contentious,[50] but there is evidence that both occupational,[51] and non-occupational,[52] renovation activities can contribute to asbestos related disease, particularly mesothelioma. The disease risks of relatively low-level exposures as well as short-term high exposures are not well understood as most exposure-response estimates at the lower end of exposure have been extrapolated from studies that have only comprised workers exposed to high levels of asbestos.[53] There is no known asbestos exposure threshold below which there is no risk of disease,[54] but there are still considerable gaps in our understanding of the risks associated with non-occupational asbestos exposure, and the prevalence of that exposure within the population. For example, there is considerable uncertainty about the amount of asbestos product that remains in the built environment and the condition of that asbestos product, the levels of asbestos from *in situ* asbestos inside and outside buildings, and who or how many in the population have been exposed to asbestos from different sources in the general community.[55]

---

50 B Armstrong and T Driscoll, "Mesothelioma in Australia: cresting the third wave", *Public Health Research & Practice*, 26 (2) 2016. doi: UNSP e262161410.17061/phrp2621614.

51 G Frost, A H Harding, A Darnton, D. McElvenny and D Morgan, "Occupational exposure to asbestos and mortality among asbestos removal workers: a Poisson regression analysis", *British Journal of Cancer*, 99 (5) 2008: 822–29. doi: 10.1038/sj.bjc.6604564.

52 Olsen *et al.*, "Increasing incidence of malignant mesothelioma after exposure to asbestos during home maintenance and renovation", 271–74.

53 D W Berman and K S Crump, "Update of potency factors for asbestos related lung cancer and mesothelioma", *Critical Reviews in Toxicology*, 38, 2008: 1–47. doi: 10.1080/10408440802276167.

54 Y Iwatsubo, J C Pairon, C Boutin, O Menard, N Massin, D Caillaud, E Orlowski, F Galateau-Salle, J Bignon and P Brochard, "Pleural mesothelioma: Dose-response relation at low levels of asbestos exposure in a French population-based case-control study", *American Journal of Epidemiology*, 148, 2, 1998, 133–42.

55 A Reid, "Review of the effectiveness of predictive models for mesothelioma to identify lessons for asbestos related policy", *Evidence Base*, 3, 2016, 1–19.

Most studies of non-occupational exposure and asbestos related disease have focused on three areas: para-occupational exposure (that is, exposures of family members of an asbestos worker),[56] and environmental exposures from either industrial operations, such as asbestos factories,[57] and mines,[58] or naturally occurring asbestos.[59] These studies have demonstrated that these exposures have been associated with asbestos related disease, predominantly mesothelioma,[60] but also asbestosis.[61] There are very few studies of asbestos related disease from the third-wave exposures described above. In fact, only two studies have investigated asbestos related disease, mesothelioma specifically, from third-wave non-occupational exposures.[52] Olsen *et al.* reported an increasing number and proportion of mesothelioma cases that had their primary exposure from participating in home renovation. The first DIY case was diagnosed in 1981 and from that time there was a steady increase in cases. In the period 2005–2008, DIY exposures accounted for 8.4 per

---

56   L T Stayner, "Para-occupational exposures to asbestos: lessons learned from Casale Monferrato, Italy", *Occupational and Environmental Medicine*, 73, 3, 2016, 145–46. doi: 10.1136/oemed-2015-103233.

57   C Magnani, P Dalmasso, A Biggeri, C Ivaldi, D Mirabelli and B Terracini, "Increased risk of malignant mesothelioma of the pleura after residential or domestic exposure to asbestos: a case-control study in Casale Monferrato, Italy", *Environmental Health Perspectives*, 109, 9, 2001, 915–19. doi: sc271_5_1835 [pii].

58   A Reid, J Heyworth, N de Klerk and A W Musk, "The mortality of women exposed environmentally and domestically to blue asbestos at Wittenoom, Western Australia", *Occupational and Environmental Medicine*, 65, 11, 2008, 743–49. doi: 10.1136/oem.2007.035782. A C Whitehouse, C B Black, M S Heppe, J Ruckdeschel and S M Levin, "Environmental exposure to Libby asbestos and mesotheliomas", *American Journal of Industrial Medicine*, 51, 11, 2008, 877–80. doi: 10.1002/ajim.20620.

59   X L Pan, H W Day, W Wang, L A Beckett and M B Schenker, "Residential proximity to naturally occurring asbestos and mesothelioma risk in California", *American Journal of Respiratory and Critical Care Medicine*, 172, 8, 2005, 1019–25. doi: 10.1164/rccm.200412-1731OC.

60   Noonan, "Environmental asbestos exposure and risk of mesothelioma".

61   S M Candura, A Binarelli, G Ragno and F Scafa, "Two cases of asbestosis and one case of rounded atelectasis due to non-occupational asbestos exposure", *Monaldi Archives for Chest Disease*, 69, 1, 2008, 35–8. doi: 10.4081/monaldi.2008.410. K H Kilburn, R Lilis, H A Anderson, C T Boylen, H E Einstein, S J Johnson and R Warshaw, "Asbestos disease in family contacts of shipyard workers", *American Journal of Public Health*, 75, 6, 1985, 615–17. C Magnani, F Mollo, L Paoletti, D Bellis, P Bernardi, P Betta, M Botta, M Falchi, C Ivaldi and M Pavesi, "Asbestos lung burden and asbestosis after occupational and environmental exposure in an asbestos cement manufacturing area: a necropsy study", *Occupational and Environmental Medicine*, 55, 12, 1998, 840–46.

62   Olsen *et al.*, "Increasing incidence of malignant mesothelioma after exposure to asbestos during home maintenance and renovation". C Rake, C Gilham, J.Hatch, A Darnton, J Hodgson and J Peto, "Occupational, domestic and environmental mesothelioma risks in the British population: a case-control study", *British Journal of Cancer*, 100, 7, 2009, 1175–83. doi: 10.1038/sj.bjc.6604879.

cent of mesothelioma cases in men and 35.7 per cent of those in women. In the British case-control study by Rake *et al.*, there was no increased risk of mesothelioma from home renovation although 19 cases (3 per cent of all cases) had any DIY activity involving asbestos as their primary exposure.

There has only been one study of professional asbestos removalists.[63] In that study, compared with the general British population, removalists had increased risk of death from all-causes, all cancers, lung cancer, and mesothelioma. Furthermore, protective activities such as dust suppression techniques and respirator types used by the workers did not reduce the risks.

Conclusions

Asbestos products are widespread in the built environment and are likely to remain there for a very long time. The risk posed by *in situ* asbestos is hard to quantify but there is evidence that activities such as renovation and removal, which can cause short-term high-level exposure to asbestos fibres, can result in asbestos related disease, particularly mesothelioma.[64] Our understanding of the risk of asbestos related disease from long-term low-level exposure that could occur from the scenarios described above, however, is poor. What is known is that the number of people exposed to *in situ* asbestos in Australia is probably very large.[65] Therefore, we need to improve our understanding about the risks associated with, and the future burden of, diseases resulting from exposure to non-occupational sources of asbestos. Specifically, we need more information about exposure levels, including background levels, in the general community.[66] We need to determine if the models used to predict occupational cases of disease can be used to accurately predict non-occupational cases, and if existing information about current non-occupational exposure is sufficient to include in those models.[67] Predictions of the future burden of asbestos related disease that may emerge from low-dose asbestos exposure might provide some insight about how best to manage the remaining *in situ* asbestos in Australia.

---

63 Frost *et al.*, "Occupational exposure to asbestos and mortality among asbestos removal workers: a Poisson regression analysis".

64 Frost *et al.*, "Occupational exposure to asbestos and mortality among asbestos removal workers: a Poisson regression analysis". Olsen *et al.*, "Increasing incidence of malignant mesothelioma after exposure to asbestos during home maintenance and renovation".

65 Reid, "Review of the effectiveness of predictive models for mesothelioma to identify lessons for asbestos related policy".

66 Armstrong and Driscoll, "Mesothelioma in Australia: cresting the third wave".

67 Reid, "Review of the effectiveness of predictive models for mesothelioma to identify lessons for asbestos related policy".

Part 6
In Their Own Words:
The Witness Stories

Chapter 12

WITTENOOM'S FLYING DOCTOR

Dr Eric Saint

Dr Eric Saint (1918-1989) grew up on industrial Tyneside where the suffering caused by social deprivation fuelled his lifelong commitment to social medicine. He completed his doctorate in industrial medicine before migrating to become a district medical officer, including working for the Flying Doctor Service. He was first to warn mine management and the state's Health Department of the potential disaster posed by Wittenoom's asbestos dust, predicting "the richest and most lethal crop of cases of asbestosis in the world's literature". Although he regretted his inability to effect change at Wittenoom, he did make a difference in the wider region. He found the "all-round doctoring" demanded of him in the remote area exciting and recalled that this was "the best work I've ever done in my life". He later became foundation professor of medicine at the University of WA. He was an expert witness at the trial Barrow & Heys v. CSR Ltd 1988 in WA's Supreme Court and his letters and warnings forty years previously about the dangers of asbestos were crucial in Justice Rowland's judgement against CSR.[1]

I was appointed in 1948 as a medical officer in the [Western Australian] Health Department. There were five of us came out from England. They couldn't get Australian doctors at all, so they advertised in England and we all came out at the same time in February 1948 and we all went to north-western ports. It was quite arbitrary and I went to Port Hedland.

I arrived in Port Hedland at the high peak of summer, to encounter heat as searing and as enervating as that experienced during the war on the plains of northern India. The township then was a ramshackle collection

---

1   This account consists of excerpts from an interview with Eric Saint conducted by Lenore Layman, 27 April 1984, together with excerpts from a personal manuscript, Eric E Saint, "Port Hedland 1948–1951". Eric G Saint papers, 2003/10 Box 2 personal. University of Western Australia Archives. L Layman, 'Saint, Eric Galton (1918–1989)', *Australian Dictionary of Biography*, National Centre of Biography, Australian National University, http://adb.anu.edu.au/biography/saint-eric-galton-15614/text26817, vol 18 (Melbourne: MUP, 2012). Accessed 11 October 2018.

of dilapidated old wooden buildings inhabited by less than 500 people, who invited the attentions of a plague of flies and countless bloodsucking insects breeding happily in the surrounding mangrove swamps. An air of torpor hung over the town, which seemed to come to life only late in the afternoon when housewives emerged to do their shopping at the bakery, the butchers, and the three stores, later joining their spouses in the beer gardens or saloons of the two hotels.

The practice was a large one and part of the flying doctor network. My medical neighbours were located in Onslow to the southwest and Broome to the northeast, leaving me to look after the inhabitants of the townships of Marble Bar, Wittenoom, and Roebourne, in addition to Port Hedland, all the pastoral properties, most of which had fashioned primitive airstrips, in the area, and the Aboriginal settlement at Jigalong, well to the east on the edge of the central desert. A rhythm of life developed. On Monday I used to fly to Marble Bar, on Friday to Wittenoom Gorge, and on alternate Thursdays either to Nullagine, further inland from the Bar, or to Roebourne. Wittenoom Gorge lay an hour and a half to two hours flying time to the south of Hedland.

When I got there Wittenoom was fairly small. There were only about 50 people, I think. In that period 1948 to 1951, when I left, the population had quadrupled. So I saw it develop from fairly small when all the houses were in the Gorge itself.

Between 1949 and 1950 on the plains at the mouth of the Gorge a township was established of featureless, treeless, waterless streets of hot little asbestos boxes, the roads being sealed with tailings from the mill. They were a very slack company. They made no provisions for me at all. In the three years I was there they didn't set up any sick quarters or anything. So it was in one of the houses, by courtesy of the occupant, that I used to conduct my surgeries. In my time two fine and dedicated women manned the first aid post, dealing with the minor infections, allergies, cuts, and bruises in my absence. I was responsible for everything.

I had been a research student in a newly established Department of Industrial Health in Newcastle University, so I knew a lot about industrial health, and in fact had just been awarded my doctorate. And in the north of England we knew how dangerous asbestos was. There was a factory in Washington just outside of Newcastle where original observations had been made on asbestosis.[2] By 1948 there was a well-established medical

---

2   Newalls Insulation Co., subsidiary of Turner & Newall, made insulation products. See Grace's Guide to British Industrial History, www.gracesguide.co.uk/Turner_and_Newall. Accessed 11 October 2018.

literature on the dangers of asbestos particles. It was known that this fibre was a highly dangerous material causing progressive lung fibrosis, incurable, and ultimately leading to respiratory insufficiency, although it was not known then that asbestos also had carcinogenic properties, causing the development of tumours of the lining of the lungs and, sometimes, the abdominal cavity.

When I went to Wittenoom and saw that mill and all that brown-blue haze, I was filled with horror. I sat down and said, "You're going to have the worst catastrophe of asbestosis ever seen" and sent that to the Commissioner of Public Health. I spoke to the Company and said, "Look, you've got problems". They pooh-poohed my anxieties and in fact they labeled me as a troublemaker. I was disturbing their equilibrium. Perhaps they doubted my competence, or perhaps they did not want to hear.

I predicted that there would be an avalanche of cases of asbestosis, and my predictions were indeed borne out. Numbers affected might have been greater had not the labour turnover been so high; a majority of men chose to leave employment as quickly as they could. In 1948 when the township was confined to the upper Gorge a majority of men were single and lived in cramped, hot single men's quarters. Some were old goldfields men, escaping the eyes of the law or of wives or de factos, but a majority were non-English speaking displaced persons newly arrived at Fremantle from resettlement camps in war-ravaged Europe—Poles, Yugoslavs, Balts, Germans. They were met at the dockside in Fremantle, offered free transport and accommodation. To a majority conditions were not to their liking; after saving up the price of a single airfare back to Perth they would shoot through.

My formal letter to the Department of Health was acknowledged; but mining health problems were the concern of the Department of Mines and it was many years, a decade or more, before action was taken. At that time the Department of Health had no sector devoted to occupational medicine. There wasn't any industry in Perth at all then. It was the local experience. They'd never encountered asbestos; they'd never had occasion to look it up in the literature. It wasn't in the front of their consciousness. All they were thinking about was what they knew, that there's a certain amount of silicosis among the miners in Kalgoorlie, working siliceous rock. But in point of fact it wasn't siliceous rock there. And I was pointing out that this is a special problem. And moreover the X-ray changes in asbestosis are much more subtle than the rather obvious changes that you see with silicosis.

So I would put it this way, that there was a combination of very poor management up there who were really disinterested in this sort of thing. All they wanted to do was to make their money as quickly as possible, disinterested in the welfare of the people. That's on the industry side. The workers were coming and going. And there were the unions: there was no union activity. And then the Health Department wasn't interested because they didn't really have the expertise at the time. The mining people [in the Mines Department] were looking at the morbidity among miners; what interested them was silicosis.

They didn't listen. I was just a young man, a Flying Doctor. They weren't listening. I could speak with the voice of authority—I hadn't got a doctorate and worked in the Department of Industrial Health for nothing. But I was a young person. I'd only just come out from England and they thought, "Who's this jumped-up fellow; who's this Johnny-come-lately?" That was the attitude.

I suppose if I'd been more politically active myself I really should have gone to Trades Hall and banged on the table. But by and large doctors don't behave like that. You had to work with these people. It's hard to re-capture. It was very interesting; I was encountering what were for me a whole series of quite unique situations.

Chapter 13

A PUBLIC HEALTH CAMPAIGNER'S STORY

Dr Jim McNulty, Occupational Health Physician

Dr Jim McNulty gained his medical degree at Queen's University of Belfast and worked as a chest physician in England before migrating to Western Australia in 1956 to a position in the Public Health Department in Kalgoorlie. His responsibility was the diagnosis of tuberculosis and dust diseases in miners. He fought the general assumption that "miners get dust disease", seeking to persuade the powerful Mines Department to utilise more effective dust sampling equipment in order to enforce tighter dust controls. The Mines Department's authority over occupational health in the mines to the virtual exclusion of the Public Health Department was a major concern. He recalls feeling "like John the Baptist bleating in the wilderness". In 1963 he moved to Perth where he joined the new, small Occupational Health Branch of the Department. He remembers the attitude at the time that disease was a natural consequence of working in industrial trades and the resultant "laissez faire" approach to workplace health dangers. The Branch focused on the areas of dust control, noise abatement, more careful handling of chemicals, and clean air control. In 1975 he was appointed Commissioner for Public Health (titled Commissioner for Health from 1979). In the 1980s and 1990s he was frequently called to give evidence in litigation seeking compensation for people who had contracted asbestos related diseases.[1]

I came out from the United Kingdom when invited to take a position as Mines Medical Officer, chest physician at the Kalgoorlie Regional Hospital. We operated a mines mobile X-ray caravan that went to all the outlying mining centres and took chest X-rays and occupational histories of the miners. And it went to Wittenoom every year.

---

1   This account consists of edited excerpts of interviews with Jim McNulty conducted by Lenore Layman, 10 May 1984, 5 August 2008 and by Criena Fitzgerald, 7, 15 November 2002; 10, 20 December 2002; 3, 21 February 2003; 18 April 2003.

The mobile unit's tour took about three months. It would go from Kalgoorlie to Leonora, Gwalia, across to Leinster, Cue, all through the mining towns, up to Wittenoom, and around Hedland and down again. Until you got to a mine there was no way of knowing who actually was working there because they were a transient group, particularly in the outlying group of gold mines, so when you got there they would give you a list of the men who were working on the mine and the mobile unit would X-ray them. The X-ray images were always developed in the bush in those days; hung in the trees to dry. They would come back in bulk with the unit when it came back.

Wittenoom

The first intimation I had [of the presence of asbestosis] was a letter to say that a Wittenoom miner had been admitted to Wooroloo [Sanatorium] for tuberculosis and had lung surgery. It was proved through a biopsy that he had asbestosis and quite progressive—a fair bit of it. Coincidently—this was in 1958—the mobile unit returned to Kalgoorlie from its tour, which had included Wittenoom, and, on looking at the X-rays, five of them showed early signs of asbestosis. The X-rays often had asbestos fibres clinging to them when they came back to Kalgoorlie.

I arranged to personally visit Wittenoom [in 1959]. It was a dreadful place. I got off the plane and was appalled at the empty scenery. It had been stripped of everything really, little vegetation; it was stinking hot in November and I was met by a blast of heat off the tarmac. Wittenoom pub wasn't a particularly desirable place but, anyway, it was a haven. I had arranged to meet 30 or 40 people I wanted to see individually to examine but, unfortunately, MacRobertson Miller Airlines had mislaid all the X-rays and files, so I had to see them without any information whatever as to their previous history or their X-ray appearance, so it was very difficult. There were severe language barriers.

I examined all of them clinically but in those years, although I found extensive disease in some of the men and I advised them strongly to get out, I don't know of a single person who took my advice. It's a bit heartbreaking; it damps your enthusiasm. But some people might have got out later because of my advice.

I went to Wittenoom four times during that period [1959–66]. I talked to everybody I saw in the bar or the pub and I talked casually to people. I talked to anybody who'd stop me. I went to homes and talked to people. I talked to the company and the mines. In all that time I interviewed dozens and dozens of miners, perhaps hundreds of them, and each one I told the same story. Short of hiring a hall and having a public meeting, which would never have happened, they didn't do things like that in those days. What didn't happen in those days and would happen now is that you would go on *Today Tonight* or some program, or you would burst free in the press. It wasn't that you were hiding from the limelight, it just wasn't seen as a role. You were always talking. I never had a parental, patronising attitude; it was up to individuals. You would talk to them and persuade them to leave, but that was their decision if they wanted to stay. It was their lives to lead.

In 1959 when I went up the first time, I was appalled at the use of mine tailings in the town. They were everywhere—at the racecourse, the golf course, and around the recreation areas, the parking areas and the pub. I complained then that the men were exposed to enough dust at work, that they shouldn't be exposed to it at home, at rest. And then in 1960, I drew attention to my worry about families and the exposure of children, because I remember driving up to a house and there was a little girl standing outside, a child standing outside with a nappy, on the sort of gateway. And when the car stopped, the dust rose up and enveloped the child and then hung around and gradually dissipated with the wind.

The tailings were done by the company on public areas and done by the men themselves, who took utes out and filled them up. They put it around the houses as a sort of blue metal. It was done by Main Roads Department for road surfacing. It was done even by a contractor who was building the hospital. It was a very handy crushed material for building purposes and for road surfacing. But the mining company allowed it, permitted it, and it took me many years to persuade them to stop.

The staff had better houses up in the gorge, and they lived right up against the mine. There was gross air pollution from the mill where they lived; blown off the road, off everything, from the workings. The general managers who once worked in Wittenoom have died of mesothelioma, and some of their children, and they couldn't not have accepted when I told them it was dangerous. In 1959 when I talked to them I told them the names of the people who had been affected and showed them the X-rays and talked about their history and they knew them all personally. They knew what jobs they did, because it was very small—a couple of hundred men—and yet they continued to live in the staff quarters with trucks full of asbestos rubbish going past the houses, dropping asbestos everywhere, and continued with the roads tailings on top of the roads.

So it was an absolutely, totally, and complete uphill task to try and influence them in any respect. The local mines inspectors were quite receptive and interested, but the primary purpose of the Department of Mines was and is the promotion of the mining industry, and that's what it lives for; health and safety come along as a second string.

When Cassandras like Professor Eric Saint, myself, Public Health, several Commissioners, advised that dust was a problem and predicted the development of disease it didn't ring any alarm bells in the people concerned in the mining industry because they were used to it, they expected it. I think there was a communication barrier between us. I did not seem to produce an effect. I never was quite sure why not, whether it was just inertia in the system or a sort of barrier.

A good example is when I proposed to send Gersh Major from the Commonwealth's School of Public Health and Tropical Medicine in Sydney, who was an expert in dust sampling, to Wittenoom to do testing. I did that through the Mines Department because I couldn't impose it on them because he had to have their help. And they were very reluctant to permit it, and only permitted it eventually because the Public Health Department paid all his expenses. The Commonwealth agreed not to charge us for his services and we paid his travelling expenses and his residency and whatever fees were due. He did a marvellous job of work in dust sampling but it took him twelve months to produce his report, by which time the mine was virtually closing anyway.

There were references to my reports which were damning—in 1959—in the press, but no-one paid any attention. The point I made in that report was that men of much younger age were getting more extensive disease in Wittenoom after three, four, and five years of mining, compared to gold miners who were a much older age group taking 20 or 30 years to develop dust disease. To my mind, to see a man of 35 or 40 with extensive lung disease after three or four years in the mill was completely appalling, but that didn't register at the top levels. I sat back waiting for some action to occur, and nothing happened. Nothing. It wasn't debated in parliament. Nobody even raised it as a matter. It was just closed minds.

Perth and Kwinana

Asbestos was handled shockingly here [in Perth]. In the 1960s there was liquid spraying of asbestos on roofs for acoustic purposes to deaden noise and also on girders above for fire protection—and that was a requirement

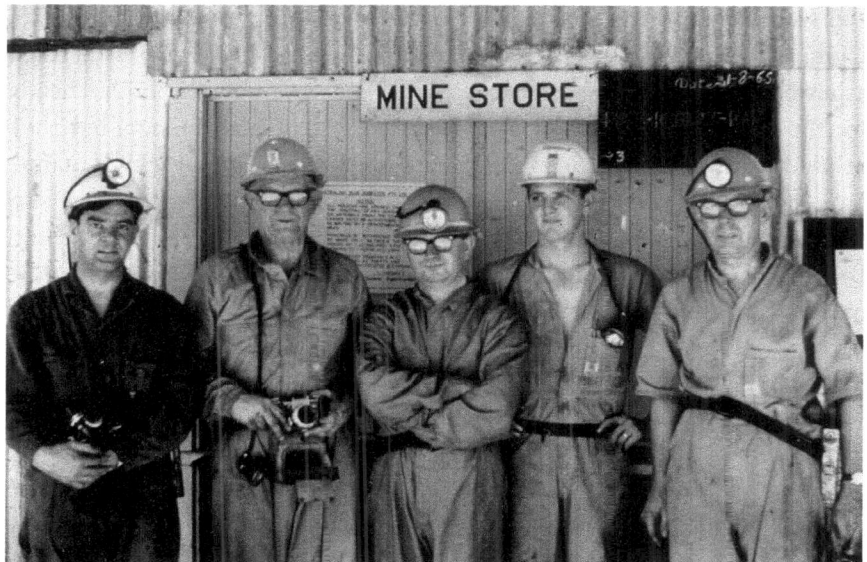

Figure 13.1: Testing dust levels at Wittenoom's mine and mill, 1966. L to R: Assoc. Prof. Bryan Gandevia, Industrial hygienist Gersh Major, Dr Jim McNulty. The two men on the right are not known.
Courtesy: J McNulty

in many places. Dumas House[2] was being constructed; I went up there and it was open floor—the third or fourth level—when I saw it, and men were spraying the asbestos. It came from out of a jet of water and asbestos and it would adhere to the ceiling, in a completely open third floor—no walls, nothing in it, and men were moving about, carpenters, people doing their own work while this was being sprayed. The asbestos sprayer was dressed in a helmet with a gown and an air supply hood, while every other Tom, Dick and Harry was moving about doing their own work around this. And the pollution, the spillage, was enormous. Half would be on the floor in clumps, and that was blowing all over West Perth. I said, "Look, there are three miners over there in Parliament that I know personally who have got silicosis—gold miners from Norseman and Kalgoorlie. I am going across there now to tell them that they are going to get asbestosis as well from the bloody dust that is falling over here". Anyway, we put such clean air restrictions that the practice of spraying was abandoned, but it continued in other ways for quite a while afterwards.

---

2   The new fourteen-storey Public Works Department office building in West Perth was completed in 1965.

I went down to Kwinana when they were building the State Electricity Commission power station [in the late 1960s]. And they were using blue asbestos—it might have been even later—to spray on the boiler heads for the huge boilers to make power. I tried to tell them to stop, but they produced the specifications from the company in England which manufactured the boilers, and if you go away from the specifications, you lose your warranties. We had to go back to England and take it up with the big British boilermaker to get them to lift their specifications and allow ordinary asbestos to be used—which they did.

Memories and regrets

There were terrible things. A little Aboriginal boy on the back of a truck getting a lift into Point Samson, lying on top of the hessian bag reeking of asbestos fibres. Because the fibres all came through the hessian bags. Things like that. Or James Hardie recycling sacks by whacking them on the ground. Dust ... God almighty, yes.

Perhaps I was too nice a guy, I don't know really. I wasn't forceful enough or something, or I didn't communicate very well. I don't really know. It has haunted all my life. It's been a black cloud all the time because you have got to ask yourself—what could I have done at that stage, or something I should have done.

Chapter 14

THE STORY OF THE ASBESTOS DISEASES SOCIETY OF AUSTRALIA

Robert Vojakovic, President

Robert Vojakovic, with Melita Markey

Australia's foremost advocate for victims of asbestos diseases is Robert Vojakovic AM JP, foundation president and spokesman for the Asbestos Diseases Society of Australia (ADSA), which is located physically in Western Australia but helps people who have had asbestos exposure and are suffering from asbestos related disease from all over Australia. Rose Marie, Robert's partner and wife, is also counsellor and carer at the Society. Together they have built the ADSA into Australia's major asbestos public health advocacy organisation.[1]

I am going to tell you a story that begins with a handful of people like myself who worked at CSR's Wittenoom mining and milling operation in the Pilbara, Western Australia. Croatian-born in 1940 I worked in Wittenoom, from October to December 1961.

The Asbestos Diseases Society of Australia Inc.—the early years

The Asbestos Diseases Society of Australia Inc. (ADSA) started from humble beginnings initially comprising a small number of former Wittenoom

---

1   This text has been compiled from Robert Vojakovic's address at the Slater & Gordon Witness Seminar, 1 October 2009, 11th biennial conference, Australian & New Zealand Society of the History of Medicine, University of Western Australia; and Robert Vojakovic's interview with Mia Lindgren, 7 September 2010 for the Australian Asbestos Network. Also from Michael Cannon, *That disreputable firm* (Melbourne: Melbourne University Press, 1998) and Ben Hills, *Blue murder* (South Melbourne: Sun Books, 1989).

workers and families concerned about their friends and family members becoming ill. By 1978 many more people were starting to get sick and newspaper stories about the lethal threat of asbestos related diseases were appearing, but advice and assistance for injured workers were not available. So a small group formed, with a nucleus of about 40 people, mostly former miners, who met once or twice a week for three hours in the afternoon at the North Perth Migrant Resource Centre.

From this small office the group began to provide help, including self-help for each other, as well as counselling, economic assistance, fundraising for the people who were doing it tough, people disabled by these then mysterious asbestos diseases and unable to work. We delivered food parcels during the year and hampers for Christmas. One member of our team drove to Mandurah to help chop wood for a family. He thought it was going to be for only a couple of hours but he chopped all afternoon and went back for the next couple of days.

We also started to fundraise money for medical research and began a community awareness program because at the time nobody in the community knew very much about asbestos related diseases. Little information was available on the safe handling of asbestos and the dangers of exposure. Many public meetings were held in city and country areas and in various workplaces. We went to construction sites, factories, universities, and to the Perth Royal Agricultural Show—undertaking approximately 2,000 lung function tests at the first show we attended. We also gave out a lot of literature.

Further to this we raised awareness on Perth City streets every second Friday. Information was disseminated at every opportunity. Our handouts were reproduced in Italian, German, and some Slavic languages, most often in Serbo-Croatian which was used throughout Yugoslavia at the time.

In 1983 I was elected President of the Asbestos Diseases Society of Australia Inc and we were finally in a position to establish our own premises at 483 Charles Street, North Perth. From here we continued to raise awareness of the dangers of asbestos and the need for fair and just compensation, treatment, and medical research for victims.

Our new North Perth premises became a drop-in centre for people to come in for a chat. It was a non-threatening environment and sometimes we were supported by trained counselors. As well, up to 30 volunteers worked on a daily basis going to people's houses and visiting patients in hospital. Some of them spent time all night there. Between 1979 and 1984 we slowly gathered momentum as a force for change.

The fight for justice

At this time compensation for asbestos related diseases was limited to the statutory entitlements under the Workers' Compensation Act which were low weekly payments. People were unsuccessful in winning more compensation because of the strong defenses mounted by Colonial Sugar Refining (CSR) Company which owned the Wittenoom mine and mill.

Cornelius Maas was the first ex-Wittenoom worker to issue a writ for civil damages against Midalco Pty Ltd (formerly Australian Blue Asbestos Ltd, a subsidiary of CSR), but he died shortly after, in 1977. Joan Joosten in 1979 was the first ex-Wittenoom worker to take Midalco to court. She had worked in the office close to the contaminated old mill in Wittenoom Gorge and she developed mesothelioma. Bear in mind that it was very hard to win any compensation for the people who worked in the mine or mill, let alone the office, situated about 50 metres from the dusty mill. Midalco vigorously defended itself.

Joan Joosten had support from others who had worked at Wittenoom and from members of the WA Trades and Labor Council. Sadly she lost her case, and it would take legislative changes to mount the next set of cases. Our North Perth premises were dedicated to Mrs Joosten and her courageous battle.

Lobbying governments for legislative changes

The *WA Workers' Compensation Act* was amended in 1981 to include asbestos related lung cancer as a compensable disease and to allow immediate lump-sum compensation for those diagnosed with mesothelioma. Through successful lobbying of the newly elected Labor government further gains began to be made. Up to this time victims of asbestos diseases faced a bar, a six-year statute of limitation to report an injury from the time they stopped work. As asbestos diseases have a latency period of 20–40 years this was a grave injustice and of great benefit to CSR and others. After failed discussions with previous governments under Charles Court and Ray O'Connor, new Labor Premier Brian Burke along with Attorney General Joe Berinson and Mining Minister Peter Dowding amended the Act to allow WA workers to proceed with an action beyond six years from leaving their employment. Further to this, they were granted access to legal aid in order to mount cases. There was more successful lobbying for the entitlement of wives to compensation when husbands died. In 1985 Peter Dowding was instrumental in finding "missing" Mines Department and Health Department files from the previous government which then became available to those preparing litigation.

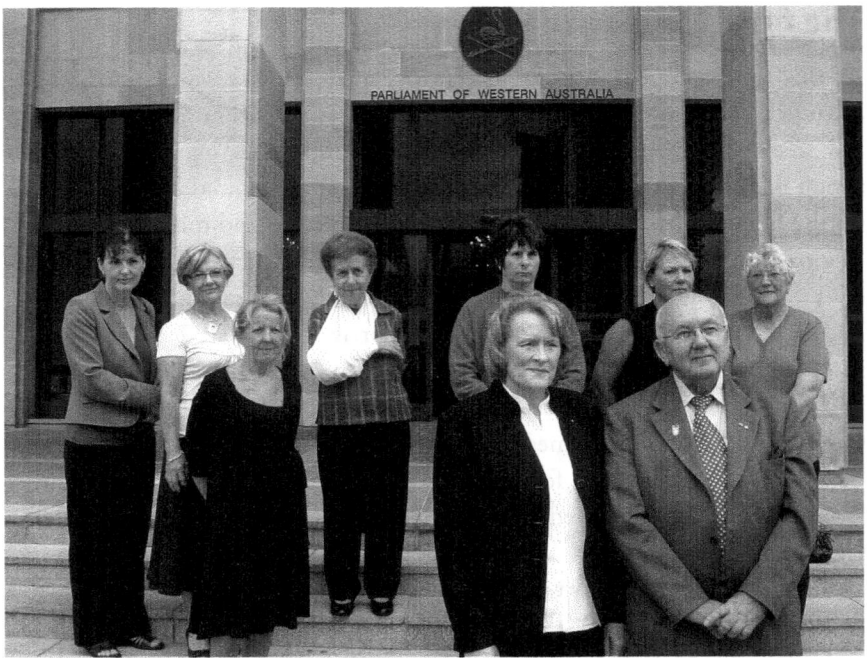

Figure 14.1: Robert and Rose Marie Vojakovic standing outside Parliament House, Perth with some of the widows of Wittenoom.
Courtesy: Asbestos Diseases Society of Australia

In 1986 ADSA mounted a test case with Rino Pedrotti who sadly died in hospital on the day he was to give bedside evidence to lawyers and a judge. The law firm Lavan and Solomon decided that they would not pursue further cases so I decided to move on and commence working with law firm Taylor Smart. This is where I connected with a young lawyer John Gordon (no relation to Slater & Gordon).

I read an article in the paper about Slater & Gordon's success in Melbourne with the case Harold Plimer v Mc Pherson's Ltd, so I rang Peter Gordon to ask if he was interested in our cases in WA. Fortunately he was and he immediately flew to Perth to meet myself and our committee. It was agreed that Slater & Gordon (S&G) would set up a branch in Perth on the no win/no fee basis and the ADSA would sign over all cases.

It was the start of an epic battle of big business against a group of sick and dying people and one small law firm in WA consisting of two lawyers: John Gordon and Luisa Formato (whose brother- in-law had recently died from mesothelioma) supported by Peter Gordon and the team in Melbourne. The costs were extraordinary and still S&G led by Peter Gordon invested to achieve justice for the victims of Wittenoom leaving themselves millions of dollars in debt. With everything ready to go, a small office, a few PCs and telephones, the fledgling S&G and the ADSA set about issuing writs for complaints. However, despite the amendments made by Brian Burke's Labor government, all claims for illnesses before 1 January 1934 had to be lodged by 18 January 1987.

So started a vicious and frightening campaign against the ADSA, myself, committee members, and our families. Especially targeted were my children with threatening calls to the home. I believe it was an industrial conspiracy to frustrate the process to issue these writs in time. The campaign consisted of a series of raids by police on the ADSA offices, my home, and committee members' homes looking for recording devices, guns, and documents. The warrant suggested our organisation had made a threat to the government. This was not true and we believed it was a ploy to discredit the ADSA.

Legal victories

Since those early days when CSR fought savagely there have been many legal victories, one of the early ones being that of Wally Simpson in 1986. In this case Justice Peter Brinsden failed to accept the medical evidence and suggested the plaintiff was exaggerating his symptoms. The case was successfully appealed and a retrial ordered based on the acceptance of the epidemiological evidence—now growing in Perth with so many cases starting to present to physicians. Mr Simpson accepted an out of court settlement.

Many lessons were learnt from the Simpson case and it was the bravery of Klaus Rabenault which enabled Peter Gordon and the team to deliver a compelling judgement in a Victorian Court that would enable victims to finally get some justice. Klaus Rabenault was a former Wittenoom worker who was living in Melbourne when diagnosed with mesothelioma in 1987. In 1988 in addition to awarding compensation for negligence the jury added a further amount for punitive damages. (See chapter 16 for Peter Gordon's account of this case.)

Counselling and support services

While the battles raged for fair and just compensation there was a compelling need to support the victims and their families both emotionally and financially. We realised early on that many were battling to live day to day and it was often necessary to assist with food parcels and work closely with what is today Centrelink and the Department of Housing to ensure people were adequately housed and fed while they and their families battled to exist with these terrible diseases.

My wife Rose Marie was a tiger in these days fighting for the civil rights of these victims in the face of an unsympathetic social services system which was still coming to terms with the growing epidemiological evidence of the diseases. With more victims finding their way to the Society we realised that we needed a system of monitoring people and their potential symptoms.

Rose Marie started an amazing file system which still exists today. We already had 500 files in our office, not only of people from Wittenoom but also of Port Authority workers who had handled asbestos, at Port Sampson, Fremantle, James Hardie, and Westrail which was still using asbestos in 1984. By 1994 we had more than 250 files just relating to Wittenoom.

People who come to us because they are worried about their past exposure to asbestos have come into contact with the material in many different ways—a housewife helping her husband by holding planks while he cut asbestos cement sheeting or sweeping up after the job; someone who had played in an asbestos cubby made from old, deteriorating boards as a child; people who had worked as plumbers, carpenters or electricians; renovators; those who had worked for James Hardie, Westrail, on the wharfs or in transport; people who had lived at Wittenoom or visited it; pilots, people from the armed forces, newspaper workers—a myriad of people. And often their exposure was a long time ago, up to 40 years, sometimes long forgotten.

Fear of asbestos disease was everywhere and people were being ridiculed for their fears. Many became socially isolated. It was frustrating for them, especially the boredom as they were used to working and now they couldn't do anything around the house. And so eventually they came to believe they were useless. There was limited income, loss of self-esteem, isolation, and guilt. So we increased our social activities. We had one or two meetings every week just to get people out of their houses and do something with them to re-orientate them. We believe that it is positive if people are no longer just languishing at home; instead that they're taking action, they are doing something for themselves or the family. Most importantly we tried to assist people with their grief and also respect them. Members of the ADSA see it very much as a family. We found how we could best help people to live and we continue to do that. This included providing access to a GP who understood the complex symptoms of asbestos diseases. This was Dr Greg Deleuil who had a specialist knowledge of lungs through his expertise in diving medicine. (See chapter 15 for Dr Deleuil's story).

Increasing community awareness

Sadly, despite the Wittenoom mine closing 52 years ago, the death toll from asbestos diseases still climbs. Western Australia has the highest incidence of malignant mesothelioma in Australia and indeed the world. One person in Australia dies every 12 hours from mesothelioma.

The ADSA continues to bring attention to the dangers of asbestos still so prevalent in our community. We have a new wave of victims, not just the miners and tradesmen, but the home handymen and women and their children who played nearby while their parents renovated an old kitchen or put up a new asbestos fence.

The safe removal of asbestos is poorly overseen and regulations rarely enforced in our communities and the ADSA deals with numerous complaints. Despite laws banning asbestos products it is still being imported in goods from countries where it is used. As a recent example, close to 500 workers were exposed to asbestos through the use of contaminated ceiling panels in the construction of the new Perth Children's Hospital which opened in 2018. There is still much work to do in legislation and enforcement in these matters.

The present day

Thirty-five years on from the founding of the ADSA there is still much work to be done in protecting the legal rights of victims and indeed finding life-saving treatments for them. With regard to the legal situation WA still lags behind other states in terms of compensation, despite ongoing attempts by successive state governments to pass similar legislation to other states regarding provisional damages for asbestos victims.

The ADSA and health professionals agree that treatment and cure is the most expedient solution to the issue of asbestos diseases in Australia. While total removal of asbestos from the environment is a worthy goal sometimes removal may increase the hazard from asbestos dust. The ongoing cost burden of compensation and medical treatment to our community is projected to increase well into the future. To improve treatments and find a cure the ADSA now funds the Asbestos Diseases Society of Australia

Mesothelioma Research PhD Scholarship every three years. This is administered by the National Centre for Asbestos Diseases Research based in the University of WA and is leading the world in mesothelioma treatment.

Remembering victims

For the last 22 years the ADSA has held an ecumenical memorial service on the last Friday of November so families can grieve and remember lost ones. We pray for justice, medical research, and fair and just legal remedies, and for the families and their suffering. For the families of Wittenoom, Australia's greatest industrial disaster, it has been particularly hard as they cannot go back to their homes at the site of the crimes against their loved ones. Wittenoom remains a contaminated and deadly ghost town.

In August 2018 after 30 years of campaigning a permanent memorial was created for the victims of Wittenoom opposite Parliament House in Solidarity Park in West Perth as a lasting memorial to past victims and reminder of the ongoing challenges to ensure the community is protected.

The year 2018 was the 30th anniversary of the Rabenault (Melbourne) and Hays and Barrow (Perth) legal victories. These cases continue to serve as reminders of the lessons of the asbestos experience, and the long tragic chain of adverse medical, legal, and social consequences. The experience has underscored the well-recognised principle that the employer, the producer of asbestos products, has always had the inherent responsibility not to endanger workers or communities. This responsibility, when ignored or covered up by management, as evidenced within the asbestos industry, has brought about an irreversible legacy of human tragedies in the succeeding decades.

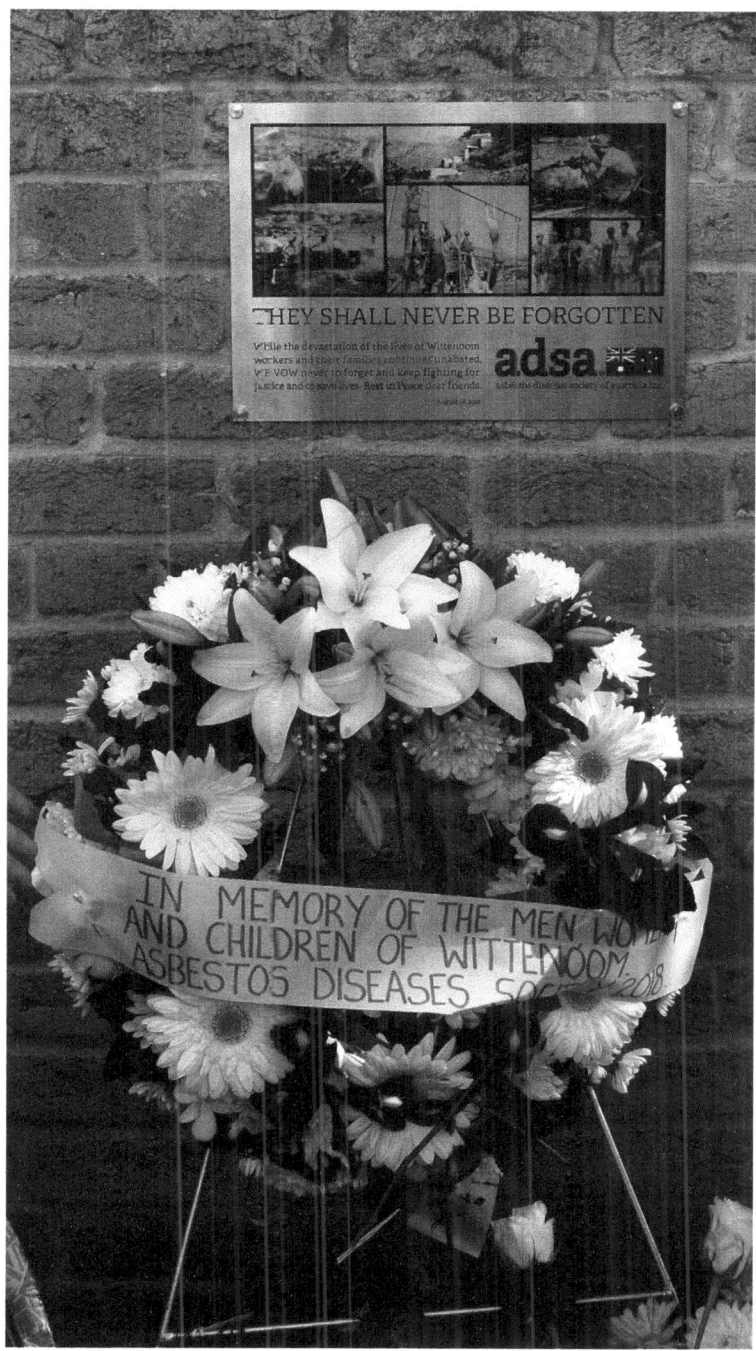

Figure 14.2: Remembering the dead
Courtesy: Asbestos Diseases Society of Australia

Chapter 15

A LIFE RECAST BY ASBESTOS

Dr Greg Deleuil, General Practitioner

Dr Greg Deleuil AM RFD is a general practitioner whose professional and personal experience has taken him from a position in which asbestos related diseases were not in the forefront of his mind to one where these diseases have become his primary focus—both as a general practitioner and as a public advocate warning of the ongoing risks of asbestos exposure. Over thirty years he has been resident at the Asbestos Diseases Society of Australia assisting people newly diagnosed with an asbestos related disease as well as those presenting who are fearful as a result of their history of asbestos exposure. This involvement has become his life's work. Greg was a member of the first intake of medical students at the University of Western Australia's newly created medical school in 1957, the first to be fully trained in Western Australia. He graduated in 1962 and has worked as a general practitioner throughout his career. In 1965 he married and in 1970 moved to work in a practice in his home town, Darwin.[1]

The starting point for this story is Darwin at dawn on 25 December 1974. Cyclone Tracy has just hit, causing enormous destruction. The cloud at dawn was an evil green colour. I was there with my wife Maris and three children. Our house was very close to the coast at Alawa and we were told to shelter in the bathroom. In fact the bathroom, bath, and toilet disappeared—they were blown away—so if we'd gone where we were supposed to go we probably would have been blown away as well. Instead we sheltered with friends. Our house was destroyed, Darwin's northern suburbs gone.

---

1   This account is an edited amalgamation of Dr Greg Deleuil's address at the Slater & Gordon Witness Seminar, 11th biennial conference, Australian and New Zealand Society of the History of Medicine, University of Western Australia, 1 October 2009; and Dr Greg Deleuil, interview with Lenore Layman, 7 April 2008; interview with Criena Fitzgerald, 21 January and 14 February 2017.

On Christmas Day 1974 the whole place was full of debris. You couldn't identify the streets, there was so much junk. Darwin had become a city-sized asbestos-contaminated demolition site which had to be cleaned up. It was a fibro asbestos city of 48,000 people with hundreds and hundreds of houses most of which were destroyed, and they were all fibro asbestos, the majority built in the 1950s and early 1960s. At that time Darwin wasn't a painted place—our house wasn't painted—so the asbestos was exposed. But it was fortunate that the cyclone occurred in the middle of the wet season which dampened down much of the asbestos dust, and therefore the clean-up teams handled much wet asbestos, which is not nearly as potentially harmful as dry.

Teams of workers—navy and army personnel and quite a few civilians—did the clean up and their uniform was a soft hat, a pair of shorts, a pair of boots, and a pair of leather gloves, that's all. They wore no protective gear against asbestos fibre inhalation. This was how the whole city was cleaned up. It was only later that I reflected on what might have happened with the asbestos; nobody thought about it. I wasn't tuned in to asbestos in those days. Although I had a case of asbestosis in my [medical examination] finals, I never thought of that.

Maris and the children were evacuated. I stayed on for about six weeks providing medical assistance and then followed them to Perth. I had a young family so I had to get out and it broke my heart because I loved it there. Darwin was my home town.

My family had moved there in 1946. I was a nine-year-old; I left when I was sixteen and went to further schooling in Melbourne. Our family's Darwin home, like so many, was a fibro asbestos house built in 1938 to withstand cyclones after the 1937 devastation. But it was unpainted. While house interiors were painted, exteriors were not, and this included the moulded asbestos louvres. I can remember how friable the louvres were: you could rub the corners and they would fray away. I can remember touching them with my hands and the dust came off in my fingers. My mother was a meticulous housekeeper and dusted the louvres regularly. It was the only exposure she had to asbestos. In 1995 my mother became ill and I was absolutely stunned when her pathology diagnosis was faxed through. She had peritoneal mesothelioma. I had to tell my father that she was dying, and I had to tell my brother. Thinking back to our asbestos house in Darwin I knew where she'd got it from—it was domestic exposure. She died in March 1996.

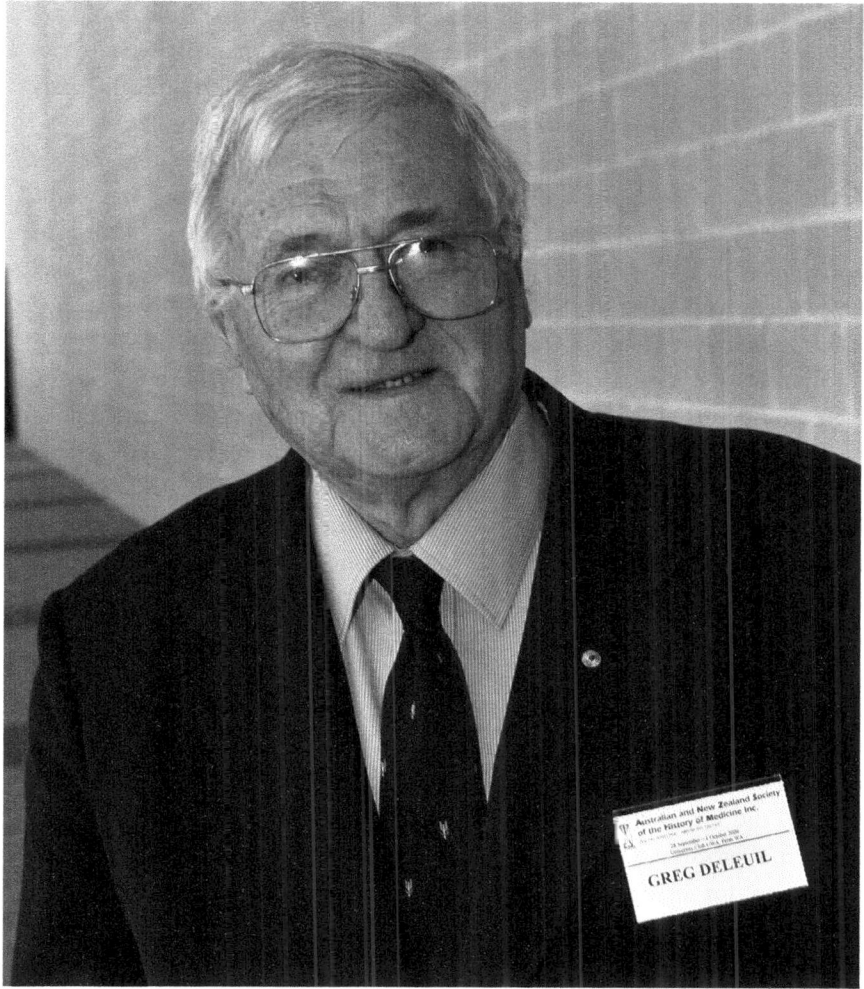

Figure 15.1: Dr Greg Deleuil
SOURCE: ANZSHM Witness Seminar, 2009.

The irony in this story is that I had worked in the field of asbestos related diseases for ten years, yet never gave a thought to the circumstances of my own and my family's life. When my mother got sick I realised then that Darwin was an asbestos city that had been destroyed by a cyclone, and I realised that we were going to see people from the clean up here [at the Asbestos Diseases Society of Australia] at some stage. That has happened and we've had asbestosis cases where the only asbestos exposure was the Darwin clean up after Cyclone Tracy. And people are still being exposed.

In more than forty years since Cyclone Tracy Darwin has expanded to 130,000 people and the new satellite town of Palmerston has encroached on burial sites for Tracy's debris which has been exposed in building works. The clean up of Australia's asbestos contamination is not complete.

Following Cyclone Tracy Greg moved to Perth where the Commonwealth Health Department declared that any doctor who was blown out of Darwin could obtain employment with the Department. So he began work there but he missed general practice and, with encouragement from a long-standing local pharmacist, Cyril Hywood, opened a new general practitioner's surgery in Dunedin Street, Mt Hawthorn, in Perth on 11 April 1975.

There was a huge area from North Perth to Mt Hawthorn where there were no doctors and I was enthusiastic about creating my own practice and so I set up by myself. The practice grew slowly. My professional involvement with asbestos arose from my involvement with diving medicine. In 1976 I joined the Army Reserve as a medical officer, and three years later I was asked to join the Special Air Service Regiment (SAS) as the regimental medical officer. Because the SAS has water operations—that is, some of its personnel were divers—I was sent to the School of Underwater Medicine at *HMAS Penguin* at Balmoral in Sydney and trained in Diving and Hyperbaric Medicine. I took this knowledge back to Perth and spent 1979 and 1980 in the regiment. When I was posted out, the new commanding officer asked me to come back and work as a civilian (with my officer rank), which I did for 27 years. I retired in 2007. The training I received in diving medicine encouraged me in 1980–82 to purchase hearing and respiratory equipment for testing civilian divers in my slowly growing medical practice. Even today not many practices have spirometry equipment and in those days it was a rarity. I did medicals for divers and then saw them with their injuries from diving.

In 1984 Robert Vojakovic from the Asbestos Diseases Society of Australia (ADSA), which was located in Charles Street near my practice, asked me to see his members who had been exposed in one way or another to asbestos. He knew that I could do lung function testing and I would be able to coordinate their scans and pulmonary function studies, dealing only with asbestos diseases. I did not take them over as patients; I facilitate these things for people. According to Robert, over approximately 33 years that I have been doing this work I have seen about 20,000 people. And it doesn't take long when you work with asbestos to develop fire in your belly. When my mother died asbestos became a personal issue and my work with asbestos related diseases has continued in her memory.

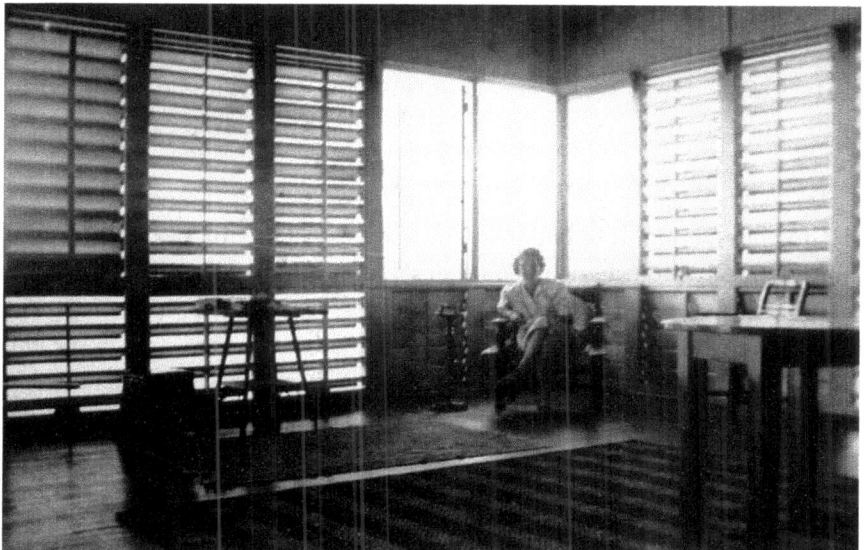

Figure 15.2: Alice Deleuil, in the family home in Darwin surrounded by asbestos louvres.
Courtesy: Greg Deleuil

At medical school [1957-62] occupational medicine and diseases such as silicosis and asbestosis came under the umbrella of respiratory diseases rather than tackling them from their industrial causes. I knew Robert [Vojakovic] was seeing people from Wittenoom. I'd read about Wittenoom and a book called *Blue murder* came out and I accumulated knowledge.[2] In those early years I saw a lot of people who had worked in the Wittenoom mill and they had dreadful asbestosis, and I can remember a firm named Ceiloyd that sprayed limpet asbestos as an insulation in roof cavities and on ceilings—dreadful. I remember when I was a young medical student in the early 1960s seeing cases of asbestosis in people from Wittenoom, and many of the patients I have seen, especially in the early years, previously lived in Wittenoom. There are photographs of the Wittenoom children playing in the asbestos tailings and having sack races in asbestos sacks. The company was very generous with the tailings. If you wanted a children's sand pit they'd bring down a big pile of blue sand. The race track was blue because it was made from blue tailings and you could see the horses kicking up blue dust. Then there was the asbestos tailing shovelling competition

---

2   Ben Hills, *Blue Murder: two thousand doomed to die, the shocking truth about Wittenoom's deadly dust* (South Melbourne: Sun Books, 1989).

where the winner was the first man to fill a 44 gallon drum with tailings; clouds of blue surrounded competitors and spectators. In my work I now deal with the deadly consequences of this exposure. Wittenoom closed in 1966 and we're not seeing, at least I don't see, the dreadful cases of asbestosis we used to see.

The ADSA sent me to a silicosis conference in San Francisco in 1993 and to the World Mesothelioma Conference in Paris in 1995. Six weeks after my return from Paris my mother's diagnosis came through. The irony was that I had been working in the asbestos field for ten years or so and never thought about my childhood and the asbestos exposure. What my mother's mesothelioma did was give me validity in the asbestos field in my own mind; it was sign that this was the work I must continue to do. It also cemented my acceptance by members at the Society: instead of being a doctor who works there I was also one of them. The changes were subtle but they were there. The last work I will phase out as I am growing older is my asbestos work which is in memory of my mother.

When I went to the United Kingdom in 1997 to attend a diving conference Robert suggested I take some photographs [relating to asbestos exposure in Western Australia] that had been collected over the years by the ADSA. I had met journalist Laurie Kazan-Allen who edits and publishes the British Asbestos Newsletter at the 1995 Paris conference and she organised for me to show the photos to a small meeting of solicitors and asbestos doctors. As a result, I was asked to present at a large conference a week later. I quickly phoned Perth to ask them to make up 38 slides for me to use and I spoke to those slides. I received accolades for the outstanding lecture of the day and Laurie asked me to develop it, which I did and talked at many different places—in Slovenia, Poland, the Netherlands, Belfast, Scotland and several times in London, including appearances at the House of Commons at the All Parliamentary Group on Occupational Safety and Health. From 1999 I went back to the United Kingdom every year and have been invited to present the asbestos story to groups around the United Kingdom. I give it to different groups, for instance in Manchester to a group of widows, and several times at different places for the solicitors Irwin Mitchell. I do it because I want to tell people the story, and it always has a powerful impact. I gave it in Thailand at an asbestos disease conference. I believe we should tell people to stop using the stuff. I feel the talk is really helpful.

I use slides in every lecture I give and they have a substantial impact. I show British people photographs because they live in a country where no asbestos was mined; all the asbestos they used was imported. I give my potted history of Wittenoom: the distribution of fibrous minerals within Western Australia, the mine, the haze of dust and dirty miners, the blue roads made entirely from tailings, the mill workers coated with dust, the bags of asbestos handled by lumpers [waterside workers] with dust permeating the fabric of the hessian; and the tailings, millions of tons of them, big tailings dumps which are highly contaminated with asbestos fibre. Dust storms instead of being brown were blue. Above all, I use Wittenoom's children as a theme and tell of the number who have died of mesothelioma. The mine closed in 1966 so the children of Wittenoom have now had post-exposure time of 40-plus years. And we have seen since 1980 many cases of Wittenoom children who have developed mesothelioma. That is what I talk about. Then I usually finish with a slide from my childhood, back to the fibro asbestos house with asbestos louvres, I return to my own experience.

So what perspective do I have on asbestos disease from my vantage point as a GP? People realised I had started to take an interest in asbestos related diseases much more so than I had before. I used to fit people in; people didn't have to make appointments, I'd always see the asbestos people. I was seeing them in my own practice and at the ADSA, but I don't treat anything at the Society apart from their asbestos exposure. I don't take them over as patients; in fact I refuse to because they have their own GPs. And GPs realise that is all I do and, if I find something [unconnected to asbestos related disease], I send them back.

My role as a GP is being able to talk to people. Everyone who walks through the door has an asbestos exposure and from that can emanate four different diseases, so you are talking about a narrow field of medicine, and, having done it for over 33 years, I can talk about it very readily. The fear of asbestos disease is quite substantial and patients are frightened. Many have recently been diagnosed with mesothelioma and that's basically the worst news they will ever get in their lives. Anyone who gets this cancer is going to die from it, not with it; it's universally fatal and everyone knows that. They are shattered and their wives are shattered and they have difficulty coping. I feel a pang for them; having gone through it myself I know how they feel. They need support and that's part of my role. I can't change it for them, but I can help them manage their situation better. The mesothelioma support group at ADSA includes carers, relatives and patients, and I encourage them to attend to meet others because people with mesothelioma are lonely. A diagnosis of imminent death is a very lonely way to be.

Both patients and carers need information they can understand. So I think that if I will have any legacy it will be my part in the creation of an Australian version of *The Mesothelioma handbook*, adapted from Dr Helen Clayson's English publication and produced by the ADSA. Helen Clayson is a very experienced GP and palliative physician who started a local support group in Cumbria and then researched and lectured to try to improve the care of those with mesothelioma. She wrote *The Mesothelioma handbook* and, when I read her book, I realised that we had to have something like that here. So, with her agreement, we worked on that at the ADSA and produced our version that we give to those affected, patients and carers.[3]

Sometimes a person's asbestos exposure is difficult to understand and accept. It is not so difficult to understand where there is an occupational history [of exposure], but females have been exposed through their husbands' working clothes or helping their husbands sawing or drilling asbestos products. That's usually unexpected. When I meet anyone with asbestos exposure who smokes I show them the graph [of their increased risk of lung cancer]. You just want to get the message through: if you continue smoking you run a very real risk of lung cancer. Their own doctors will tell them too, but I have authority to say it because of my background with asbestos related diseases. We pick up a few very early lung cancers with our screening so these people have a chance of cure. As well we have had early detection of other cancers (kidney and thyroid) as accidental findings.

Many people are dying when they come to the Asbestos Diseases Society and the Society's role is critical. There is no other society like it; they have developed expertise, care, and organisational skills. Robert has become an expert in the medico-legal field and his wife Rose Marie does counselling, visits to hospitals and assists patients with personal matters. Western Australia has close to the highest incidence of mesothelioma in the world, so where else would such a society be?

Unfortunately we pick up disease but we cannot cure any of them. However I think their life quality and quantity has improved with developments in chemotherapy skills, with the support groups, and, in a small number of cases, with surgery. As with any disease, we must remove the causes [of asbestos related diseases] and undertake research to render the diseases harmless.

I had been working in the asbestos field for ten years or so and never anticipated, never thought about my own childhood. Quite clearly I've been

---

3   H Clayson, *The Mesothelioma handbook* (Perth: Asbestos Diseases Society of Australia, 2016).

exposed but not to the degree my mother had. My chest is clear, I have no sign of anything at this stage, but you just never know. Instead of being simply the doctor who worked for the ADSA, however, I became one of them, one of those whose lives have been badly affected by asbestos. I know the circle has not yet closed because the clean up of Australia's asbestos-contaminated urban environments has not been done.

For his work in the asbestos field over three decades Greg Deleuil has been awarded the Eric Saint Memorial Award (1999) and the Centenary of Federation medal (2001) and been made a Member of the Order of Australia (2006).

Chapter 16

THE LITIGATOR'S STORY

Peter Gordon, Slater & Gordon Lawyer

Peter Gordon started working in asbestos litigation in 1981 when he was then with the legal firm Slater & Gordon, and he was involved in some of the earliest litigation against the asbestos manufacturer James Hardie. In 1984 and 1985 he ran the first successful negligence claim for damages for someone with mesothelioma. The Harold Pilmer case attracted attention and he found himself involved in more asbestos cases. This led him to Perth where, joining forces with Luisa Formato and John Gordon, he was at the forefront of landmark compensation cases against CSR and others over the following decades. Peter's story covers the period of intense litigation from the 1980s to the 2000s.[1]

I got a call out of the blue one day from Robert Vojakovic who told me that he ran the Asbestos Diseases Society in Western Australia and they were facing a formidable fight with CSR over the operations of the Wittenoom mine. He had hundreds of members, many of whom were dying from mesothelioma, and they faced a deadline to get proceedings underway, and could we help.

So I very quickly went over there with a few colleagues and we decided that we could and should help, and we did so. Over the course of two or three weeks we had to get about 360 writs issued before a statutory deadline expired. So I'd have to say that knowing that almost from day one we had 360 cases, many of whom were for people who'd been suffering from asbestos disease for many years, we were in no doubt that it was a very substantial undertaking for a large number of people. I guess we probably had no idea of the length and complexity of the litigation which was involved, because CSR certainly did leave no stone unturned in their efforts to distance themselves from any responsibility for what had gone on at Wittenoom.

---

1 This account consists of edited excerpts of an interview with Peter Gordon conducted by Mia Lindgren for the Australian Asbestos Network, 3 September 2008.

1987: Wally Simpson

The first case that we ran, which we lost, was for a fellow called Wally Simpson, and by today's standards it was a very straightforward case of very significant asbestosis. It went for 55 days, they ran every point, and convinced the judge at first instance that all of the 16 or 17 symptoms of asbestosis that he suffered from could be accounted for by some other pathology, either that he was overweight or that he had once smoked, or various other things, that the X-ray changes in his lungs which weren't consistent with either being overweight or with smoking were some kind of fibrosis which was idiopathic or which had no known cause at all, rather than the obvious fact that he'd worked in the mill at Wittenoom for several years. It was later a decision which was overturned on appeal, but having run it for 55 days and incurred all of the expenses, I think we were about $2 million in debt by the time the Simpson case finished.

1987–1988: Peter Heys and Tim Barrow

When Simpson finished, our second cases of Peter Heys and Tim Barrow were underway, and those cases went for 133 days.

Tim Barrow had worked in the mill at Wittenoom between 1948 and 1951, and Peter Heys, who when I first met him was a parking inspector for the City of Perth, had worked there only for about six months in 1955. They were both suffering from mesothelioma, they both therefore had limited life expectancy, and they both very much tested the envelope because they took on not only the subsidiary to CSR (which when they were employed there was known as Australian Blue Asbestos, but its name was later sanitised to Midalco), but these two men also took on CSR as the parent company and said that they had a direct liability to do so. They needed to do that because CSR only provided Australian Blue Asbestos with about $1,000 or $2,000 worth of insurance cover for its pre-1960 exposure, and both of these blokes had worked there prior to 1960s. So even if they'd won against their direct employer, they may never have recovered complete damages. So they needed to take on the parent company, and they did.

Of course mesothelioma, it's often said, was only discovered as a discrete consequence of asbestos in about 1959, 1960 due to the publication of work with South African miners by Wagner in 1959, 1960. So these two men had the added burden of showing that the sort of asbestos disease from which they suffered was a foreseeable consequence of exposure to asbestos, even if mesothelioma itself wasn't known. That is to say, they needed to show that it was dangerous to inhale asbestos and that it was known to be dangerous to inhale asbestos back in 1948, 1951 and 1955, and that it caused lung damage which was sufficiently similar to mesothelioma to make mesothelioma itself compensable.

So the degree of difficulty in the two cases was great, and that's without superimposing onto that the "scorched earth" tactics that CSR imposed. I well recall halfway through the trial an event where we sought to tender a letter from a mines inspector who was deceased, and under the evidentiary rules at that time you're entitled to tender a written document signed by someone who was dead but you needed to prove that he was dead. Now, everybody knew this bloke was dead, they knew he was dead, we knew he was dead, and so we sought by agreement to put it in, but they objected, rose to object, and said that we hadn't gone through any of the proper legal channels to establish by admissible means that in fact this long-dead mines inspector was dead. And so we needed to get a delay, incur some expenses, turn up the evidence, the death certificate, which took some time to do.

We found a yellow post-it note that one of the CSR lawyers, [Julie Bishop], now quite a well known politician, had passed to one of the CSR executives there to say "of course we knew this person was dead, it's all part of the principle of stuffing them up", which was a fair insight into the sort of tactics which were being visited upon us at that time.

When Justice Rowland delivered his verdict in that case, it was a verdict not just against a subsidiary company but against CSR. It established that in fact asbestos was known to be dangerous back in 1948 when a young Flying Doctor, Eric Saint, had first sent a note to the managers of CSR saying that you are going to produce "the richest crop of asbestosis cases ever seen in the world's literature" unless you do something about the conditions in this mine. Justice Rowland in the Heys and Barrow decision properly held not only the subsidiary company but CSR to account.

It did a number of things. It meant that all of the families and the mesothelioma sufferers themselves who were waiting in line all of a sudden had a verdict in their favour. It meant that CSR couldn't stand behind the corporate shell of its subsidiary company and the limited insurance in order to evade liability. It was probably one of the most significant developments in occupational health and safety and compensation law in the history of the country.

1988: Klaus Rabenault

After we lost the Simpson case there was quite a deal of media and public relations work done by the State Government Insurance Office of Western Australia [SGIO] and CSR to say that everyone has been put to a large expense and the hopes of asbestos victims are being falsely inflated by these lawyers for no good reason because these cases can't be won and would never be won. It was really, at that time, quite a conservative legal and judicial culture over there and it was not at all easy. And for that reason, when Klaus Rabenault walked into my office in the western suburbs of Melbourne, in Footscray, and we had the opportunity to run a Wittenoom case in front of a jury in Melbourne, it was quite a special event.

Klaus Rabenault had, as a very young man, come out to Australia and landed in Fremantle in about 1960 and gone straight out to Wittenoom. Like many young men coming to Australia at that time he sought to make his fortune, and he thought that the chance to get ahead and earn some decent wages may have existed in this outback town and he went up there. He only stayed there for the mandatory six months until he could afford the plane fare back, and he spent three months in the mill and three months in the mine at Wittenoom before coming to Melbourne and running a number of successful businesses, including a quite well known furniture shop in Prahran, before one day feeling some strange pains in his chest and getting the terrible news that his exposure those many years ago to asbestos at Wittenoom had come back to haunt him in the most horrible of ways and he had mesothelioma.

We brought the claim against CSR and its subsidiary, Australian Blue Asbestos. The claim went to trial only against the subsidiary, Australian Blue Asbestos. In many ways it suited us to do that because their insurance cover wasn't so limited for the 1960 period. It went for 28 days, and somewhat unusually for a claim at the time it included not just a claim for negligence but a claim for punitive damages. And the allegation that we made in that case was that the conduct of the CSR subsidiary company was not just negligent but it was so grossly reckless and insulting and arrogant towards the plaintiff and his right to a healthy working environment that they should be punished in addition to the compensation for negligence.

The jury considered that and came back after four or five hours of deliberation to a packed courtroom telling the judge they had a question. The question they had to ask was how they assess the punitive damages aspect of the claim. I'll always remember in my legal career that moment because we had no idea whether the question was going to be one which meant that we were going to lose the case altogether, which truly would have been the end of the campaign to get compensation for all asbestos victims, but it would have some very serious consequences for my law firm, but instead of that it was a question which went to effectively vindicate the decision we'd taken not just to sue for negligence but for punitive damages as well.

It was quite a watershed moment. I remember Klaus and his partner being very emotional at that point, and within the hour the jury had returned with a verdict for $425,000 for compensatory damages, the ordinary damages for negligence, and a further $250,000 in punitive damages. It was a verdict and a judgment which sent a very loud message across Australia, and in particular I think to the legal establishment in Western Australia, that this really was a standard of corporate conduct which could not be abided. It was a very important moment.

2000s: James Hardie

Why does a company ever seek to act in a particular way? Because there was profit in it. What James Hardie's board of directors was seeking to achieve throughout the 1990s and the early 21st century was to minimise its payout. Hardie fought like stuck pigs to avoid any liability to asbestos victims for many years. The compensation fund that it set up in 2001 was in fact an apportionment of what it knew its legal liabilities to be. There was no element of giving or largesse or generosity in the establishment of this fund, it was simply a provisioning of its legal liabilities, and it was of course a fundamentally dishonest apportionment of its liabilities because it was in fact an assessment of about one-tenth of what its true liabilities were.

It had worked hand-in-glove with a firm of actuaries called Trowbridge, a firm that no longer exists, partly because of the besmirching of the reputation of Trowbridge, to come up with a set of figures based on a number of assumptions which were demonstrably false, and they came up with an initial assessment of $293 million for the future liabilities of James Hardie. Of course we now know that the real figure was close to ten times that amount.

So what we know about James Hardie in many ways reflects the attitude of most of the asbestos corporations and their behaviour in Australia over the past 50 years. I think this is a point that's important. There are many common features to what James Hardie did that CSR in various guises has done, and many other companies as well. James Hardie Asbestos used to be the name of one of the principal James Hardie companies and they used to operate from a building called Asbestos House. Well, one night in the dead of night in the late 1970s, once they knew that the asbestos problem was going to be a big PR and legal problem for them, they changed the name of the building by dead of night and the "Asbestos House" moniker was removed.

Over time the name "James Hardie" changed from James Hardie Asbestos to James Hardie Industries. And then in 2001 the sanitised renaming of the company became the Medical Research and Compensation Foundation. In the same way CSR didn't want to be saddled with the subsidiary company Australian Blue Asbestos because of everything that name connotes, so they changed it to Midalco.

James Hardie was the biggest manufacturer of asbestos products in Australia for most of this period. The second biggest was Wunderlich Asbestos, now known as Seltsam. What do all of these new names have in common? Of course they're all sanitised names to take the asbestos out and confuse people in relation to the former true history. It was, I guess, a necessary predicate to the managing director of James Hardie whilst the Netherlands fiasco was going on, Peter McDonald actually circulating public relations in the early part of this decade to say that asbestos was really only a minor part of the James Hardie business activities which also included selling budgerigars or canaries. That sort of real dishonesty was only possible with the elaborate set of steps. It started with the renaming of the company and the sanitising of the name to take out things such as "asbestos".

What we saw with the reorganisation of the James Hardie companies in 2001 was a shifting of assets from the company which brought a legal liability into a company which could allege in court that it had no such legal liability. Again, history repeated itself in a telling way because that's precisely the form of legal manoeuvre that CSR engaged in with Australian Blue Asbestos back in the 1970s when it stripped the assets of Australian Blue Asbestos before circulating public relations propaganda to say that CSR itself had no liability for Wittenoom and that the subsidiary company which was the employer of people and the seller of products, Australian Blue Asbestos, had no insurance and had no assets left. It had no assets left because they'd been stripped by CSR.

So the point that I seek to make in relation to that is that we've seen with James Hardie corporate conduct which was disgraceful but by no means unique to a group of malevolent directors over a period. This was the standard *modus operandi* of the Australian asbestos industry which learned from each other tactics in a desperate bid to maximise the profits for their shareholders at the expense of those who worked for them and used their products.

2007: David Hannell and Dennis Moss

Mr Hannell and Mr Moss were two people who originally ran and won their cases in the Western Australian Supreme Court and then had their verdicts overturned and taken away from them. They had them taken away for different reasons, Mr Moss on the basis that his weekend exposure was so light that it could not be differentiated in terms of the amount of the exposure from the background exposure that everyone else has. Mr Hannell was in a slightly different position in that it was found by the court of appeal that in fact his weekend exposure to James Hardie asbestos had been the cause of his disease, but that given what James Hardie knew or could have known, or what was available to be known or done in terms of effective mass marketing or media communications as to the dangers of asbestos, on a cost benefit analysis it didn't justify the sort of measures which we were arguing would have been appropriate for James Hardie. The sort of risk that was run by Mr Hannell in terms of the chances of him getting mesothelioma, which of course he actually got, justified the sort of media campaign that we were suggesting might have been appropriate.

And the sort of media campaign that we were suggesting might have been appropriate stemmed from the proposition that if a manufacturer is putting out a product which they know may have fatal consequences, may kill you, if it's used in an improper way, there is in fact a very heavy onus to communicate by effective means what ought and ought not to be done in the safe handling of that product. We allege and we continue to allege that by the time these products were being used in the late 1970s and early 1980s, big companies like James Hardie knew very well that mass marketing techniques including communication via television and radio and effective marketing and communications strategies could be very effective in raising community awareness.

It's our position and it will be our position in future cases in relation to this that not only could James Hardie have ascertained that, that in fact James Hardie did know that. And our position in future cases is going to be that not only did they know that but in fact they did engage in mass marketing, but it wasn't a form of mass marketing designed to alert the public to the dangers of asbestos, rather it was a campaign to obfuscate or deny people a proper information or understanding about the dangers of the very uses of asbestos which Mr Hannell and Mr Moss did.

So, there is a fair bit more water to go under the bridge in relation to this particular point, and I'm convinced that not all of the evidence which ought to have seen the light of day in those two test cases has yet been seen by courts in relation to this very important question. I think that in the next cases which are to come there will be a lot more information which the courts will have to assess what the true position of James Hardie really was.

Chapter 17

THE JAMES HARDIE STORY

Gideon Haigh, Historian

Historian Gideon Haigh drew extensively on both documentary records and oral interviews in order to write his acclaimed book Asbestos House: the Secret History of James Hardie Industries *(2006, rev. ed. 2007). Here the author reflects on the changing circumstances and culture of the Company he observed so closely and on the long-running compensation saga in which it engaged.*[1]

I have always thought of the James Hardie story as covering a century over which Hardies has been involved in asbestos—and 70 years of that history was in asbestos, and the next 30 years was trying to get out.

A successful asbestos company

What distinguished James Hardie from other asbestos manufacturers in Australia such as CSR and Wunderlich is that it was a genuine one-substance company. The company itself was called James Hardie Asbestos; it had a headquarters in Sydney called Asbestos House; it was comparable to the big integrated asbestos combines overseas like Turner & Newall in the UK, Johns Manville in the US, Cape Asbestos in South Africa. In fact it was closely linked to all of them. It had for many years a large shareholding in Cape, it had strong technical links with Johns Manville and Turner & Newall, and was involved in joint ventures with both companies. And it was a big shareholder in Canadian asbestos mines, associated with Turners.

Hardies was not unusual for most of its history in being a relatively paternalistic kind of company. It prided itself on looking after its employees,

---

1   This account consists of edited excerpts of an interview with Gideon Haigh conducted by Mia Lindgren for the Australian Asbestos Network, 1 September 2008.

ironically so. It was particularly proud of never having fired a worker during the Great Depression; it kept jobs open for men who went off to serve during World War Two; it had, for its age, quite advanced health and superannuation benefits. And it's remarkable how long a lot of people stayed with the company. It had a thriving quartile of workers who'd served 20 to 25 years. There was a vigorous social scene within the factories themselves. I think because it had origins as a family company through both the Hardie and the Reid families, it tended to look upon its workers as kind of extensions of its own family.

That began to change after World War Two. It became difficult to acquire labour; employment conditions were tight with low levels of unemployment. So Hardies began to acquire workers virtually straight off the boat, in the waves of post-war immigration. It had relatively high turnover, but maintained that paternalistic character, and it was one of the only jobs that you could get, one of the key employers of people at the very bottom levels of the social strata and in the first stages of acquiring Australianness; a lot of workers with non-English speaking backgrounds.

Looming health problems

There were individuals in Hardies who took dust and disease very seriously indeed, some plant managers both in Sydney and Melbourne who tried to do their best to engineer the risk to minimise exposures by workers, mainly I think for reasons of cleanliness rather than necessarily because they understood there to be a significant health risk, but these individuals were isolated. Hardie's board and senior managers seemed to have been untroubled about dust. They regarded it as an occupational hazard, and it was always a problem whose consideration you could defer. When the Hardie asbestos business was at its height, occupational health and safety was not considered a paramount concern of business.

There were efforts made from the mid-1960s to try to remediate or at least to monitor the health problems that might be developing, and in particular after the 1964 US conference by the New York Academy of Sciences. We know that James Hardie executives were forwarded copies of the conference papers by colleagues at Turner & Newall, and we also know that they were concerned by what they read. We know that James Hardie executives went overseas to study what Johns Manville, the big American manufacturer, was doing with its own health program. Hardies instituted a series of checks on the health of workers in the second half of the 1960s, and made efforts to ameliorate working conditions in their factories. But it was mainly—not window dressing because I think some people did take it seriously—but it was always subordinate to the desire of the Company to continue earning profits.

Terry McCullagh, who became the first full-time medical officer at the Company in 1967, was an absolute pragmatist; he never, ever needed to be reminded that Hardies was a Company first and foremost rather than a welfare organisation.[2] Peter Russell, who was the chief safety officer in the 1960s, once said to him that the only way to eliminate dust risk was to stop using asbestos and McCullagh simply said to him, "Asbestos pays yours and my salary". McCullagh even proposed at one stage that Hardies should use older men for the dustiest jobs because the older men wouldn't live long enough for cancer to develop. In the end Hardies didn't pursue that policy, but it does suggest that he was the kind of doctor with whom you could do business.

I think the efficacy of the health program was limited because with asbestos, where the diseases are progressive and have long latency periods, up to 40 years in the case of mesothelioma, the current health of your workers is only going to be a guide to how you were doing 20, 30 years earlier, not how you were doing at the time.

From the 1970s Hardies tried to get away from asbestos when the news media and health authorities begin to become extremely concerned about asbestos' long-term health effects. The Company changed its name on a purely cosmetic basis and also the name of its headquarters; it became James Hardie Industries and the headquarters became James Hardie House. It revived long-dormant experiments with asbestos substitutes, and eventually found some successful and durable technology with which to replace asbestos in fibre cement. And it undertook a major diversification by buying a conglomerate called Reid Consolidated Industries, which led Hardie into different areas of industry.

Moving overseas

In the 1990s when Hardies took its new post-asbestos building products to the US, it proved well positioned to benefit from a huge housing boom that was taking place, and became a high performance industrial. And in doing so its identity changed, even though people were unaware of it because the name didn't change and it was identified as a

---

2   His official name was Dr Stanley Forster McCullagh.

blue chip Australian industrial. I think from the mid-1990s Hardies was an American company with an Australian board, but a diminishing Australian presence and a diminishing sense of attachment to the country that had given it birth.

In a sense there was a change of culture at James Hardie that entailed another stage in the separation of the Company from its own past. There was a steady seepage of executive power from Australia to the US which was at the time becoming the overwhelming contributor to group earnings. The Company began to fall in line with the expectations of American investors and the American capital market in general. That process was mostly lost on Australian shareholders, institutions, and private investors alike, and certainly on potential tort claimants.

Managing its asbestos liabilities

The funny thing about Hardies is that, if you'd been asked to name an evil asbestos company perhaps even ten years ago, the chances are that it would have been CSR. Hardies very successfully remained out of the public eye, and that was because it was able to settle cases on terms of confidentiality; it courted no publicity. As the compensation market got hotter, Hardies took a tougher line and fought some cases to verdict and mostly lost, but it was able to almost divorce itself from its asbestos past. What happened in the 1990s was that ghost of the asbestos company that it had been turned up to haunt it again.

Hardies was confident that it could manoeuvre its way out of the dilemma it found itself in and it did it in a couple of ways. One was the Medical Research and Compensation Foundation, which was a closed-end fund created for the purposes of finalising compensation to people suffering from asbestos related disease, and a re-domicile in the Netherlands.

I think we have to understand this in terms of a kind of cultural change. I need hardly say that the American system of compensation, like the corporate culture over there, is pretty Darwinian. I think over the last 30 years about 70 companies have gone into "Chapter 11".[3] Techniques for minimising tort compensation are very common in the US. We don't have quite the same legal and corporate culture in Australia and we were

---

3   A provision in the US Bankruptcy Code which enables the debtor to retain control of its business operation while corporate re-organisation takes place.

surprised and even appalled to be confronted by it. It was as though an American solution was imposed on an Australian corporate problem, and the results speak for themselves.

I think that it is true that by the time the James Hardie Board and management were deliberating on these problems in the early 21st century there was no one at the Company even vaguely associated with Hardie's asbestos past. This had always been a risk when you are dealing with diseases that have such long latency periods. It was always going to be the possibility that the next generation or the next generation but one was going to be left to clean up the misdeeds of the previous ones, and as a result people didn't feel obligated towards the past. I don't think that they wanted to escape their obligations entirely, but they certainly didn't feel responsible. I think there was a sense of irritation that they'd been left to clean up this mess, this mess that had been deferred by previous managements.

There was a draft paper prepared for the board at the height of the discussion about the various solutions: "... there is no 'silver bullet' solution available. The asbestos position is not one created by the current management or Board—but it is here and needs to be dealt with. This decision is a 'Beauty contest between warthogs' and the decision is which option is least ugly".[4] Obviously the Board in the end backed the wrong warthog. But I think the key phrase is "not one created by the current management or Board". No one seems to have grappled with the ramifications of the failure of the Foundation they were creating despite, I think, their cognisance that it was a possibility. It's as though morality has been stripped back until it is an exact fit with legality. And there's an assumption that what we need in all cases is for self-interest to prevail.

I think they were keen for the problem to go away. They'd pretended for a long period that James Hardie's asbestos problems were, if not at an end, they were certainly over the hump, and all of a sudden they found the problem recrudescing in front of them. There was a desire for finality because the future for James Hardie, especially in the United States, was extremely promising. A long decade of painstaking and methodical investment in the right places by a very able management had turned Hardies into a bit of a stock market darling. And, if you could sever that residual connection to asbestos, which in the United States is a significant disincentive for

---

4   G Haigh, *Asbestos House: the secret history of James Hardie Industries* (Melbourne: Scribe, 2006) ch. 18, especially 252.

investors because so many asbestos companies have gone to the wall, then you could really begin to reap the benefits of that investment. And that was the grail that kept drawing the company on.

It didn't take long for it to be revealed to the directors of the Foundation that they were not within a bull's roar of being able to satisfy claims that were coming in. And certainly in the long term, because asbestos is going to be a problem in Australia for generations, there may even be potential claimants who haven't yet been exposed to asbestos. The time horizons were so mind-boggling that I think they outstripped the corporate imagination. When the degree of under-funding became public, the Foundation finally went to the media and laid it open for all to see.

At Hardie's new headquarters at Mission Viejo on the west coast of the US, there was a general level of ignorance about the public odium that enveloped the Company once the story became known. I think the Hardie executives got a very big and unpleasant surprise by how quickly they became public enemies. They thought that they could brazen it out from the US, but of course the directors themselves were in Sydney and they, I think, felt the level of public scorn more emphatically than the executive.

When the NSW government empowered the ACTU and its secretary Greg Combet to negotiate the terms of the settlement in the wake of the Jackson Inquiry, it was a process of one step forward, two steps back while the negotiating was taking place, with periodic attempts to use the media in order to build up the pressure on the other antagonist.[5]

Bernie Banton's presence

Bernie was a fascinating figure in this. Bernie turned up in the middle of the Jackson Inquiry and attended most days. He had been a worker at the old Hardie insulation joint venture, Hardie BI, in the 1970s and had developed asbestos cancer in the late 1990s, had proceeded through the courts and had received certain levels of compensation. But his health had continued to deteriorate. And he was intent on the inquiry not simply becoming a question of the analysis of various corporate finance transactions: he wanted David Jackson QC overseeing the inquiry to understand that this had an enormous and grievous human cost. So he sat there, on some occasions quite hauntingly because when the hubbub

---

5   Greg Combet discusses the Jackson Inquiry and Bernie Banton in Chapter 18, below.

died occasionally you could hear the sound of Bernie's respirator rasping towards the back of the room. There was absolutely no possibility of anyone pretending that this was anything other than a public health disaster that was being analysed rather than the analysis of just a series of business deals.

A distinctively Australian story

One hundred years spans a lot of Australian history and a lot of changed attitudes to public health and safety, to working-place conditions, to commercial and financial risk, and also changing attitudes to the idea of saying sorry. It's interesting that it should have happened in the Australia of the early 21st century which is struggling to come to terms with aspects of its past and is constantly wondering whether it should have known more at various stages in its history, whether it was as enlightened as it could have been at various times. So the idea of a company wrestling with its own vestigial presence in the past is actually, I think, a distinctively Australian story.

Chapter 18

THE BERNIE BANTON STORY

Greg Combet, ACTU Secretary

Greg Combet was the secretary of the ACTU when in 2004 he was the lead negotiator of the settlement with James Hardie that delivered a long-term compensation outcome for victims of James Hardie asbestos products. The landmark Bernie Banton case was the culmination of a long involvement with the struggle for compensation for victims of asbestos disease.[1]

My own history with asbestos compensation efforts goes back to the early 1980s when I was working in an occupational health and safety centre in the western suburbs of Sydney. At that time we were still having to argue the case that asbestos mining and manufacturing companies had known about the harmful health effects of asbestos on people's health in order to try and assist compensation cases, gain ground through the compensation system and at common law. So a lot of work was still being done as recently as the 1980s and 1990s, and companies were vigorously resisting it, including James Hardie, in compensation tribunals and at common law because they recognised at the time just what significant liabilities there may in fact be for them.

In the late 1990s and in the early part of this decade, James Hardie had a very close look at the liability that it was carrying within Australia and into the future for its exposure to people of their asbestos products, and clearly its very serious liability, one that we now know in present value terms is around $1.5 billion.[2]

---

1   This account consists of edited excerpts of an interview with Greg Combet conducted by Mia Lindgren for the Australian Asbestos Network, 23 September 2008.
2   In 2018 the estimated liability has risen to $1.853 billion. See S Letts, "James Hardie profit tumbles on mounting asbestos claims", ABC, 22 May 2018. http://www.abc.net.au/news/2018-05-22/james-hardie-profit-tumbles-on-mounting-asbestos-claims/9786850. Accessed 11 October 2018.

The company at that time decided to restructure and this was clearly, in my view, in an effort to avoid the full extent of their potential liabilities. They created a trust fund into which they put about $293 million and argued that this was sufficient to meet their future liabilities, and then reincorporated the company in the Netherlands where, I believe, the company knew that it would be difficult for Australian-based asbestos victims to pursue them for further liability if the trust fund proved to be inadequate. It was these circumstances, once it became evident that the trust fund was insufficiently financed, that led to the Jackson Inquiry in 2004.

The Jackson Inquiry 2004

It was very important that the Jackson Inquiry was established. I worked with the Premier of NSW at the time, Bob Carr, on the issue, and Bob Carr was a tremendous supporter of the union cause in this regard and a supporter of asbestos victims. And he set up the Jackson Inquiry and, to his great credit, once the Jackson Inquiry had reported, he in fact called me and said, "I want you to represent the NSW government in negotiations with the company to try and achieve some justice now that we've seen the findings of this inquiry." So he demonstrated very clearly that he was right behind the broader community and union campaign to bring the company to the table, and it would have been very difficult to achieve without the power and authority of the state government.

I remember the evidence that was given in the Jackson Inquiry was quite horrifying in many respects, from a moral point of view more than anything else, I think that's what shocked people. A lot of evidence was given about the way in which the company went about restructuring, the motivations they had, the internal advice, the emails and the like. It was the moral outrage that people felt that was most compelling, and it wasn't very pretty listening to some of the evidence. It's as if people just had no heart at all when they were sitting considering making these decisions, and I felt that myself when I sat across from some of these directors and executives, that they just did not seem to understand what life was like and how exposure to their products really affected people.

Bernie Banton

Bernie Banton, along with a couple of his brothers, had worked at the James Hardie manufacturing facility at Camellia in the inner western suburbs of Sydney in the 1970s. I've seen some photographs of Bernie at that time working at the factory covered in white asbestos dust, as were all of the other workers. He of course first contracted asbestosis, which is a degenerative process in your lungs and you lose lung capacity as the scarring from the asbestos damage grows. He'd had that condition for quite some time when I met him.

I met him during the Jackson Inquiry in Sydney in 2004. As we got towards the end of that enquiry and it was evident that a very large public campaign would need to be mounted to bring the company to justice, I thought that Bernie would make a great public advocate, which he certainly proved to be. And we ensured that in mounting a public campaign in my role as the leader of the union movement, that Bernie was a key element and public spokesperson for victims of asbestos diseases.

I've been around media issues for quite a while in my working life but rarely have I met someone who could communicate so easily and quickly with people through the electronic media and reach out to them in an emotional way and convey what the issue really was and reduce it to its very simple basis. In this particular campaign that was essentially about morality and the morality of corporate behaviour in trying to avoid obligations to people who were going to die and live vastly debilitated lives for the time that they would continue to live. Bernie was able to cut through all of the guff, the complexity, the legal argument, the technical arguments, the procedural things around a commission of inquiry, and cut to the chase and communicate with people what this was really all about.

It's not to be underestimated, the importance of that in the campaign to bring James Hardie to justice because the fact of the matter was that the company of course had used all of the top legal brains in the country and internationally to restructure in a way where they felt they would have insulated themselves from their obligations to people in the Australian community, and at least it looked very difficult to us to achieve justice by using the legal system. We needed to utilise massive public pressure on the directors and executives of the company to bring them to the table and negotiate a solution, and Bernie's role in helping build that pressure was immense.

Negotiating with James Hardie

The negotiations with James Hardie and their corporate and legal advisors in 2004 were the most complex negotiations that I have been involved in, and as a union leader over 25-odd years I've been in plenty of difficult ones, but this was extremely complex. We had to deal, for example, with not only Australian commercial, constitutional, and corporate law and compensations systems, but we also had to deal with international corporate and commercial law in the Netherlands and the US in particular in order to try and pull a solution together. We had to get across compensation systems across every state and territory and try and ensure that we had a coordinated effort to deal with compensation in each of the jurisdictions. We made reforms to the NSW dust diseases compensation processes to try and achieve some efficiencies and take some of the legal and administrative costs out of the system in the NSW jurisdiction in particular, and that was because so many cases are prosecuted in the NSW system.

We also had to look at the evidence about the incidence of disease and the time frame in the future over which claims would be made. In fact all of the best information available to us indicated that the peak in asbestos related diseases from James Hardie products may well be ahead of us over the next five to ten years and then start to taper off.[3] We had to give consideration to how we could prevent disease in the future and put greater emphasis into prevention and safe removal of fibro from houses and the like, and to contemplate what sort of building regulation changes needed to be made.

We had to look at different financing mechanisms for the finance to be made available by the company from the cash flow that is generated in its US activities, and the list could go on. One of the other elements that I was pleased to be able to achieve in the settlement was to gain the commitment of James Hardie to make a significant amount of money available not just for community education about asbestos diseases and their prevention but also into medical research, because we need to put a lot of effort in that regard to see if there are better ways for us to be able to treat people with asbestosis and mesothelioma.

One very difficult element of the negotiations was the difficulty of obtaining a serious approach from James Hardie. They tried so many different manoeuvres to try and frustrate the process, in my opinion.

We also had to thoroughly assess the projections for the James Hardie business, because the point needs to be made that in order to be able to compensate people James Hardie needs to be a viable commercial entity, and most of its operations are in the US now. So we also had to work on the

---

3   In fact according to KPMG's 2018 assessment of James Hardie's future liability, far from mesothelioma claims peaking in 2014–15 as originally predicted, the projected date has blown out to 2025 (Letts, "James Hardie profit tumbles on mounting asbestos claims"). This is the result of the so-called third wave of exposures amongst home renovators. See above, Chapter 11.

company on the business strategy and the financial outlook to ensure that we made available through the settlement a sufficient amount of the company's cash flow to finance its liabilities to asbestos victims in Australia, and that was complex as well.

But the company wiggled and wormed around and did not make the process easy or short, it took a long time. In fact, once we'd achieved an in-principle settlement by Christmastime in 2004 they are another good 12 to 18 months in converting the in-principle settlement into a detailed and enforceable document. I have as much confidence as I could possibly have about the capacity of that settlement to be able to ensure that there's sufficient finance available in the years to come. We can't guarantee it, but it's about as rigorous and robust a settlement as I think we could have achieved.

Who was responsible?

I know from my own involvement in this area that going right back to the 1930s there was evidence that the asbestos products caused health problems. Certainly by the 1950s it's known that James Hardie and other manufacturers knew that serious health effects were being incurred by people. In fact they continued to produce in Australia asbestos related products in James Hardie until 1986, and even in recent years, as we've been discussing, it's been difficult to get the company to face up to things.

So this is a very complex issue for our economic system, our forms of governance, the responsibilities of directors. And one of the arguments that the directors of James Hardie were always putting across the table in the negotiations in 2004 was that it was their statutory duty as directors to protect the interests of shareholders and they felt that they were properly discharging those duties by trying to minimise the liability of the company. So we've got lots of work to do on all these fronts, in corporate governance, and not just in compensation arrangements. I would like to see a far greater examination of what really gave rise to these things and why, under our legal arrangements in this country for such a long period of time this was able to continue to be pursued.

Obviously governments and regulators, health and safety authorities, I think they were probably intimidated with the knowledge that was available at the time, intimidated by the scale of the problem and what could be done. For example, in the early 1980s, I think it was about 1983, 1984, I was writing some leaflets for unions at the time to distribute in workplaces. The debate was about what a safe level of exposure to asbestos might be, and I couldn't reconcile in my own mind that there was any safe level of exposure. But to put that argument around in an industrial context to business at that time, they looked at you rather strangely, and it was because of the scale of the issue that had to be dealt with, whether it be asbestos lagging around pipes, in power stations, on naval vessels, asbestos filters used in different industries. It just seemed that it was such a large issue that the authorities and the business community couldn't contemplate how they could possibly address it and therefore they buried their heads in the sand to a significant degree. But I still don't think there's a safe level of exposure to asbestos.

Did the unions do enough?

I hear occasionally people say, well, the unions could have moved faster as well. Maybe that's the case in some circumstances, however it is really only the unions that have ever brought this issue to the fore, fought for justice, fought to get asbestos out of workplaces, fought for compensation, and there is a long history of unions having played that role. A lot of my work as a union official was dealing with asbestos related issues, even up until I think 2001; we discovered that a firm in Victoria in the automotive manufacturing area was still importing asbestos products for use in brake linings. So I and my colleagues in the maritime union had to work very, very hard to put an end to those asbestos imports and to ensure that the company found an alternative product that it could use. That's the sort of work that unions do.

It may not surprise you to learn that I'm not going to accept criticism of the unions in this regard. Unions weren't manufacturing and marketing this stuff in a way that exposed people to fatal diseases. But unions over time, as they learnt about it too, stepped up the pressure. I know that in Sydney at the James Hardie manufacturing plant, for example, the union was working on these issues and trying to ensure that there were safer work practices and the like. They were being assured all of the time in the 1950s, 1960s and 1970s that it was safe and there was no real evidence that it caused health diseases. All those arguments were being put to the union representatives at the same time that the company was doing medical screenings of the employees to identify just how badly some of their lungs may have been affected. The unions were deceived like the rest of the community.

Really Australia's unions over many years deserve a lot of credit for bringing this issue to the forefront, so too do the often maligned plaintiff lawyers who have taken on these cases over the years, firms like Slater & Gordon and Maurice Blackburn Cashman, but there are many others who have taken up the cause of representing people with asbestos diseases and fighting compensation cases through the court system, often very difficult times.

So people like that in the broader labour movement and union representatives who've fought very hard for justice deserve a lot of credit because they have brought the ordinary stories and suffering of people to the fore, they've taken it through the legal and compensation systems, they've fought in workplaces and industries to have asbestos removed and the hazard eradicated, they've fought to stop mining in places like Wittenoom, and a lot has been achieved over many years. We've still got a way to go but the labour movement deserves a lot of credit for representing people who really suffer.

Lessons for the future

What this (and similar to the tobacco industry) demonstrates is just the extent to which companies over a long, long period of time are oftentimes prepared to frustrate justice in an attempt to ensure that they don't have to meet their financial liabilities to victims of their products in whatever form that may occur. There's a long history of that happening, there's a long history therefore of people campaigning for justice. That's never been an easy thing to achieve, there are still plenty of challenges on that front in this country and internationally.

But at least the settlement with James Hardie that was achieved in 2004 was as robust as we could achieve; in any event, a settlement that will see people who tragically may contract an asbestos related illness from a James Hardie product, that at least there will be some compensation available to them in the future. And just on that point, the negotiation that we had to have with the company at the time contemplates a 40- to 50-year time horizon for many billions of dollars over that period of time in compensation. We had to take into account, for example, the fact that there may well be, on the projections available to us, people who were not even born in 2004 who could well contract an asbestos related illness from a James Hardie product in the years to come, and we wanted to ensure that they would have access to compensation as well. So that's how difficult and complex and long-term the settlement was.

I think they misjudged many things. I think they misjudged their moral commitment to the Australian community for a start, and I do think that they misjudged the intensity of feeling that there would be in the community about what at least could be perceived to be an attempt by a company to avoid its obligation to people who were contracting very serious and oftentimes of course fatal diseases. It's a very awful disease, a disease like mesothelioma, and it's a shocking way for people to die. And for people to be dying without a prospect of achieving compensation from the company that had exposed them to the disease was always going to be an extremely emotive and powerful issue in the community, and I don't think the James Hardie directors properly understood it.

In our society it's people who have been working people that largely contract asbestos related disease, that is whether they worked on the waterfront carrying bags of asbestos dust onto and off ships, or working in a manufacturing facility or working at Wittenoom or cleaning brake linings in a service station or an automotive repair facility, or working in a power station on lagging, it might be an electrician, might be a plumber, might be a manufacturing worker, but they're basically working people who disproportionately contract these diseases. And those people don't have as much of a voice in our society as many others do who are in more influential positions in the institutions of power in our country. So in large part the suffering that's been caused by asbestos diseases is an untold story.

The work needs to continue. We need to work at the prevention of people getting these diseases, that's a first and foremost priority. And for people with asbestos fibro homes they have to be very, very careful. If there are any renovations that are being done or you're knocking down an old fibro garage, don't do it, get advice, learn about safe removal processes, get professional people in, and make sure that it is done without any harm to your health, or your family's health. That's extremely important. We've got a lot of houses made out of fibro across this country and so you can see that it's going to take many decades, I think, to achieve the necessary outcome on the prevention front, but we've also got the medical research aspect of asbestos diseases that needs greater investment and attention.

And we have to remain vigilant, not just in relation to James Hardie of course, but in relation to every other company, CSR and others, that has mined and manufactured and retailed asbestos products and to ensure that they meet their responsibilities to people who tragically, one way or the other, have contracted or may contract an asbestos related disease. This is something that has been a feature of my working life for at least 25 years, and I think it will be a feature of my working life for some years to come and in the working lives of many others who wish to stand up for justice in this area.

Asbestos isn't the only area where these sorts of problems have occurred or will occur in the future, but we need to learn some lessons out of it because the damage to people in the community is so significant.

INDEX

Page locators containing 'n' indicate notes, for example "26n103" means page 26, note 103.

ABA *see* Australian Blue Asbestos Ltd
ABC (Australian Broadcasting Commission), 102, 117, 119–22, 216
Aboriginal people *see* Baryulgil, New South Wales
  asbestos mine workers, 18, 87, 205–21
  housing, 57–8, 67
Adam, Ray, 246, 251
Adelaide Stevedoring Co Ltd v Forst (1940), 239, 248
ADSA *see* Asbestos Diseases Society of Australia
adverse publicity about asbestos *see* media reporting
advertising *see* marketing
airborne asbestos *see* asbestos dust/fibre counts; asbestos exposure standards; asbestos tailings; health hazards of asbestos
Alies-Patin, A M, 162
amateur builders *see* home renovation and maintenance; owner building
amosite *see* brown asbestos (amosite)
amphiboles *see* blue asbestos (crocidolite); brown asbestos (amosite); Libby amphibole; tremolite
Anderson's Creek, Tasmania, 7–8, 16, 17, 87
asbestic wall plaster, 7–8, 11
Asbestolite sheets and slates, 12, 14, 17, 25, 39, 44
asbestos *see* blue asbestos (crocidolite); brown asbestos (amosite); white asbestos (chrysotile)
Asbestos Awareness Healthy House Checklist, 259
asbestos building materials *see* building materials
asbestos cement insulating boards, 23, 68
asbestos cement pipes, 19, 26, 33, 37–8, 39 *see also* coverings; lagging
asbestos cement products, 15–22, 25, 44, 61
  blue asbestos in, 28, 29, 34–5, 36
  building uses *see* building materials; fibro houses
  catalogues, 12, 13, 21–2 *see also* marketing
  demand for, 32, 36, 64
  manufacturing hazards, 78, 81–5, 100
  see also health hazards of asbestos
  product innovations, 23, 38–9, 61–6
  see also asbestos cement pipes; asbestos cement roofs; asbestos cement sheets; asbestos insulation products
asbestos cement roofs
  corrugated fibro, 47, 59, 63, 65–6, 67
  degradation, 66, 260, 261
  health dangers, 66, 67
  management of, 261
  school buildings, 67
  slates, 12–14
asbestos cement sheets, 12–22, 43–5
  fencing, 32, 40, 47, 66
  imports, 11–17
  manufacturing, 15–22, 24–6, 31–2, 38–9
  present but not visible, 39, 64–5
  see also fibro houses
Asbestos Diseases Society of Australia, 120, 126, 203, 245, 252
  Deleuil's work, 297, 299–305
  Vojakovic's account, 287–94
asbestos dust/fibre counts, 81–5, 138
  ambient air levels, 260
  at Baryulgil, 212, 213, 218
  during demolition activities, 265
  equipment and methods, 81, 95, 96, 144–5, 146
  at Hardies' plants, 77, 81–2, 83, 84, 234
  during renovation activities, 263–4
  in small workplaces, 82–3
  at Wittenoom, 70, 91, 95–9, 138, 144–6, 170–1, 243, 284, 285
asbestos exposure
  Baryulgil *see* Baryulgil, New South Wales
  in the built environment, 257–69
  everyday activities, 292, 330
  during renovation and maintenance *see* home renovation and maintenance
  risk and risk management, 260–1, 272
  Wittenoom *see* Wittenoom, Western Australia
  see also asbestos related diseases; health hazards of asbestos; public health response to asbestos hazards
asbestos exposure standards, 138, 211, 212
  Australian jurisdictions, 103, 145–6, 234, 243

Dreesen standard, 81, 83, 84, 85, 95–6, 100, 134
NHMRC recommendations, 103, 145–6
safe removal of asbestos, 263
soil contamination investigation guidelines, 269
US, 81, 124, 145
WHO/IARC statement, 225, 235
see also health hazards of asbestos
asbestos fibre imports, 18, 25, 30–5, 40
bans, 41, 148, 257
consumption, 31–3, 102
prices, 18, 34, 35
statistics, 30–1, 41
tariff rules, 19, 35–6
asbestos-free fibre cement, 40, 102, 317
asbestos health hazards *see* health hazards of asbestos
asbestos houses *see* fibro houses
asbestos industry in Australia (overview)
demise, 40–1, 163, 257
history, 5–15, 22, 315–21
interwar market, 18–24
postwar, 30–41
responses to reports of asbestos danger, 107, 109–10, 122, 125–6 *see also* media reporting
vested interests, 122
wartime, 15–18, 24–30
see also Australian Blue Asbestos Ltd; Colonial Sugar Refining Company (CSR); James Hardie & Co.; Wunderlich Ltd
asbestos industry in United States
asbestos exposure standards, 81, 124, 145
asbestos related diseases, 33, 108–9, 110, 113–15, 154–5, 159, 162
deprecation of medical practitioners, 226–7
litigation, 226–30
responses to reports of asbestos danger, 107, 111, 115, 122–7 *see also* media reporting
vested interests, 122
see also Johns Manville Inc
asbestos insulation products, 19, 32–3, 257
coverings, 11–12, 22–3, 32, 68, 82–3
electrical insulating boards, 23, 68
fire-proof properties of asbestos, 9–10, 21
in industrial workplaces, 11–12, 22–3, 68
lagging, 11, 32, 68, 82, 86, 100, 234, 246
location in homes, 259 *see also* fibro houses
loose-fill asbestos, 70–1
manufacturing dust counts, 82–3, 84
removal of, 68–71
sprayed insulation, 33, 68, 69–70, 115, 284–6, 301
Asbestos Management Review 2012, 67
asbestos milling, 87, 88–92, 94, 97 *see also*

Baryulgil, New South Wales; Wittenoom, Western Australia
asbestos mining *see* mining
Asbestos, Molybdenum and Tungsten Company, 24
asbestos pipes *see* asbestos cement pipes
"asbestos pleurisy", 143–4
asbestos products, 9–15, 257
19th century manufacturers, 9
consumer danger warnings required, 234–5
consumption of imported fibre, 31–3, 102, 257
damage and degradation, 258–61
interwar market, 18–24
in situ management, 257–72
litigation concerning, 227–9, 244–6, 311–14 *see also* litigation
location in typical homes, 259 *see also* fibro houses
postwar demand, 30–3
wartime demand, 15–18, 24–5, 28
see also asbestos cement products; asbestos insulation products; building materials; friction products
Asbestos Products Pty Ltd, 20, 26, 28, 32, 39, 83
dust levels and worker health, 83–5
Johns Manville Inc as model, 226
asbestos registers, 67, 74
asbestos related diseases
asbestos removalists' risk of disease, 272
Canada, 159, 160–1
compensation cases *see* litigation
and different asbestos types, 111, 124–5, 133, 135, 136–41, 157–65
France, 162
and *in situ* asbestos, 269–72
latency *see* latency of disease
medical knowledge milestones, 100–2, 114, 131–48
South Africa, 101, 110–11, 124–5, 136–7, 150–1, 153
third wave, 67, 269–72, 293, 326n3 *see also* home renovation and maintenance
treatment, 147–8
UK, 78, 111–13, 152–9, 161, 162, 272
US, 33, 108–9, 110–11, 113–15, 154–5, 159, 160, 162–3
warnings of *see* McNulty, Dr Jim; Saint, Dr Eric; Selikoff, Dr Irving J
see also specific diseases: asbestosis; mesothelioma; benign asbestos pleural effusion; diffuse pleural fibrosis; lung cancer, asbestos related; pleural plaques; rounded atelectasis
asbestos removal programs, 68–74, 293
Central Australia, 67

INDEX

commercial buildings, 70, 104, 118–19
factory and mine sites, 71–3
illegal dumping of asbestos, 67, 72, 265–7
industrial sites, 68–73
residential buildings, 66–7, 70–1, 261–4
school buildings, 67
union activism, 104–5
see also health hazards of asbestos
asbestos removalists' risk of disease, 272
asbestos roofs *see* asbestos cement roofs
asbestos rope, 11, 33, 68, 82, 237
Asbestos Slate and Sheet Manufacturing Company Ltd., 16
asbestos tailings, 72–3
Barraba, 73, 102
Baryulgil, 72, 206–9
Wittenoom, 72–3, 158, 169, 194–5, 199, 234, 283, 301–2
asbestos types
amphibole variety *see* blue asbestos (crocidolite); brown asbestos (amosite); tremolite
and asbestos related diseases, 111, 124–5, 133, 135, 136–41, 157–65
serpentine variety *see* white asbestos (chrysotile)
asbestosis, 132–4, 146
asbestos cement plant workers, 78, 83, 84–5, 100
asbestos health hazard exposed, 33
Baryulgil, NSW, 87, 215–16, 217
clinical description, 131–2, 133
compensable disease status in UK, 78, 145, 230 *see also* compensation
CSR/ABA knowledge of, 93, 98, 236, 241, 243
and different types of asbestos, 133
first diagnoses, 77–9, 97–8, 131, 236, 243, 282
latency, 105, 289, 317, 319
length/amount of asbestos exposure, 78, 100–1, 133
litigation, 235–9, 241–4, 246–51, 308
and lung cancer, 134–6, 146
medical understanding of, 100–2
and pleural plaques, 142
treatment, 147
Victoria, 77, 85, 101
Wittenoom *see* Wittenoom worker and resident asbestosis cases
X-ray as diagnostic tool, 85, 93, 97, 99, 101, 279, 282
Ausbestos Ltd, 20, 23
Australasian Asbestos Company, 7–8, 11, 16
Australian asbestos industry *see* asbestos industry in Australia (overview)
Australian Asbestos Network, 186

Australian Blue Asbestos Ltd (ABA), 26–30, 34–7, 109, 138
assets stripped by CSR, 312
company records, 101–2, 137, 169–70, 242, 249
dust control efforts, 89–91, 98–9
duty of care, 249–50
incompetence, 88, 89
Johns Manville Inc as model, 226
knowledge of asbestosis, 93, 98, 236, 243
knowledge of mesothelioma, 248
litigation (ABA/Midalco), 238–9, 241, 242–4, 245, 246–50, 251, 289, 308–11
litigation defence, 145
mine and mill official inspections, 89–90, 98–9, 215, 243
workforce, 93, 93, 167, 169, 186–7
see also Colonial Sugar Refining Company (CSR); Midalco Ltd; Wittenoom, Western Australia
Australian Blue Asbestos Pty Ltd v Rees (1981), 238–9
Australian Broadcasting Commission (ABC), 102, 117, 119–22, 216
Australian Capital Territory
house building practices, 48, 49
residential properties containing asbestos, 67, 70–1
Australian Council of Trade Unions, 41
Australian court cases *see* litigation
Australian Paper Manufacturers Ltd, 246
Australian Workers Union, 97, 104, 219–20
awards (recognition), 305

Badham, Dr Charles, 80–1
bagasse, 25
Balangero chrysotile mine, Italy, 160
bans on asbestos mining, import and use, 41, 148, 163, 257
Banton, Bernie, 320–1, 323, 324–35
Barraba, New South Wales, 18, 73, 102
Barrow and Heys v CSR LTD and Midalco Pty Ltd (1988), 236n11, 244, 248, 249–50, 277, 308–9
Barrow, Tim, 249–50, 308–9
Baryulgil, New South Wales, 205–6
asbestos tailings in township, 72, 206–9
asbestosis diagnoses, 87, 215–16, 217
living conditions, 206, 209–10, 220–1
media reports, 120, 121
mine and mill inspections, 214–15, 218–19
mine and mill work, 212–14
Mundine family memories, 206–8
ownership, 18, 25, 40n149, 218
production for James Hardie, 39
regulatory and institutional failures, 214–15, 218–20

– 333 –

worker unawareness of risks, 216–17, 218
workers' compensation, 217–18
workforce, 18, 210–11
workforce illness, 87, 206–8, 215–18
working conditions, 87, 211, 214–15, 220
Bates, John H, 14
Bell, Dr Alan, 84
Bell's Asbestos, 9, 12–13
benign asbestos pleural effusion, 143–4
Benson v James Hardie & Co Pty Ltd (1975), 241
Berry, Geoffrey, xvi, 149
Bestic Plaster, 11
Better Brakes Holdings Ltd, 39
Bishop, Julie, 309
blankets *see* coverings
Blesovsky, infolding lung syndrome of, 144
blue asbestos (crocidolite), 24, 25, 125, 153
    adverse publicity, 102, 104–5
    in asbestos cement products, 25, 26, 28, 29, 34–5, 36
    and asbestosis, 92–5, 234, 236 *see also* Wittenoom worker and resident asbestosis cases
    bans on new use, 163
    carcinogenity and deaths, 163
    CSR mining venture *see* Colonial Sugar Refining Company (CSR); Wittenoom, Western Australia
    dust and fibre measurement, 144–5 *see also* asbestos dust/fibre counts
    exports/exports planned, 26, 27–8, 34, 37
    and lung cancer, 153 *see also* lung cancer, asbestos related
    and mesothelioma, 136–41, 145, 150–9, 162–5 *see also* mesothelioma
    price comparisons, 34–5
    railway workers' exposure, 87, 104
    South African, 26, 29–30, 150–1, 153
    sprayed insulation, 286
    see also Wittenoom, Western Australia
Blue Heaven neighbourhood, Charlotte, North Carolina, 108
Bonnington Castings v Wardlaw [1956], 230
Borel v Fibreboard Paper Products (1973), 228
brake linings, 19, 25, 32, 37, 41, 84, 328 *see also* friction products
Breen, T, 220
Brewer, W H, 11–12
Broadhurst, C H, 243
Brodeur, Paul, 113–15, 117, 121, 228
bronchial cancer, asbestos related *see* lung cancer, asbestos related
brown asbestos (amosite), 124, 153
    bans on new use, 163
    carcinogenity and deaths, 163
    imports, 31–2, 34–5, 257
    and mesothelioma, 137, 139, 159, 162–3
    South African, 18, 25, 31–2, 34–5, 153
Brown, K O, 226, 243, 249–50
Bryce v Swan Hunter Group plc [1987], 231–2
Builders Labourers' Federation, 104
building materials, 14–15, 17
    alternatives to asbestos, 17, 19
    asbestic wall plaster, 7–8
    asbestos cement pipes *see* asbestos cement pipes
    asbestos cement sheets *see* asbestos cement sheets
    asbestos-free, 40, 102, 317
    blue asbestos in, 25, 28, 29, 34–5, 36
    consumption of imported fibre, 32
    damage and degradation, 66–7, 258–61
    imports, 12–15
    manufacturing output, 18
    owner building, 56
    paint, 9–10
    specialised and customised products, 23, 38–9, 61–6
    state differences in house building practices, 47–51
    see also Colonial Sugar Refining Company (CSR); fibro houses; home renovation and maintenance; James Hardie & Co.; Wunderlich Ltd
built environment, asbestos in *see* asbestos cement roofs; asbestos insulation products; building materials; fibro houses; fibro in industrial and commercial buildings; fibro sheds; home renovation and maintenance; industrial buildings
The Bulletin, 115–17, 126
Bundjalong Aboriginal people, 18, 205–21
Burrows v WA Government Railways Commission (1982), 237–8
Byrne, Dr Alfred, 112–13, 117

"Cabin Homes", 49–50
Canada
    asbestos expertise, 8
    asbestos mines, 154, 160–1, 315
    asbestos related diseases, 159, 160–1
    chrysotile imports to Australia, 18, 31–2, 34–5
Canberra *see* Australian Capital Territory
cancer
    latency, 135, 152, 289
    notifiable disease, 139
    registries, 101, 139
    treatment, 140–1, 147
    WA population, 175–6, 178–9
    see also lung cancer, asbestos related; mesothelioma
Cancer Registry (Western Australia), 139

INDEX

Caneite wallboard, 25, 26
Cape Asbestos Co., 18, 26n103, 29–30, 39, 315
Cape Blue Asbestos mining, 150–1 *see also* blue asbestos (crocidolite)
Carr, Bob, 324
Carroll, Jack, 191, 192, 194
Carter, Dr B N, 109
Cartier, P, 152
Cartledge v E Jopling & Sons Ltd [1963], 230
Castleman, Barry, 108, 111
catalogues (product catalogues), 12, 13, 21–2
see also marketing
Cave, Angus, 213–14
Central Asbestos Co Ltd v. Dodd [1973], 231
Central Australia, asbestos removal programs, 67
Charlotte, North Carolina, 108
chemotherapy, 140–1, 147
children
 childhood at Baryulgil, 206–9
 childhood at Wittenoom, 187, 198–9
 exposure to asbestos, 72, 115, 150, 169–72, 206–9, 251
 health outcomes of Wittenoom children, 72, 176–80
 home renovation exposure to asbestos, 293
 mesothelioma susceptibility, 177–3
chrysotile *see* white asbestos (chrysotile)
Churg, J, 33, 155
Cirkel, Fritz, 8, 10
Clayson, Dr Helen, 304
Clough, E L, 11
Colonial Sugar Refining Company (CSR)
 asbestos operations, 20, 25–30, 83, 134
 blue asbestos mining, 26–30, 34–7, 87–100
 see also Australian Blue Asbestos Ltd; Wittenoom, Western Australia
 company records, 101–2, 137, 169–70, 242, 249
 corporate conduct, 312
 duty of care, 249–50
 knowledge of asbestosis, 93, 98, 236, 241, 243
 knowledge of mesothelioma, 241, 248
 lack of worker education on hazards, 103
 litigation (CSR/ABA/Midalco), 238, 240–51, 308–11
 litigation defence, 145
 manager visits to Johns Manville, 226
 Silbestos sprayed asbestos insulation, 33
 warned of asbestos danger, 92–5, 234, 243, 248, 250, 309
 Wittenoom Group Settlement, 241, 244, 245, 246, 251
 Wittenoom Trust, 102, 244
 Wunderlich acquisition, 38

Combet, Greg, 122n43, 320
 on Bernie Banton and compensation, 323–30
commercial buildings
 asbestos cement construction materials, 39, 63–5
 asbestos removal, 70
 sprayed asbestos insulation, 284–5
 see also industrial buildings
common law cases *see* litigation
Commonwealth Department of Health, 234
 Division of Industrial Hygiene, 79
 miners' X-ray program, 79, 91–2, 93, 97, 281–2
community asbestos mapping programs *see* asbestos registers
community awareness *see* public awareness of asbestos hazards
compensation, 74
 ADSA role, 289–94
 Baryulgil miners, 217–18
 ILO recommendations, 109
 NSW workers, 77, 217–18
 trust funds, 102, 244, 318–20, 324
 UK, 78, 113, 145
 US, 108
 WA legislation, 238, 289, 293
 see also workers' compensation
compensation cases, 225, 251–2
 Australia, 234–52, 290–1, 307–14, 323–30
 UK, 113, 230–3
 US, 226–30
Condor, Hartwell, 87
Conference on the Biological Effects of Asbestos, New York, 1964, 33, 40, 111, 155, 316
confidentiality agreements, 122–3, 127
contaminated sites, 268–9 *see also* site remediation
Cooke, W E, 132–3, 226
corporate sponsorships, 38, 64
counselling and support services, 288, 291–3, 303–4 *see also* mental health
country area housing, 57–9, 67
court cases *see* litigation
Court, Sir Charles, 118–19
coverings, 11–12, 22–3, 32, 68, 82–3 *see also* lagging
crocidolite *see* blue asbestos (crocidolite)
CSR *see* Colonial Sugar Refining Company (CSR)
CSR Ltd v Young (1998), 251
Cunningham v Wunderlich Pty Ltd (1972), 240–1
cyclones, 66, 258, 267–8, 297–300
Czarnikow Ltd v Koufos [1969], 233

– 335 –

D Jansen & Co. Pty Ltd, 70
Dahl v Grice (1981), 239
Daily News (Perth), 109–10, 117–19
Danville Asbestic Plaster, 9
Darnton, A, 163
Darwin
  fibro houses, 48, 57, 298–9
  post-cyclone clean up, 66, 298, 299–300
Deleuil, Dr Greg, xvi, 293
  his story, 297–305
Delpero, Celestina, 188, 193, 196, 197
demolition of buildings, 265
diffuse pleural fibrosis, 142–3, 144
Dignam, Ian, 236, 243
display homes, 20, 44–5, 65
do-it-yourself (DIY) renovations *see* home renovation and maintenance
Doll, Sir Richard, 135, 136–7, 153, 163
Donnelly, Andy, 216
Dreesen standard, 81, 83, 84, 85, 95–6, 100, 134
Driscoll, T, 163
Duffus, Robert Luther, 108
Dugan, Bernard, 227
dumping of asbestos waste, 67, 72, 265–7
Durabestos asbestos cement sheets, 16, 20–1, 44
dust control measures, 82–4, 105–6, 132, 133, 219
  at Wittenoom, 87–100, 145–6
  see also asbestos exposure standards; mining regulation shortcomings; public health response to asbestos hazards
dust counts
  asbestos *see* asbestos dust/fibre counts; asbestos exposure standards
  in gold mines, 96
dust diseases
  experts in, 92, 95, 131, 149 *see also* McNulty, Dr Jim; Musk, Dr A W (Bill); Saint, Dr Eric; Selikoff, Dr Irving J
  in gold miners, 79, 93, 96, 284, 285
  monitoring *see* asbestos dust/fibre counts; public health response to asbestos hazards
  research, 80–1
  see also asbestos related diseases; asbestosis; pneumoconiosis; silicosis
Dust Diseases Board (New South Wales), 216, 217, 219
dust exposure standards *see* asbestos exposure standards
duty of care, 75, 218, 245, 247, 249–50, 251

education programs *see* public awareness of asbestos hazards; worker education, lack of
effusion *see* benign asbestos pleural effusion
Elder, Dr Janet, 100, 101, 139, 239, 242

electrical insulating boards, 23, 68
Elizabeth, South Australia, 50
Ellis & Clark Ltd, 23
Elmes, P C, 155
Elphick, Dr, 242
endothelioma of the pleura *see* mesothelioma
Eternit brand, 13, 39
exports of asbestos fibre, planned, 26, 27–8, 34

factories *see* industrial buildings
Faichney, Jack, 96
Favelle Mort Ltd v Murray, 239
fencing sheets, 32, 40, 47, 66
Ferodo friction products factory, England, 156–7, 162
fibre cement, asbestos-free, 40, 102, 317
fibre imports *see* asbestos fibre imports
fibres *see* asbestos dust/fibre counts; asbestos fibre imports
Fibro-Cement, 12, 13, 14
fibro houses, 18, 21, 43–7, 60, 62, 298
  advantages of fibro, 32, 44, 57
  advertising, 20–1, 44–6
  construction costs, 49
  in country areas, 57–60
  Darwin, 48, 57, 298–9
  demand, 32, 38
  display homes, 20, 44–5, 65
  holiday houses, 32, 60
  owner-built, 56
  Perth, 52–4
  public image, 61, 65
  safety, 66–7
  social difference marker for suburbs, 52–5, 61
  state differences, 47–55
  statistics, 18, 43, 46–8, 53–5, 60
  Sydney, 32, 52–5, 61
  see also asbestos cement sheets; building materials; residential properties containing asbestos
fibro in industrial and commercial buildings, 32, 39, 59, 63–5 *see also* asbestos cement sheets
fibro pipes *see* asbestos cement pipes
fibro roofing *see* asbestos cement roofs
fibro sheds, 32, 59
Fibrobestos sheets, 20
Fibrock asbestos cement products, 36
Fibrolite
  pipes, 38
  sheeting, 16, 19, 20, 38–9, 44–5
  Show Home, 20, 45, 65
fibrosis
  asbestosis *see* asbestosis
  diffuse pleural fibrosis, 142–3, 144
  rounded atelectasis, 144
fire, fear of, 10

INDEX

fire-proof properties of asbestos, 9–10, 21 *see also* insulation
fires, 258, 267–8
floods, 258, 267–8
Flying Doctor, 92, 93, 96, 277–80, 309 *see also* Saint, Dr Eric
Footner v Broken Hill Associated Smelters Pty Ltd (1983), 245
Formato, Luisa, 290, 307
France, mesothelioma cases, 162
Francis, Dr Eva, 219
friction products, 32, 37, 39, 41
    manufacturing health risks, 156–7, 162–3
    see also brake linings

Gaensler, E A, 143
galvanised iron, 13–15, 19, 48, 57, 58, 60n79
Gandevia, Assoc. Prof. Bryan, 148, 285
Gas & Fuel Corporation of Victoria, 241–2
gas mask manufacturing, 28, 154, 158–9
gestational trophoblastic diseases, 174–5
Gilbert, Neil, 84
Gilson, Dr John C, 153–4
Gloyne, S R, 134, 142, 152
Gold Coast, Queensland, holiday houses, 60
gold miners, dust risk and disease, 73, 93, 96, 284, 285
Goliath Portland Cement Company, 32, 63
Gordon, John, xvi, 290, 307
Gordon, Ken, 208–9, 215
Gordon, Pauline, 208–9, 216, 221
Gordon, Peter, 245, 290, 291
    his story, 307–14
    see also Slater & Gordon
government assistance for asbestos industry, 35–6
government contracts, 25, 37–8
government housing
    for Aboriginal people, 57–8
    industry housing needs, 32, 58–9
    regional areas, 57–9
    state differences in fibro use, 47–51
    Sydney and Perth suburbs, 53–5, 61
    see also fibro houses; housing demand
government records, 170, 243, 249
government regulation, 40–1, 103
    in Australian states *see* New South Wales; Victoria; Western Australia
    see also mining regulation shortcomings; public health response to asbestos hazards
Grant, Ted, 193, 195, 198–9, 200, 203
Green Valley, New South Wales, 55
Griqualand Exploration and Finance Company (Gefco), 26n103, 29–30
Gunn v Wallsend Slipway and Engineering Co Ltd (unreported, 1988), 233
Gyprock wallboard, 25–6

Hall, Tim, 116–17, 126
Hammond, Dr E Cuyler, 33, 111, 154–5
Hancock, Lang, 116, 117 *see also* L G Hancock Asbestos Company
Hannell, David, 313–14
Hansen, J, 138, 158
Hardie-Ferodo Pty Ltd, 39
Harries, Peter, 154, 155
Harrington, Greg, 212
Hawker Britton, 125
Hawker, South Australia, 8
health hazards of asbestos, 234–5, 243–4
    asbestos removalists' risk of disease, 272
    by asbestos types, 111, 124–5, 133, 135, 136–41, 157–65
    fibro houses, 66–7
    first public documentation of, 33, 40
    home renovation and maintenance, 66, 116, 140, 163, 261–4
    in situ products, 257–61
    loose-fill asbestos, 70–1
    manufacturing hazards, 81–5
    media coverage *see* media reporting
    occupations and activities, 292, 330
    in remote communities, 67
    research *see* medical research
    safe level of exposure non-existent, 137, 225, 270, 327–8
    "safe" level of use promotion by industry, 123
    sources of exposure (WA), 140–1
    WHO/IARC statement, 225, 235
    see also asbestos exposure standards; asbestos removal programs; litigation; public health response to asbestos hazards
heart complaints, asbestos treatment for, 109–10
Heath, Robert L, 125
heavy industry, 11–12
Henderson v State Electricity Commission of Victoria (1987), 246
Herculite, 17
Heys, Peter, 244, 249–50, 308–9
Hill and Knowlton, 115, 123
Hills, Ben, 117
Hobbs, Professor Michael, 102
Hodgson, J T, 163
holiday houses, 32, 60
home renovation and maintenance
    airborne asbestos fibre concentrations for selected activities, 263–4
    asbestos exposure hazard, 66, 116, 140, 163, 257–8, 261–4, 271–2
    and asbestos related disease, 67, 269–72, 293, 326n3
    fibro building materials, 32, 39, 65, 66–7
    popularity, 262

house building practices, 47–59
  construction costs, 49
  renovation *see* home renovation and maintenance
  social differences markers, 52–5
  see also fibro houses
housing demand, 32, 36, 38, 44, 49, 58–9 *see also* government housing
Hueper, Wilhelm, 227
Hummerston, David, 118, 119
Hunter, Cecily, 86
Hyslop v Australian Paper Manufacturers (1986), 246

illegal dumping of asbestos, 67, 72, 265–7
imports
  asbestos fibre *see* asbestos fibre imports
  asbestos sheets and slates, 12–17
  goods for heavy industry, 11–12, 23
  tariffs, 12, 16–17, 19, 22–3, 35–6
  tons imported, 31, 41, 257
in situ asbestos
  and asbestos related disease, 269–72
  in the built environment, 257–69
  risk and risk management, 260, 272
  see also asbestos insulation products; asbestos products; building materials; commercial buildings; fibro houses; home renovation and maintenance; industrial buildings; residential properties containing asbestos
industrial buildings, 32, 39, 59, 63–5 *see also* commercial buildings
industrial medicine *see* asbestos related diseases; health hazards of asbestos; occupational health; public health response to asbestos hazards
industrial sites
  asbestos uses, 11–12, 22–3, 68
  site remediation, 68–73
"infolding lung syndrome of Blesovsky", 144
insulation *see* asbestos insulation products
International Agency for Research in Cancer statement on asbestos, 225, 235
international companies *see* Cape Asbestos Co.; James Hardie & Co.; Johns Manville Inc; Turner & Newall
International Labour Organisaton, 109, 116, 243
investigative journalism *see* ABC (Australian Broadcasting Commission); *The Bulletin*; *Daily News* (Perth); media reporting; *New York Times*; *New Yorker*; *Sunday Times*; *West Australian*
Irving, N E, 241, 242
Italy, 160

Jackson Inquiry and consequent settlement, 320, 324–7
Jackson v Johns Manville (1982), 228–30
James Hardie & Co., 12, 14
  corporate conduct, 125, 311–21, 323–30
  and CSR/ABA Wittenoom operations, 27, 36–7
  failure of duty of care, 218, 220, 234–5
  head office, 19, 40, 312
  history, 315–21
  insurance policies, 244
  Jackson Inquiry and settlement, 320, 324–7
  joint ventures, 25, 39, 206, 315
  legal liabilities, 216, 311–12, 318–20, 323–4, 326, 327
  litigation, 235–6, 241, 242, 244, 311–14
  mining, 18, 25, 39–40
  sponsorships, 38, 64
  success, 37–40
  takeovers, 38, 39
  trust fund for victims, 318–20, 324
James Hardie & Co. manufacturing, 16, 17, 19, 37, 39, 312, 315–17
  blue asbestos use, 28, 34–5, 36
  consumption of imported fibre, 32
  dust levels and worker health, 76–7, 78, 81–5, 234, 316–17
  tailings distribution, 72
  war-time growth, 24–5
  workforce, 17, 25
James Hardie & Co. products
  elimination of asbestos, 40, 102, 317
  marketing, 16, 20–2, 40, 64
  product types, 19, 23, 37–9, 40, 61–6
  see also specific products: asbestos cement pipes; asbestos cement roofs; asbestos cement sheets; asbestos insulation products
James Hardie Civil Liabilities Bill 2005 (NSW), 216
James Hardie Project 72, 64
John Sanderson & Co, 13
Johns Manville Inc, 28, 37, 115, 315
  bankruptcy, 230
  deprecation of medical practitioners, 226–7
  lawsuits, 226–30
  statement on asbestos, 5–6
  visits from CSR/ABA representatives, 226
joint ventures, 25, 39, 206, 315
Jones Creek, New South Wales, 7
Jones, Dr Stephen, 154, 158
Jones, Robert H, 8
Jones v James Hardie & Co Ltd [1939], 235–6
Joosten, Joan, 242–4, 249, 251, 289
Joosten v Midalco Pty Ltd (1979), 242–4
journalism *see* ABC (Australian Broadcasting Commission); *The Bulletin*; *Daily News*

INDEX

(Perth); media reporting; *New York Times*; *New Yorker*; *Sunday Times*; *West Australian*

Kalgoorlie, Western Australia
  Commonwealth Health Laboratory, 79, 91–2
  miner dust diseases, 94, 95, 279, 285
Kaplan, A L, 143
Kemp v EMF Electric Co. Pty Ltd (1956), 236
Kennedy, Trevor, 116, 117
King, M G, 226, 243, 249–50
Kwinana, Western Australia, 50
  power station, 286

L G Hancock Asbestos Company, 24, 26, 29, 134 *see also* Hancock, Lang
labour movement *see* International Labour Organisaton; trade unions
lagging, 11, 32, 68, 82, 86, 100, 234, 246 *see also* coverings
Landrigan, P J, 269–70
latency of disease, 105, 110, 289
  asbestosis, 105, 289, 317, 319
  lung cancer, 135, 152, 289
  mesothelioma, 101, 110, 138, 152, 163–5, 178, 289, 317, 319
Laurie, Ffloyd, 207, 208
Lawrence, Chris, 220
Le Mesurier, C J R, 22
LeGrande, Frederick, 227
Leicher, F, 152
Leigh, J, 163
Leith, Russell, 102
Leopold Barnett & Co, 9, 13n33
Letham, Dr Don, 92, 97–8
Libby amphibole, 139, 142, 147
Libby, Montana, 141, 143
limpet asbestos, 33, 70, 301
litigation, 225, 251–2
  ADSA role, 289–91
  Australian common law litigation, 240–51
  Australian workers' compensation cases, 234–40
  "Chrysotile Defence", 125
  defendants' behaviour, 136, 145, 243, 309
  Peter Gordon's account, 307–14
  UK, 113, 230–3
  US, 226–30
loose-fill asbestos insulation, 70–1
Lovenfosse, Phil, 188–9
Lovenfosse, Silvia, 186, 188–9, 194, 195–6, 197, 200, 201, 202
lung cancer, asbestos related, 134–6, 152–3, 155, 239, 243
  and asbestosis, 134–6, 146
  compensable disease status, 289, 309
  and different types of asbestos, 135

latency, 135, 152, 289
litigation, 236, 237–40, 246
  and pleural plaques, 142
risk, 136
and smoking, 135–6, 155, 225, 237–8, 246, 304
treatment, 147
Wittenoom workers and residents, 173, 178, 238–9, 246
workers' compensation cases, 236
see also mesothelioma
lung diseases *see* asbestosis; pneumoconiosis; silicosis; tuberculosis

Maas, Cornelius, 241, 244, 251, 289
Maas v Midalco Ltd (1977), 241
Major, Gersh, 70, 91, 96, 138, 144–5, 284, 285
malignant mesothelioma *see* mesothelioma
Malloch Bros, 13, 17
manufacturing
  asbestos products *see* asbestos cement products; asbestos insulation products; asbestos products; friction products
  building products *see* building materials
  see also Colonial Sugar Refining Company (CSR); James Hardie & Co. manufacturing; Wunderlich Ltd manufacturing
Marchand, P, 101, 150–1
Margereson v J W Roberts Ltd (unreported 1995), 233n6
marketing, 9–15, 41, 64
  asbestos-free fibre cement, 40
  fibro houses, 20–2, 44–6
  "safe" level of use promotion by industry, 123
Marshall, Rex, 210
Martin, Catherine, 119
Martiny, O, 151
McCullagh, Dr Stanley Forster (Terry), 213, 317
McDonald, A D, 151, 161, 162
McDonald, Dr J C (Corbett), 151, 154, 158, 160, 161
McDonald, S, 133
McGhee v National Coal Board (1972), 238
McNulty, Dr Jim, 92, 95–102, 106, 117, 234, 248
  first diagnosis of mesothelioma, 97–8, 101, 117, 139, 234
  his story, 281–6
  warnings of asbestos danger, 282–4
media reporting, 33, 40, 103, 325
  on dangers of asbestos dust, 104–5, 109, 110, 216
  early-20th century, 107–10
  media attitudes in Australia, 121–2, 127

on mesothelioma, 110–18
newspapers post-1960, 110–19, 121
radio and television, 102, 119–22, 216
suppression and management by industry, 109–10, 111, 115, 122–7
medical knowledge of asbestos disease (milestones), 100–2, 114, 131–48
medical practitioners, deprecation of, 226–7
medical research
 ADSA scholarship, 294
 asbestos related diseases knowledge and treatment, 131–48
 asbestos related diseases (mesothelioma), 112, 149–65
 dust diseases (coal mining and quarrying), 80–1
 media reports, 107–17 *see also* media reporting
 personnel records provided by CSR/ABA, 101–2, 137, 169–70
 public relations response by industry, 111, 115, 122–6
 Wittenoom epidemiological and clinical studies, 132, 138–42, 167–80
Medical Research and Compensation Foundation, 312, 318–20
medical services *see* Flying Doctors; public health response to asbestos hazards; X-ray programs
Melbourne, "blue" trains, 87, 104, 121
Meletis v James Hardie, 242
mental health, 179–80 *see also* counselling and support services
Merewether, E R A, 78, 100, 133, 152, 243
 report on effects of asbestos dust, 78, 82, 133, 225, 230, 234, 236, 237
mesothelioma, 71–2, 136–41, 163, 301–5
 ADSA scholarship, 294
 and asbestos exposure intensity and duration, 156–7
 and asbestos types, 111, 135, 136–41, 157–65
 Canada, 159, 160–1
 causes, 137–9, 163
 compensable disease status, 289, 309
 CSR/ABA knowledge of, 241, 248
 diagnostic methods, 143
 distinct pathological entity recognised, 136–7, 151–2
 early diagnoses, 97–8, 101, 117, 137, 139, 149–57, 234
 fatalities, 140, 293
 France, 162
 incidence in Australia, 164–5, 293
 Italy, 160
 latency, 101, 110, 135, 138, 152, 163–5, 178, 180, 289, 317, 319

litigation, 231–4, 239, 240–6, 248–51, 289, 290–1, 307–14
media reports, 110–18
and non-asbestiform fibre, 139
and pleural plaques, 141–2
research, 110–11, 136–41, 149–65
sources of asbestos exposure (WA), 138–40
South Africa, 111, 124–5, 150–1
susceptibility, 172–3, 177–8
from third-wave exposures, 271–2
treatment, 140–1, 147
UK, 111–12, 152–9, 161, 162, 272
US, 110–11, 113–15, 154–5, 159, 160, 162–3
Wittenoom *see* Wittenoom worker and resident mesothelioma cases
The Mesothelioma handbook (Clayson), 304
mesothelioma registers, 101, 139
Midalco Ltd
 formerly Australian Blue Asbestos Ltd, 308, 312
 litigation, 241, 242–4, 245, 246–50, 251, 289, 308
 see also Australian Blue Asbestos Ltd
Midalco Pty Ltd v Rabenault [1989], 248–9
milling, 87, 88–92, 94, 97 *see also* Baryulgil, New South Wales; Wittenoom, Western Australia
mine, definition (Western Australia), 94
mine site remediation, 71–3
Mines Department, Western Australia
 purpose and responsibilities, 79, 88–91, 146, 279, 280, 281, 285
 and Wittenoom, 87–99, 117, 134, 243
 Wittenoom dust exposure surveys, 91, 95–9, 146, 170–1, 243, 284
Mines Inspectorate (New South Wales), 218–19
Mines Regulation Act and Regulations (Western Australia), 94, 146
mining, 6–9, 17–19, 24, 73
 asbestos dust control, 87–100
 bans, 41
 by CSR *see* Colonial Sugar Refining Company (CSR)
 dust diseases (coal mining and quarrying), 80–1 *see also* asbestosis; mesothelioma
 by James Hardie, 18, 25, 39–40
 last Australian asbestos mine, 73
 NSW *see* Baryulgil, New South Wales; Woodsreef mine, Barraba, New South Wales
 site remediation, 71–3
 South Africa *see* South Africa
 Tasmania, 6–9, 16, 17, 26, 87, 88
 WA *see* Kalgoorlie, Western Australia; Wittenoom, Western Australia
 by Wunderlich, 17, 18, 25, 87

INDEX

mining regulation shortcomings, 105–6
  NSW, 102–3, 218–19
  WA (Wittenoom), 87–99, 117, 134, 145–6
Monaghan, Scott, 209
Montana, US, 141, 143, 160
Montpelier Foundry Pty Ltd, 39
Mooney (factory inspector), 78
mortality, Wittenoom residents and WA population compared, 176, 179
Moss, Dennis, 313–14
Mount Druitt, New South Wales, 55
Mr Fluffy (company), 70–1
Mundine, Michael (Mick), 206
Mundine, Tony, 206–7
Mundine, Warren, 207
Murdoch v SG Sayer Pty Ltd [1961], 236–7
Murray, Dr Montague, 131
Murray v Wunderlich Ltd (1961), 237
Musk, Dr A W (Bill), xvi–xvii, 131, 158, 238, 240, 242, 248

Napolitano, Liborio and Angela, 187, 201–2
National Centre for Asbestos Diseases Research, University of Western Australia, 294
National Health and Medical Research Council (NHMRC), xvi
National Health and Medical Research Council (NHMRC) recommendations, 103, 145–6
National Occupational Health and Safety Council (NOHSC) Code of Practice for the Safe Removal of Asbestos, 263
natural disasters and release of fibres, 66, 258, 267–8
naval dockyard workers, 152, 154, 155, 234
New South Wales
  asbestos hazards investigation and regulation, 77, 79–85, 102–3, 145, 218–19
  country area housing, 57–9
  fibro houses in Sydney, 32, 52–3, 61
  holiday houses, 60
  house building practices, 36, 48, 49, 51, 53, 54–5
  owner-built houses, 56
  residential properties containing loose-fill asbestos, 70–1
New South Wales Department of Health, 77, 219
  Division of Industrial Hygiene, 79–85, 100, 219
New South Wales Dust Diseases Board, 216, 217, 219
New South Wales Mines Inspectorate, 218–19
New York Academy of Sciences conference on the biological effects of asbestos 1964, 33,
40, 111, 155, 316
New York Times, 108–11, 113
The New Yorker, 113–15
Newhouse, Dr Muriel (Molly), 112, 149, 154, 155–7
newspaper reports *see* media reporting
Newton v Cammell Laird & Co (Shipbuilders & Engineers) Ltd [1969], 231
Nicholson v Atlas Steel Foundry [1957], 230
Nordmann, M, 152
Northern Territory
  asbestos mapping programs, 67
  fibro houses, 48, 57, 298–9
  post-cyclone clean up, 66, 298, 299–300
Nottingham, England, 154, 158–9
Noyes Bros, 13, 17

occupational health, 75–6, 89–100
  monitoring, 79–80
  neglected, 78–9, 91–5, 148
  union role *see* trade unions
  see also asbestos related diseases; mining regulation shortcomings; public health response to asbestos hazards
Oliver, Sir Thomas, 133
Olsen (Young) v CSR Ltd (1994), 251
Owen v IMI Yorkshire Copper Tube (unreported, 15 June 1995), 233
owner-building, 44, 56

P C Jones & Co, 13n33
packings, 11–12, 22–3, 26, 32, 82–3
Page, Margaret, 194, 195, 196, 197–8, 199, 200–1, 202
paint, 9–10, 11
palliative care, 147
Park, E K, 262–3
patents, 11, 19
Peacock, Matt, 102–3, 117, 119–22, 216, 217
Pedrotti, Rino, 245, 251, 290
Pedrotti v Midalco, 245
Perth
  contaminated ceiling panels, 293
  fibro houses, 32, 52–5
  James Hardie plants *see* James Hardie & Co. manufacturing
  sprayed asbestos insulation, 284–5
  use of asbestos tailings, 73
Peto, J, 163
Pilbara, Western Australia, 8, 15, 24 *see also* Wittenoom, Western Australia
Pilmer v Mcphersons LTD (1985), 245
pipe coverings *see* coverings
pipes
  asbestos cement, 19, 26, 33, 37–8, 39
  asbestos-free, 40
pleural effusion, 143–4, 246–8

– 341 –

pleural fibrosis, 142–3, 144
pleural plaques, 139, 141–2
pneumoconiosis, 78, 80, 83, 85
   conferences, 109, 136, 144–5, 149–50
   experts, 95, 149
   parliamentary inquiry, 96
   research, 153–4
   worker compensation entitlement, 109
   see also asbestosis; silicosis
Pneumoconiosis Research Unit, Penarth, South Wales,, 153–4
Poilite sheets, 12–13
Powell, C W, 226
Powell, Rod, 188, 189–91, 192, 197, 200
power stations, 68–9, 86–7, 234, 240, 246, 286
Price, C W, 78, 82, 133, 225, 230, 234, 236, 237
product catalogues, 12, 13, 21–2 see also marketing
products see asbestos cement products; asbestos insulation products; asbestos products; building materials; friction products
prospecting, 6–7, 24 see also mining
public awareness of asbestos hazards, 73, 74, 111, 116, 121, 293, 313, 325 see also media reporting; worker education, lack of
public health response to asbestos hazards, 75–106
   communication with workers, 103–4, 219
   industrial medicine neglected, 78–9, 91–5, 148
   initial responses, 76–9
   mesothelioma registers, 101, 139
   NSW, 77, 79–85, 100, 216, 218–19
   regulatory failings, 87–95, 96–7, 102–6, 117, 327–8
   trade union role, 103
   Victoria, 77, 85–7
   Western Australia, 77, 78–9, 91–2, 117
   at Wittenoom, 88–102, 279–80
   see also asbestos related diseases; health hazards of asbestos; and specific diseases: asbestosis; lung cancer; mesothelioma; pleural plaques
public housing see government housing
Public Interest Advocacy Centre, Sydney, 209–10
public relations response by industry to criticism, 109–10, 111, 115, 122–7 see also media reporting
publicity see adverse publicity about asbestos; marketing

QBE (insurer), 244
Queensland
   country area housing, 57
   holiday houses, 60
   house building practices, 48, 49, 51

Rabenault, Klaus, 248–9, 291, 310–11
Rabenault v Midalco Pty Ltd (1988), 248–9, 291, 294, 310–11
radio and television reports see media reporting
radiology see X-ray programs
Raftos, Dr John, 237
railway workers exposure to asbestos, 87, 104, 121
Raybestos-Manhattan, 122
recordkeeping
   company records, 102, 137, 169–70, 242, 249
   government records, 170, 243, 249, 289
Rees v Australian Blue Asbestos (1981), 238–9, 240
regional areas
   housing, 57–9
   remote community asbestos registers and remediation, 67
regional development housing support, 67
registers
   asbestos, 67, 74
   mesothelioma, 101, 139
regulation, 40–1, 103
   in Australian states see New South Wales; Victoria; Western Australia
   see also mining regulation shortcomings; public health response to asbestos hazards
removal of asbestos see asbestos removal programs; asbestos removalists' risk of disease; site remediation
Rennie, Dr H M, 98, 243
Report on Effects of Asbestos Dust on the Lungs and Dust Suppression in the Asbestos Industry (Merewether and Price), 78, 82, 133, 225, 230, 234, 236, 237
reproductive cancers, 174
research see medical research
residential properties containing asbestos, 23, 66–7, 69, 70–1
   asbestos locations in typical home, 259
   asbestos removal programs, 66–7, 70–1, 261–4
   see also fibro houses; home renovation and maintenance
Robens principle of tripartite responsibility, 105
Rockhampton district, Queensland, 8
roofing material see asbestos cement roofs
rope, 11, 33, 68, 82, 237
rounded atelectasis, 144
Russell, Peter, 234, 317
Rutty, Clive, 186–7, 193, 195, 203

Index

Saint, Dr Eric, 106, 284
   award named for, 305
   his story, 277–80
   warns CSR of asbestos danger, 92–5, 234, 243, 248, 250, 309
Salamanderite, 10
Sales v Dicks Asbestos & Insulating Co Ltd (unreported 1967), 230
Salisbury, South Australia, 49–50
Sarna v Wunderlich Ltd (1967), 237
school buildings, 67, 197–8, 259
Schrott, Josef, 192, 194, 199–200
secrecy agreements *see* confidentiality agreements
Seidler, Harry, 61
Seidman, H, 159
Selikoff, Dr Irving J, 33, 110–11, 114, 126, 137, 154–5, 227
sense of control and wellbeing *see* mental health
serpentine variety of asbestos *see* white asbestos (chrysotile)
sheds, fibro, 32, 59
Shiels, Dr Douglas, 85–7, 106, 234
shivers *see* asbestos tailings
Silbestos sprayed asbestos insulation, 33
"Silex" boiler covering, 11–12
silicosis, 152, 301
   causes, 97
   clinical description, 133
   and coal dust fibrosis, 80, 95
   compensation litigation, 108, 230, 235–6, 243
   experts, 95
   incidence, 79, 94, 97–8, 100n115, 108, 152, 285
   management and regulator preoccupation with, 94, 97, 279–80
   X-ray diagnosis, 92, 101, 279
Simpson, M J C, 155
Simpson v Midalco Pty Ltd (1987), 246–8, 291, 308
Simpson, Wally, 246–8, 291, 308
Sindanyo (imported product), 23
site remediation, 265–6
   contained sites, 268–9
   Darwin clean up, 66, 298, 299–300
   industrial sites, 68–73
   Wittenoom, 72–3
Skingsley v Cape Asbestos Co Ltd [1968], 230
Slater & Gordon
   litigation, 241–2, 245–6, 248–9, 251, 290–1, 307–14, 328
   negotiated settlement with CSR, 245, 251
Slater & Gordon Witness Seminar, 2009, xvi
   addresses, 287–94, 297–305
Sleggs, C A, 101, 150–1

Sluis-Cremer, G K, 159
Smeaton, T H, 13–14
Smith v Central Asbestos Co Ltd [1972], 231
smoking and asbestos exposure in lung cancer causation, 135–6, 155, 225, 237–8, 246, 304
social differences, fibro estates as marker of, 52–5
soil, asbestos-contaminated, 72, 268–9 *see also* asbestos tailings
South Africa
   asbestos related diseases, 101, 110–11, 124–5, 136–7, 150–1, 153
   blue asbestos (crocidolite), 26, 29–30, 150, 153
   brown asbestos (amosite), 18, 25, 31–2, 34–5, 153
   mining history, 150–1, 153
   white asbestos (chrysotile), 153
South Australia, house building practices, 48, 49–50
spin *see* public relations response by industry to criticism
Spivak, John L, 108
sprayed asbestos insulation, 33, 68, 69–70, 115, 284–6, 301
Spriggs, F A (company), 12, 14, 17
standards *see* asbestos exposure standards
state differences in fibro use for houses, 47–55 *see also* fibro houses
State Electricity Commission of Victoria, 86–7, 240, 246
steam engine insulation, 11–12
Stokes v Guest, Keen and Nettlefold (Bolts and Nuts) Ltd [1968], 232
Stretton, Hugh, 55
suburban developments, 32, 52–5, 61
Sunday Times, 111–13 *see also* media reporting
Super-Six corrugated sheeting, 19, 66
Sydney
   fibro houses, 32, 52–5, 61
   James Hardie plants *see* James Hardie & Co. manufacturing
   use of asbestos tailings, 73

tailings *see* asbestos tailings
tariffs, 12, 16–17, 19, 22–3, 35–6
Tasbestos asbestos cement sheets, 32, 44
Tasmania
   asbestos mines, 7–8, 16, 17, 26, 87, 88
   house building practices, 48, 51
Taylor, Clarence, 202
Taylor Smart (law firm), 245, 290
Taylor v CSR & Midalco (1992), 251
television reports *see* media reporting
third wave of asbestos related disease, 67, 269–72, 293, 326n3
Thomas, Dr D L Gordon, 77, 85, 101, 106

Thomas v Gas & Fuel Corporation of Victoria (1978), 241–2
Thompson, Hilda, 112, 156
Tilux decorative board, 19, 62
"Toope" patent, 11
Torrens, Greville, 211
trade unions
 activism, 41, 86, 87, 104–5, 120, 328–9
 concerns about silicosis, 97
 dust money increases rather than safety, 104, 117
 inaction, 122, 219–20, 280
 no role in industrial health regulatory model, 103
trains, asbestos in, 87, 104, 121
tremolite, 7, 153, 160–1
Trowbridge (actuaries), 311
trust funds, 102, 244, 318–20, 324
tuberculosis, 97, 99, 108, 133, 142, 143, 282
 screening, 79, 92
Tuck & Co, 12
Tucks Asbestos Ltd, 33
Turner & Newall, 30, 33, 39, 70, 278n2, 315
Turner Bros, 9, 23

unions *see* trade unions
United Kingdom
 asbestos exposure control, 145
 asbestos litigation, 113, 230–3
 asbestos related diseases, 111–13, 152–9, 161, 272
 asbestosis diagnosis and compensation, 78, 145
 media reports on asbestos danger, 111–12 *see also* media reporting
 research, 153–4, 155, 156–7
United States
 asbestos exposure standards, 81, 124, 145
 asbestos litigation, 226–30
 asbestos related diseases, 33, 108–9, 110–11, 113–15, 154–5, 159, 162
 industry deprecation of medical practitioners, 226–7
 industry media strategies concerning asbestos danger, 111, 115, 122–7
 media reports on asbestos danger, 108–11, 113–15 *see also* media reporting
 vested interests, 122
US Gypsum, 123
Valleron, A J, 162
Van der Schoot, H C M, 152
Van-Zyl v State Energy Commission (1983), 240
vermiculite, 139, 160
Vic Rail, 87, 104
Victoria
 asbestos hazards investigation and regulation, 77, 85–7, 145, 234, 243
 asbestos related diseases, 77, 85–6, 101
 house building practices, 48, 50–1
 litigation involving government bodies, 240, 241–2, 246
 Melbourne's "blue" trains, 87, 104, 121
Victoria Division of Industrial Hygiene, 85–6
Victoria Gas & Fuel Corporation, 241–2
Victoria State Electricity Commission, 86–7, 240, 246
Vojakovic, Robert, xvi, 126–7, 192, 203, 252, 287, 290, 307
 on ADSA, 287–94
 Deleuil on, 300–2, 304
Vojakovic, Rose Marie, xvi, 203, 252, 287, 290, 292, 304

Wagner, Dr J C (Chris), 101, 111, 137, 150–1, 153–4, 308
Wagner, Dr Percy Albert, 153
Walker, Linda, 215, 220
Walker, Neil, 210, 211, 214, 215, 217
wartime demand for asbestos, 15, 16–17, 24–5, 28, 158–9
water pipes *see* asbestos cement pipes
Water Research Foundation of Australia, 38
water supply schemes, 11
Watkins, Jack, 104
Watson, Colin, 250–1
Watson v State of Western Australia (1988), 250–1
weatherboard houses, 21, 49, 51
Wedler, H W, 136, 152
Weiss, A, 152
wellbeing *see* counselling and support services; mental health
West Australian, 110, 119
West Australian Blue Asbestos Fibres Ltd, 30
Western Australia
 asbestos hazards investigation and regulation, 77, 78–9, 87–99, 117, 145–6 *see also* Western Australia Mines Department
 cancer incidence, 175–6, 178–9
 country area housing, 57–9
 fibro houses (Perth and Kwinana), 32, 50, 52–5
 holiday houses, 60
 house building practices, 36, 48, 50, 51, 53–4
 litigation involving the state, 250–1
 mesothelioma register, 101, 139
 mortality, 176, 179
 owner-built houses, 56
Western Australia Mines Department
 purpose and responsibilities, 79, 88–91, 146, 279, 280, 281, 285

Index

and Wittenoom, 87–99, 117, 134, 243
   Wittenoom dust exposure surveys, 91, 95–9, 146, 170–1, 243, 284
Western Australia Public Health Department, 77, 78–9, 97–100, 139, 146, 279–80, 281, 284
Western Australia v Watson (1990), 250–1
Western Australian Asbestos Manufacturing Company, 22
Western Australian Goldfields Water Supply Scheme, 11
white asbestos (chrysotile), 153
   Australian deposits, 7, 8–9, 15, 17–18, 25, 26, 88
   bans on new use, 163
   Canadian, 18, 31–2, 34–5, 154, 160–1, 315
   carcinogenity, 163
   deaths (ratio), 163
   health hazard downplayed by industry ("Chrysotile Defence"), 124–5
   imports, 18, 35, 257
   Italy, 160
   and lung cancer, 153
   and mesothelioma, 137, 139, 157, 160–3
Williams, A E, 33
Williams, George, 117–19
Williams, Lillian, 207–8
Wilson, Laurie, 217
Winters, J, 212
Witness Seminar 2009 (Slater & Gordon), xvi
   addresses, 287–94, 297–305
Wittenoom Group Settlement, 241, 244, 245, 246, 251
Wittenoom Trust, 102, 244
Wittenoom, Western Australia, 26, 27, 185
   asbestos clean up, 72–3
   asbestos dust control failure, 89–100, 138
   asbestos dust/fibre counts, 70, 91, 95–9, 138, 144–6, 170–1, 243, 284, 285
   asbestos tailings in township, 72–3, 158, 169, 194–5, 199, 234, 283, 301–2
   asbestosis incidence, 93, 97–8, 100–1
   closure, 72–3, 101
   CSR blue asbestos venture, 26–30, 34–7, 87–91 *see also* Australian Blue Asbestos Ltd (ABA); Colonial Sugar Refining Company (CSR)
   Deleuil's account, 301–3
   living conditions, 167–9, 187–8, 192, 195–9
   McNulty's account, 281–4
   media reports, 116–19, 126 *see also* media reporting
   medical services, 92–3, 96, 97–8, 99, 277–80, 281–4
   mine and mill inspections, 89–91, 98–9, 215, 243
   mine and mill work, 186–94
   Saint's account, 277–80
   union response to dust levels, 104
Wittenoom worker and resident asbestosis cases, 92–101, 134, 199, 234, 236, 282, 301
   litigation, 238–9, 241–4, 246–51
Wittenoom worker and resident mesothelioma cases, 138–40, 180, 199–203, 302–3
   children, 176–9
   first Australian case, 137
   group settlement, 251
   increase in cases, 157–8, 163–5
   litigation, 241, 242–4, 245, 248–50, 251, 289, 290–1, 307–11
   women and men contrasted, 172–3
   see also mesothelioma
Wittenoom workers and residents
   ABA workforce, 93, 98, 167, 169, 186–7
   asbestosis *see* Wittenoom worker and resident asbestosis cases
   epidemiological and clinical studies, 132, 138–42, 167–80
   health outcomes, 167–80, 199–203
   lung cancer, 173, 178, 238–9, 246
   memorial to, 294–5
   memories of Wittenoom, 185–203
   mesothelioma *see* Wittenoom worker and resident mesothelioma cases
   personnel records provided for medical research, 101–2, 137, 169–70
   support for, 126
Wm Adams & Co, 9, 12
women
   domestic exposure to asbestos, 156, 158, 196, 200, 207–9, 233, 240–1
   exposure to asbestos at Wittenoom, 169–72, 200
   factory workers' exposure to asbestos, 158–9
   health outcomes of Wittenoom residents, 172–6, 180
   home renovation exposure to asbestos, 271–2, 293
   mesothelioma susceptibility, 172–3
Woodsreef mine, Barraba, New South Wales, 17–18, 73, 102–3
Woodsreef Mines Ltd, 40n149, 206, 218
worker education, lack of, 103–4, 107, 122–3, 216–17, 218
workers' compensation
   ADSA role, 289–94
   Australian cases, 235–40, 290–1, 307–14
   Baryulgil miners, 217–18
   ILO recommendations, 109
   NSW workers, 77, 217–18
   UK cases, 113, 230–3
   US cases, 226–30
   see also compensation

Workers' Compensation Act (Western Australia), 238, 289
World Health Organisation statement on asbestos, 225, 235
Wragg, George, 86
Wright v Dunlop Rubber Co (1971), 232–3, 243–4
Wunderlich Hume Asbestos Pipes Pty Ltd, 38, 39
Wunderlich Ltd, 17
   CSR acquisition of, 38 *see also* Colonial Sugar Refining Company (CSR)
   joint ventures, 25, 39, 206
   litigation, 237, 240–1
   marketing, 20–2
   mining, 17, 18, 25, 87
Wunderlich Ltd manufacturing, 16, 17, 19, 20, 24–5, 72, 312
   blue asbestos use, 25, 28, 34–5, 36
   consumption of imported fibre, 32
   dust levels and worker health, 83–5
   products, 16, 20–1, 39, 44, 62–3

X-ray programs, 79, 91–2, 93, 281–2
   asbestosis diagnosis, 85, 93, 97, 99, 101, 279, 282
   silicosis diagnosis, 92, 101, 279

Yallourn power station, Victoria, 86
Yampire Gorge, Western Australia, 24, 30
Yilgarn area, Western Australia, 22, 92
Young/Olsen v CSR, 244

Zeehan, Tasmania, 26, 88
Zelamite board, 23